Autoimmune Disease Models

A Guidebook

Autoimmune Disease Models

A Guidebook

Edited by

Irun R. Cohen and Ariel Miller

Department of Cell Biology
The Robert Koch–Minerva Center for
    Research in Autoimmune Diseases
The Weizmann Institute of Science
Rehovot, Israel

Academic Press

San Diego   New York   Boston   London   Sydney   Tokyo   Toronto

Front cover photographs: (Top) Extensive demyelination of the anterior column of the spinal cord. See p. 31 for details. (Bottom) Histology and CSF cytology in EAE. See p. 10 for details.

Academic Press, Inc.
A Division of Harcourt Brace & Company
525 B Street, Suite 1900, San Diego, California 92101-4495

United Kingdom Edition published by
Academic Press Limited
24-28 Oval Road, London NW1 7DX

Library of Congress Cataloging-in-Publication Data

Autoimmune disease models / edited by Irun R. Cohen, Ariel Miller,
      p.   cm.
   Includes bibliographical references and index.
   ISBN 0-12-178330-8
   1. Autoimmune diseases--Animal models. I. Cohen, Irun R.
II. Miller, Ariel
RC600.A825   1994
  6161.97'8027--dc20   94-17093
                                           CIP

PRINTED IN THE UNITED STATES OF AMERICA
94 95 96 97 98 99 MM 9 8 7 6 5 4 3 2 1

Contents

v

Chapter 3   Theiler's Virus-Induced Demyelinating Disease

Stephen D. Miller, William J. Karpus, Jonathan G. Pope, Mauro C. Dal Canto, and Roger W. Melvold

Chapter 4   Experimental Autoimmune Neuritis

Christopher Linington and Hartmut Wekerle

Chapter 5   Experimental Autoimmune Uveoretinitis— Rat and Mouse

Rachel R. Caspi

Chapter 6 # Experimental Autoimmune Myasthenia Gravis

Angela Vincent

Chapter 7 # The Obese Strain with Spontaneous Autoimmune Thyroiditis as a Model for Hashimoto Disease

G. Wick, R. Cole, H. Dietrich, Ch. Maczek, P.-U. Müller, and K. Hála

Chapter 8   Experimental Autoimmune Thyroiditis in
             the Mouse and Rat
             Yi-chi M. Kong and Alvaro A. Giraldo

Chapter 9   The NOD Mouse: A Model for
             Autoimmune Insulin-Dependent Diabetes
             Dana Elias

Chapter 10   The BB Rat Models of IDDM
             Peter A. Gottlieb and Aldo A. Rossini

Chapter 11   **Experimental Myocarditis**

Noel R. Rose, Susan L. Hill, and David A. Neumann

Chapter 12   **Experimental Hepatitis**

Ansgar W. Lohse and Karl-Hermann Meyer zum Büschenfelde

Chapter 13   **Adjuvant Arthritis**

Marca H. M. Wauben, Josée P. A. Wagenaar-Hilbers, and Willem van Eden

Chapter 14   Murine Models of Spontaneous Systemic
                  Lupus Erythematosus
                  Chaim Putterman and Yaakov Naparstek

Chapter 15   Experimental Systemic Lupus
                  Erythematosus: Role of the
                  Idiotypic Network
                  Edna Mozes and Yehuda Shoenfeld

Chapter 19   Assessment of Discomfort in
                  Laboratory Animals
                  H. van Herck, V. Baumans, and S. F. de Boer

Contributors

Numbers in parentheses indicate the pages on which the authors' contributions begin.

Ahmad Al-Sabbagh (15) Center for Neurologic Diseases, Brigham and Womens Hospital, and Harvard Medical School, Boston, Massachusetts 02115

V. Baumans (303) Department of Laboratory Animal Science, Veterinary Faculty, Utrecht University, 3508 TD Utrecht, The Netherlands

Stefan Brocke (1) Department of Neurology and Neurological Sciences, Stanford University Medical Center, Stanford, California 94305

Karl-Hermann Meyer zum Büschenfelde (191) Department of Medicine, Johannes Gutenberg-University, D-6500 Mainz, Germany

Rachel R. Caspi (57) Laboratory of Immunology, National Eye Institute, National Institutes of Health, Bethesda, Maryland 20892

R. Cole (107) New York State College of Agriculture and Life Sciences, Department of Poultry and Avian Sciences, Cornell University, Ithaca, New York 14853

Mauro C. Dal Canto (23) Department of Pathology, Northwestern University Medical School, Chicago, Illinois 60611

S. F. de Boer (303) Department of Animal Physiology, University of Groningen, 9750 AA Haren, The Netherlands

H. Dietrich (107) Institute for General and Experimental Pathology, University of Innsbruck Medical School, 6020 Innsbruck, Austria

Dana Elias (147) Department of Cell Biology, The Weizmann Institute of Science, Rehovot 76100, Israel

Zsuzsanna Fabry (257) Department of Pathology, Division of Neuropathology, University of Iowa, College of Medicine, Iowa City, Iowa 52242

Sandrine Florquin (291) Laboratoire Pluridisciplinaire de Recherche Experimentale Biomédicale et Service d'Immunologie, Hôpital Erasme, Université Libre de Bruxelles, B-1070 Brussels, Belgium

Koenraad Gijbels (1) Department of Neurology and Neurological Sciences, Stanford University Medical Center, Stanford, California 94305

Alvaro A. Giraldo (123) Division of Immunopathology, St. John Hospital, Detroit, Michigan 48236

Michel Goldman (291) Laboratoire Pluridisciplinaire de Recherche Experimentale Biomédicale et Service d'Immunologie, Hôpital Erasme, Université Libre de Bruxelles, B-1070 Brussels, Belgium

Peter A. Gottlieb (163) Division of Diabetes, Department of Medicine, University of Massachusetts Medical School, Worcester, Massachusetts 01655

K. Hála (107) Institute for General and Experimental Pathology, University of Innsbruck Medical School, 6020 Innsbruck, Austria

Michael N. Hart (257) Department of Pathology, Division of Neuropathology, University of Iowa, College of Medicine, Iowa City, Iowa 52242

Susan L. Hill (175) Department of Immunology and Infectious Diseases, The Johns Hopkins University, Baltimore, Maryland 21205

William J. Karpus (23) Department of Microbiology-Immunology, Northwestern University Medical School, Chicago, Illinois 60611

Yi-chi M. Kong (123) Department of Immunology and Microbiology, Wayne State University School of Medicine, Detroit, Michigan 48201

Christopher Linington (39) Max-Planck-Institute of Psychiatry, D-82152 Martinsried, Germany

Ansgar W. Lohse (191) Department of Medicine, Johannes Gutenberg-University, D-6500 Mainz, Germany

Ch. Maczek (107) Institute for General and Experimental Pathology, University of Innsbruck, Medical School, 6020 Innsbruck, Austria

Roger W. Melvold (23) Department of Microbiology-Immunology, Northwestern University Medical School, Chicago, Illinois 60611

Stephen D. Miller (23) Department of Microbiology-Immunology, Northwestern University Medical School, Chicago, Illinois 60611

Edna Mozes (245) Department of Chemical Immunology, The Weizmann Institute of Science, Rehovot 76100, Israel

P.-U. Müller (107) Institute for General and Experimental Pathology, University of Innsbruck Medical School, 6020 Innsbruck, Austria

Yaakov Naparstek (217) The Clinical Immunology and Allergy Unit, Department of Medicine, Hadassah University Hospital, Jerusalem 91120, Israel

David A. Neumann (175) Risk Science Institute, International Life Sciences Institute, Washington DC 20036

Jonathan G. Pope (23) Department of Microbiology-Immunology, Northwestern University Medical School, Chicago, Ilinois 60611

Chaim Putterman (217) The Clinical Immunology and Allergy Unit, Department of Medicine, Hadassah University Hsopital, Jerusalem 91120, Israel, and the Department of Microbiology and Immunology, Albert Einstein College of Medicine, Bronx, New York 10461

Noel R. Rose (175) Department of Immunology and Infectious Diseases, The Johns Hopkins University, Baltimore, Maryland 21205

Aldo A. Rossini (163) Division of Diabetes, Department of Medicine, University of Massachusetts Medical School, Worcester, Massachusetts 01655

Yehuda Shoenfeld (245) Research Unit of Autoimmune Diseases, Department of Medicine 'B,' Sheba Medical Center, Sackler Faculty of Medicine, Tel-Aviv University, Tel-Hashomer 52621, Israel

Lawrence Steinman (1) Department of Neurology and Neurological Sciences, Stanford University Medical Center, Stanford, California 94305

Osamu Taguchi (267) Aichi Cancer Center Research Institute, Nagoya 464, Japan

Cory Teuscher (291) Department of Microbiology, Brigham Young University, Provo, Utah 84602

Kenneth S. K. Tung (267) Department of Pathology, University of Virginia, Charlottesville, Virginia 22906

Willem van Eden (201) Utrecht University, Faculty of Veterinary Science, Institute of Infectious Diseases and Immunology, Department of Immunology, Utrecht, The Netherlands

H. van Herck (303) Central Laboratory Animal Institute (GDL), Utrecht University, 3508 TD Utrecht, The Netherlands

Angela Vincent (83) Neurosciences Group, Department of Clinical Neurology, Institute of Molecular Medicine, University of Oxford, Oxford OX3 9DU, United Kingdom

Josée P. A. Wagenaar-Hilbers (201) Utrecht University, Faculty of Veterinary Science, Institute of Infectious Diseases and Immunology, Department of Immunology, Utrecht, The Netherlands

Marca H. M. Wauben (201) Utrecht University, Faculty of Veterinary Science, Institute of Infectious Diseases and Immunology, Department of Immunology, Utrecht, The Netherlands

Howard L. Weiner (15) Center for Neurologic Diseases, Brigham and Womens Hospital, and Harvard Medical School, Boston, Massachusetts 02115

Hartmut Wekerle (39) Max-Planck-Institute of Psychiatry, D-82152 Martinsried, Germany

G. Wick (107) Institute for General and Experimental Pathology, University of Innsbruck Medical School, 6020 Innsbruck, Austria

Preface

Animal models of autoimmune disease make it possible to study how the immune system relates to the tissues of the body. As in many areas of biology and medicine, we often learn most about the physiology and genetics of health by studying disease. The complexities of biological systems, like those of social systems, are not fully appreciated until the systems fail us. Diseases demand detailed attention, and autoimmune diseases point us in the direction of the most fundamental questions in immunology. However, the aim of this book is not to discuss the fundamental questions; it is to tell the reader about the animal models themselves. This book is intended to be a concise guide for those who want to set up a particular animal model. It also aims to equip the reader with information needed to evaluate the results and conclusions described by immunologists who work with these models. We anticipate that our instructions for model building will outlast those in many of the books that review the data and opinions based on experiments with these models. Data and opinions have a short life span because, ideally, they are replaced by new information and hypotheses. The models, the subjects of experimentation, do not change as quickly. New models do not make existing models obsolete; they extend existing models.

The value of animal models of autoimmune diseases is not only in the convenience of their manipulation. There is now reason to suspect that the autoimmune diseases of rodents may provide good examples of the same immunological processes involved in the natural autoimmune diseases of humans. It appears that standard representations of autoimmunity are built into the immune systems of both animals and humans (for more discussion, see I. R. Cohen (1992a). *Immunology Today* **13**; 441–444; I. R. Cohen (1992b). *Immunology Today* **13**; 490–494). Thus the animal models may be applicable as well as illustrative.

We have tried to cover the most used and useful models and have asked our contributors to follow a common outline. This book aims to serve and we shall be pleased to modify future editions according to the comments of our readers. We have included a final chapter on ethical animal experimentation because the obligations of humanity have no limitations.

Irun R. Cohen
Ariel Miller

Chapter 1

Experimental Autoimmune Encephalomyelitis in the Mouse

Stefan Brocke, Koenraad Gijbels, and Lawrence Steinman
Department of Neurology and Neurological Sciences, Stanford University Medical Center, Stanford, California 94305

I. Introduction: Murine Experimental Autoimmune Encephalomyelitis as a Model for T-Cell-Mediated Demyelinating Disease of the Central Nervous System

In 1949, Olitsky and Yager described the induction of experimental disseminated encephalomyelitis in white mice, thus establishing murine experimental autoimmune encephalomyelitis (EAE) as a model for autoimmune inflammatory diseases of the central nervous system (CNS). EAE in the mouse shares many features with the human disease multiple sclerosis (MS), such as acute, chronic, and relapsing neurological dysfunctions, including paralysis and ataxia; a histopathology characterized by perivascular inflammatory infiltrates and demyelination in the CNS; and a link to major histocompatibility complex (MHC) class II determinants (Zamvil and Steinman, 1990). A recent study demonstrated an accumulation of T cells in brain lesions of patients with MS which share T-cell receptor (TCR) gene rearrangements with T cells specific for the most commonly used antigen for induction of EAE, myelin basic protein (MBP) (Oksenberg *et al.*, 1993). Thus, murine EAE can be considered a useful model for several aspects of the pathogenesis of MS (Steinman *et al.*, 1984).

II. Models of EAE in the Mouse

A. Induction of EAE by Immunization with Autoantigens (Actively Induced EAE)

EAE can be induced by immunization of animals with mouse spinal cord homogenate (MSCH) or myelin proteins, namely MBP or proteolipid protein (PLP). Several immunodominant epitopes in these antigens have been determined, and it is possible to induce EAE with peptides representing epitopes of MBP or PLP (Table I). Actively induced EAE allows the study and manipulation of the immunization and effector phases in a model of autoimmune disease. The usually reproducible time course of the disease allows for a study of disease induction and expression. However, owing to the severe long-term inflammation caused by the use of complete Freund's adjuvant (CTA Difco, Detroit, Michigan) containing *Mycobacterium tuberculosis*, some of the observed effects could be attributed to the mode of immunization rather than the pathogenic process of inflammation and demyelination in the CNS.

Susceptibility of mice to EAE is genetically controlled (Bernard *et al.*, 1976a). Similarly, the encephalitogeneity of MBP or PLP peptides is dependent on the expression of certain *H-2* antigens of mouse strains (Table I) (Whitham *et al.*, 1991; Zamvil and Steinman, 1990; Sobel *et al.*, 1990; Tuohy *et al.*, 1989; Sakai *et al.*, 1988; Tuohy *et al.*, 1988; Zamvil *et al.*, 1985, 1986). Thus, the N-terminal encephalitogenic epitope Ac1–11 of MBP is immunodominant in *H-2u* mice (Zamvil *et al.*, 1985, 1986), whereas peptide 89–101 is a major encephalitogenic epitope in mice expressing *H-2q and H-2s* antigens (Zamvil and Steinman, 1990; Sakai *et al.*, 1988).

To induce EAE, mice at 5–9 weeks of age are immunized by subcutaneous (s.c.) inoculation (tail base or flank) with 5 mg of lyophilized spinal cord homogenate or 200 μg of the MBP peptide in a 0.1-ml emulsion with equal volumes of phosphate-buffered saline (PBS) and CFA. In order to enhance the immunization with antigen, killed *Mycobacterium tuberculosis*, strain H37Ra (Difco) can be added to the emulsion at a concentration of 2–4 mg/ml.

Some older protocols call for the s.c. immunization in the footpads. However, this procedure is not recommended because it is painful for the animal and the resulting local inflammation can interfere with the gait and hence with EAE scoring (the same goes for injecting the emulsion at the tail base and evaluation of tail weakness).

It has been observed that the induction of EAE can be significantly improved by the administration of heat-killed whole organisms of *Bordetella pertussis* (Lee and Olitsky, 1955; Bernard and Carnegie, 1975) or a derived toxin (PTX) (Munoz *et al.*, 1984). We successfully use whole heat-inactivated organisms from the Instituut voor Volksgezondheid en Milieuhygiene, Bilthoven, The Netherlands, or pertussis toxin from List Biologicals, Campbell, California or JRH Biosciences, United Kingdom. Usually, 10^8 to 10^9 heat-inactivated pertussis organisms or 100–400 ng of PTX is given intravenously (i.v.) (dissolved in 100 µl PBS) on the day of immunization and again 48 hr later. However, each batch of pertussis should be titrated individually to determine the optimal dose for EAE induction, since the potency of batches varies widely and there is a narrow dose range between EAE-inducing potential and toxicity. The latter will be evident from sudden mortality between days 4 and

Table I
Encephalitogenic Peptides from MBP and PLP in Various Mouse Strains

Mouse strain	H^2	Peptide	Reference
		MBP[a]	
(PL/J × SJL)F1	*s,u*	Ac1-11	Zamvil *et al.* (1985, 1986, 1990)
PL/J	*u*	Ac1-11	Zamvil *et al.* (1985, 1986, 1990)
PL/J	*u*	35–47	Zamvil *et al.* (1985, 1986, 1990)
SJL/J	*s*	89–101	Sakai *et al.* (1988)
		PLP[b]	
(PL/J × SJL)F1	*s,u*	43–64	Whitham *et al.* (1991)
PL/J	*u*	43–64	Whitham *et al.* (1991)
SJL/J	*s*	103–116	Tuohy *et al.* (1988)
SJL/J	*s*	139–151	Tuohy *et al.* (1988); Sobel *et al.* (1990)
(PL/J × SJL)F1	*s,u*	139–151	Whitham *et al.* (1991)

[a] MBP peptides are prepared according to the sequence of guinea pig/rat, mouse, or bovine MBP. Consult the references for details.
[b] PLP peptides are prepared according to the sequence of murine PLP with or without substitution. Consult the references for details.

8, that is, before EAE develops. In addition, the optimal PTX dose varies in different mouse strains.

We induce EAE in a highly reproducible way in SJL/J mice by immunizing them with the $PLP_{139-151}$ peptide, without the addition of PTX (see Table I). Another advantage of this model is that 30–50% of the mice show clinical relapses after complete or partial recovery from the first attack.

Spinal cord homogenate is produced as follows: mice are euthanized by CO_2 inhalation and the skin on the back and around the neck is disinfected with 70% ethanol. They are decapitated with a pair of heavy scissors and the four limbs are fixed to a board, whereafter the skin on the back is cut longitudinally and opened. The spinal column is cut just above the pelvis, without cutting too deep and damaging the intestines. A 16- to 18-gauge needle, fixed to a 10-ml syringe filled with PBS, is put into the caudal opening of the spinal canal and the spinal cord is then flushed out at the cranial end of the mouse and collected in a 50-ml tube. After being washed in PBS, the spinal cords can be stored frozen until they are homogenized in PBS and lyophilized. The resulting powder is stored frozen. MBP peptides are prepared by continuous flow, solid-phase synthesis according to the desired sequences. Peptide purity is examined by high-performance liquid chromatography and peptide identity is confirmed by analyzing amino acid composition. Depending on the sequence, the peptide solution might require some pH adjustments before being dissolved in distilled water. After synthesis and before use, peptides should be lyophilized several times to remove volatile organic compounds. Lyophilized peptides should be stored in the cold in a desiccator until used.

Most of the classical EAE models described are monophasic, with an acute phase of the disease, after which the clinical deficit remains fixed or the animals return to normal function. Sometimes, however, animals develop new or recurrent clinical deficits ("relapses") after variable time intervals. We mentioned EAE induced with $PLP_{139-151}$ in SJL/J before and there are variants of the induction protocols in the literature that are reported to induce relapsing-remitting EAE in a reproducible way (Suckling *et al.*, 1984; Fallis and McFarlin, 1989; Baker *et al.*, 1990; Soos *et al.*, 1993; Brocke *et al.*, 1993). To exclude mere fluctuations in clinical performance without any correlation at the lesion level, it is preferable to document relapses and remissions histopathologically.

B. Induction of EAE by Transfer of Autoreactive T Lymphocytes (Adoptive or Passive EAE)

It has been demonstrated that EAE can be induced by transferring sensitized lymph node cells from mice or rats which have been immunized with MSCH or MBP (Paterson, 1960; Bernard *et al.*, 1976b; Paterson *et al.*, 1978; Pettinelli and McFarlin, 1981). This approach allows for the separate study of the effector phase of EAE, most probably without any influence on immunization and inflammation outside the CNS. Also, the prime mediators of this type of disease, MBP-specific T cells, can be studied in detail *in vitro* by standard immunological techniques such as proliferation assays for the determination of antigen specificity, surface marker analysis by fluorescence-activated cell sorter, TCR sequencing, etc.

The method for establishing long-term antigen-specific T-cell lines and clones, which was developed by Kimoto and Fathman (1980), facilitated the induction of autoimmune disease by transferring enriched autoreactive T-cell populations. Utilizing this technique, it is possible to establish MBP-specific T-cell lines and clones transferring EAE in rats (Ben-Nun *et al.*, 1981) and mice (Zamvil *et al.*, 1986). T-cell lines specific for MBP or MBP peptides can be established as described (Zamvil *et al.*, 1986, Brocke *et al.*, 1993). The following method for the generation of T-cell lines or clones specific for the N-terminal encephalitogenic peptide Ac1-11 can be used for a variety of antigens (Brocke and Hahn, 1991). The optimal concentration for each antigen, for example, protein or peptide, has to be determined both for the immunization of the mice as well as for the *in vitro* stimulation of the lymph node cells.

Mice are immunized s.c. with antigen emulsified in CFA as described in the chapter about active EAE without PTX. Seven to 12 days after immunization with 200 μg Ac1-11 in an emulsion of PBS and CFA, mice are euthanized and draining lymph nodes are harvested under sterile conditions. The lymph nodes are gently processed and washed through a steel mesh until a single-cell suspension is obtained. The cells (30×10^6) are cultured in 5 ml RPMI 1640 (Gibco, Grand Island, New York) supplemented with 2 mM glutamine, 100 U/ml penicillin and 100 μg/ml streptomycin, $5 \times 10^{-5}M$ 2-mercaptoethanol, 10% fetal calf serum (Hyclone, Logan, Utah) and 5–15 μmol antigen. After 4 days of incubation, the cells are washed and resuspended in 5 ml of the enriched medium as described earlier without antigen. Depending on cell growth, the cell culture medium can be supplemented with interleukin-2 (IL-2) or 10% (v/v) concanavalin A (ConA; Sigma Chemical Co., St. Louis, Missouri) supernatant as a source of IL-2 (and other growth factors) in between stimulations. ConA supernatant is prepared from splenocytes of BALB/c mice by incubating 5×10^6 cells/ml with 5 mg/ml ConA for 24 hr. The remaining ConA in the supernatant is removed by stirring it with 2 mg/ml Sephadex G-50 (Pharmacia LKB, Uppsala, Sweden) for 1 hr. The resulting ConA supernatant is filtered sterile and stored at $-70°C$ until used. T cells are kept in ConA supernatant-enriched medium at a concentration of 1×10^6 cells/ml and restimulated every 14 days using

5–15 μmol antigen presented on irradiated (3000 rads) syngeneic spleen cells at a ratio of 1/5 to 1/50 T cells versus antigen-presenting cells (APCs). T-cell clones from the MBP-induced T-cell lines are derived by the limiting dilution technique. Cells are diluted in medium and distributed in the wells of flat-bottomed microtiter plates at a concentration of 0.2 cells/200 μl on 5×10^5 irradiated syngeneic splenocytes as APCs. The resulting clones are maintained by techniques described for the lines.

For adoptive transfer, after extensive washing, about 5×10^6 cells of the T-cell lines or clones are injected i.v. in 500 μl PBS into naive mice of 6–8 weeks of age. The severity of EAE is dependent on the number of MBP-specific cells transferred and can be adjusted accordingly. In some cases, whole-body irradiation of mice with 350 rads facilitates the transfer of EAE by weakly encephalitogenic T-cell clones. However, this method is not always necessary and might interfere with most studies (e.g., by damaging the blood–brain barrier).

III. Evaluation of the Disease

A. Clinical Evaluation and Care of Diseased Animals

The clinical manifestations of EAE, such as loss of tail tonus and limb paralysis, are readily apparent to most observers and can be quantified according to various schemes. We evaluate all immunized animals daily for disease signs according to the scale presented in Table II.

It should be emphasized that this system scores for an ascending myelitis, that is an inflammation of the spinal cord, progressing from caudal to rostral. If the inflammation in the CNS takes a different course (most often this is in the more severe models), a different way of clinical scoring might better

Table II
Clinical Scoring of Mouse EAE

EAE score	Clinical disease
0	No clinical disease
1	Tail weakness
2	Paraparesis (incomplete paralysis of one or two hindlimbs)
3	Paraplegia (complete paralysis of one or two hindlimbs)
4	Paraplegia with forelimb weakness or paralysis
5	Moribund or dead animals

reflect the pathology in the CNS. However, clinical signs associated with encephalitis, such as a lack of activity, piloerection, and a humped back, are much less specific and can also be caused by pathophysiological processes outside the CNS. In order to exclude any subjective influence on grading of diseased mice, scoring should be performed by an observer blind to the experimental protocol and by the same observer throughout the experiment.

More severe forms of the disease are associated with an earlier onset, a higher incidence, higher scores, a slower recovery, and a more synchronized course in the different animals. In the actively induced form, disease signs will normally start from day 10–12 onward (up to day 25 in very mild cases). A significant drop of body weight usually precedes other clinical signs of EAE for about 1–2 days. Maximum severity is reached in 2–4 days and surviving animals recover slowly thereafter. Most mice recover completely in 10–20 days. Sometimes animals reach a plateau phase with a lasting clinical deficit. In adoptive EAE, onset of clinical disease depends on the number and encephalitogenic capacity of the transferred cells. Adoptive EAE in the mouse rarely results in a full recovery and tends to leave long-lasting neurological deficits. Typical courses of active and adoptive EAE are shown in Figure 1.

Since EAE in the mouse has side effects on the animal's well-being, strict guidelines to maintain animal welfare are recommended. These guidelines can include monitoring body weight, hydration status, general condition, and activity of mice during the whole experiment. If experimental effects such as paralysis or paresis are expected, animals have to be monitored several times daily and easy access to food and water should be provided by placing food pellets on the cage floor and by using long drinking tubes. Mice can become dehydrated as a result of either the CNS-directed side effects of disease induction or paralysis. Dehydrated animals should receive supplemental fluid therapy consisting of 1 ml lactated Ringer's solution or physiological saline solution s.c. a minimum of twice daily. Severely diseased animals (grades 4 or 5) whose condition does not improve after fluid therapy should be euthanized to prevent unnecessary suffering.

B. Histopathology and Cytology

1. Histology

Histopathological evaluation of the CNS is used to prove that clinical differences among treatment groups are caused by differences in the physiopathological processes, that is, differences in the extent as well as in the composition of CNS lesions.

Paraffin-embedded, formalin-fixed, 6–10-μm sections usually include four to five transverse sections of the brain (including brainstem and cerebellum);

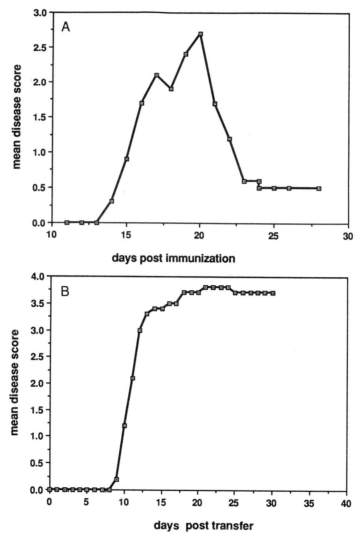

Figure 1 Disease course in EAE. (A) Actively induced EAE. EAE was induced with the N-terminal encephalitogenic epitope Ac1-11 of MBP in (PL/J × SJL)F$_1$ mice by s.c. inoculation (tail base) of 200 μg of the MBP peptide in an 0.1 ml emulsion with equal volumes of PBS and CFA. Killed *Mycobacterium tuberculosis*, strain H37Ra was added to the emulsion at a concentration of 4 mg/ml. Two hundred nanograms of PTX were given i.v. (dissolved in 100 μl PBS) on the day of immunization and again 48 hr later. EAE scores (see Table II) were recorded daily and are shown as mean disease scores on any given day after immunization. (B) Adoptive EAE. Seven to 12 days after s.c. immunization with 200 μg Ac1-11 in an emulsion of PBS and CFA, mice were euthanized and draining lymph node cells harvested under sterile conditions. Peptide-specific T cells were cultured as described (Section II,B) until a long-term line was established. For adoptive transfer, 5×10⁶ T cells were injected i.v. per mouse. EAE scores (see Table II) were recorded daily and are shown as mean disease scores on any given day after immunization.

transversal sections of the cervical, thoracic, and lumbar spinal cord; as well as a longitudinal section of the remaining lumbosacral part (since most lesions, if any, are expected in this part of the cord, but can be focal and hence missed on a single transverse section). The following stains are useful: hematoxylin and eosin (H–E, a routine stain that shows inflammatory lesions clearly), Klüver-Barrera (KB, a combination of luxol fast blue and cresyl violet stains that is ideal for demonstrating demyelination), Bielschowsky (a silver stain for axons) and Giemsa (inflammatory cells). We routinely use the H–E and the KB stains; selected sections are stained with Bielschowsky's if we are looking for axonal damage or with Giemsa if it is not possible to discriminate among the different inflammatory cells on H–E. Alternatively, fresh tissue can be snap-frozen if immunohistochemical detection of sensitive antigens is planned.

If electron microscopy is desired, it is best to fix the CNS material of interest immediately in a suitable fixative (e.g., paraformaldehyde/glutaraldehyde in cacodylate buffer). Semithin (1-μm) sections of resin-embedded tissue stained with toluidine blue can be evaluated light microscopically for fine details of the myelin sheath.

The extent of the lesions is dependent upon the severity of the disease: inflammatory lesions are almost invariably found in the lumbosacral part of the spinal cord, a patchy distribution more rostral in the cord, the brainstem and cerebellum, and in the more severe cases also in the cerebral hemispheres. A meningitis accompanies even the mildest cases. The lesions have a predilection for the perivascular areas in the white matter ("perivascular cuffs," Figure 2A). The typical infiltrate consists of T lymphocytes, a few plasmocytes, monocytes/macrophages, and granulocytes. In both actively induced and transferred mouse EAE, neutrophils as well as eosinophils are numerous. Microglial cells in the vicinity of the infiltrates become more ameboid and astrocytes acquire a "reactive" appearance. Demyelination of the tissue surrounding the perivascular cuffs is evident (Figure 2B). The axons are relatively spared, but in the more severe models there is also gross axonal loss. In the most severe cases, erythrocytes are present in the tissue surrounding the lesion, indicating intraparenchymal hemorrhage that is reminiscent of the human disease, acute hemorrhagic leukoencephalitis. After clinical recovery, the infiltrate disappears slowly and proliferating astrocytes cause astrogliosis. If remyelination occurs, it is visible on semithin sections as thin myelin sheets of variable size surrounding the axons.

2. Cerebrospinal Fluid

Cerebrospinal fluid (CSF) is taken by suboccipital puncture. After euthanasia—and preferably bleeding—the mouse is fixed with its limbs to a board and the skin of the neck is disinfected with 70% ethanol. A 1-ml Eppendorf-type tube is put under the throat for maximal exposure of the neck. The skin is opened with a longitudinal incision and the three layers of neck muscles are dissected carefully to avoid bleeding. The dura mater between the occiput and the first cervical vertebra is now visible. The dura is pierced with a pointed 50-µl capillary pipet attached by a rubber tube to a Pasteur pipet,

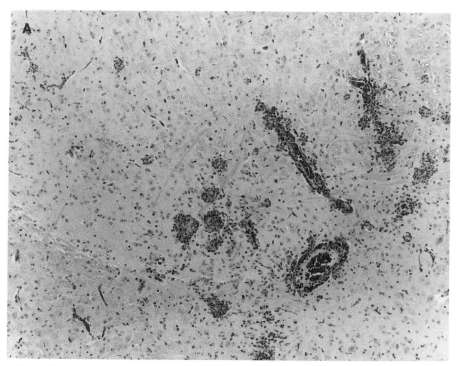

Figure 2 Histology and CSF cytology in EAE. (A) Perivascular inflammatory infiltrates in the brainstem of a mouse with adoptive EAE, clinical score grade 2, diseased for 3 days. Paraformaldehyde-fixed and paraffin-embedded tissue, hematoxylin and eosin stain. ×100. (B) Longitudinal section through the spinal cord of the same mouse as in A. Perivascular inflammatory infiltrates (arrowheads) are present in the white matter and demyelination (open arrow) is obvious near the largest infiltrate. Note the absence of infiltrates in the gray matter (bottom of the picture). Paraformaldehyde-fixed and paraffin-embedded tissue, Klüver-Barrera stain. ×100. (C) CSF smear of a mouse with adoptive EAE, clinical score grade 1, diseased for 1 day. Monocytes (open arrows), lymphocytes (arrows), and polymorphonuclear leukocytes (arrowheads) are present. CSF was obtained by suboccipital puncture, air dried on a glass slide, and stained with May–Grünwald–Giemsa. ×400. (For details concerning EAE transfer, see the legend for Figure 1.)

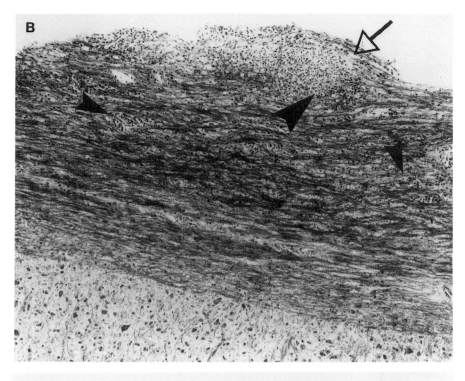

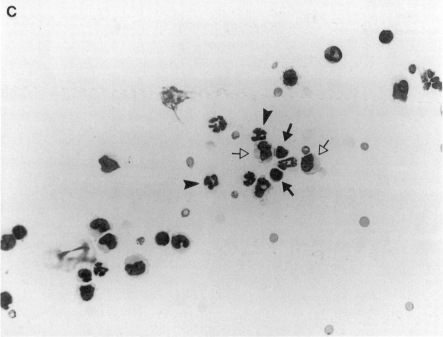

Figure 2 *(continued)*

avoiding the clearly visible blood vessels. One to 5μl of CSF can be collected by gentle suction through the Pasteur pipet. We discard any sample that is macroscopically contaminated with red blood cells, even if such samples taken from normal animals never showed an elevated nucleated cell count. The resulting CSF can be used for counting the number of cells in a counting chamber and for making a differential cell stain. One to 2 μl of CSF are spread on a glass slide, allowed to air dry, and stained with May–Grünwald–Giemsa stain as for blood smears (Gijbels *et al.*, 1993). If used for other assays (e.g., bioassay or enzyme-linked immunoabsorbent assay—ELISA), it might be necessary to pool the CSF from several animals (Gijbels *et al.*, 1990).

In EAE the number of cells in the CSF is usually in the range of $1-7 \times 10^3$ cells/μl. In actively induced as well as in transfer EAE, the pleiocytosis consists of lymphocytes, neutrophils, eosinophils, and monocytes, thereby reflecting the composition of the inflammatory infiltrate in the parenchymatous lesions (Figure 2C).

C. Statistical Evaluation

Clinical evaluation produces different variables that can be used in the statistical evaluation of the disease, such as incidence, mortality, time of disease onset and mortality, duration, relapse rate, and body weight. If the experiment results in groups of mice which are either diseased or healthy, a χ^2 test allows an easy statistical evaluation of the data. If the clinical course of the disease is compared among different groups of mice, mean disease scores can be compared on a day-to-day basis for the different groups or used as a mean cumulative score for the duration of the observation period ("area under the curve"). Since there can be quite some variation in the clinical course among animals in the same experimental group, standard deviations can be expected to be high. In addition, the data might have a non-normal distribution and hence a nonparametric statistical method has to be used.

IV. Summary

EAE in the mouse is characterized by perivascular inflammatory demyelinating lesions in the CNS and a immunogenetically determined susceptibility. Clinical expression of the disease is obvious from neurological signs and can be easily quantified. Actively induced or adoptively transferred EAE allows for the separate study of immunization and effector events in the pathogenesis of the disease. The immune system of the mouse has been extensively studied and immune reagents are readily available, making mouse EAE an ideal animal model for the study of human inflammatory demyelinating disorders of the CNS.

Acknowledgment

The authors thank Dr. Hans Lassmann, Vienna, for the expert histopathological training he gave to one of us (K.G.).

References

Baker, D., O'Neill, J. K., Gschmeissner, S. E., Wilcox, C. E., Butter, C., and Turk, J. L. (1990). *J. Neuroimmunol.* **28**, 261–270.

Ben-Nun, A., Wekerle, H., and Cohen, I. R. (1981). *Eur. J. Immunol.* **11**, 195–199.

Bernard, C. C. A. (1976a). *J. Immunogenetics* **3**, 263–274.

Bernard, C. C. A., and Carnegie, P. R. (1975). *J. Immunol.* **114**, 1537-1540.

Bernard, C. C. A., Leydon, J., and Mackay, I. R. (1976b). *Eur. J. Immunol.* **6**, 655–660.

Brocke, S., and Hahn, H. (1991). *Infect. Immun.* **59**, 4531–4539.

Brocke, S., Gaur, A., Piercy, C., Gautam, A., Gijbels, K., Fathman, C. G., and Steinman, L. *Nature,* **365**, 642–644.

Fallis, R. J., and McFarlin, D. E. (1989). *J. Immunol.* **143**, 2160–2165.

Gijbels, K., Van Damme, J., Proost, P., Put, W., Carton, H., and Billiau, A. (1990). *Eur. J. Immunol.* **20**, 233–235.

Gijbels, K., Proost, P., Masure, S., Carton, H., Billiau, A., and Opdenakker, G. (1993). *J. Neuroscience Res.*, **36**, 432–440.

Kimoto, M., and Fathman, C. G. (1980). *J. Exp. Med.* **152**, 759–770.

Lee, J. M., and Olitsky, P. K. (1955). *Proc. Soc. Exp. Biol. Med.* **89**, 263–266.

Munoz, J. J., Bernard, C. C. A., and Mackay, I. R. (1984). *Cell. Immunol.* **83**, 92–100.

Oksenberg, J. R., Panzara, M. A., Begovich, A. B., Mitchell, D., Erlich, H. A., Murray, R. S., Shimonkevitz, R., Sherritt, M., Rothbard, J., Bernard, C. C. A., and Steinman, L. (1993). *Nature* **362**, 68–70.

Olitsky, P. K., and Yager, R. H. (1949). *J. Exp. Med.* **90**, 213–223.

Paterson, P. Y. (1960). *J. Exp. Med.* **111**, 119–133.

Paterson, P. Y., Richardson, W. P., and Drobish, D. G. (1975). *Cell. Immunol.* **16**, 48–59.

Pettinelli, C. B., and McFarlin, D. E. (1981). *J. Immunol.* **127**, 1420–1423.

Sakai, K., Zamvil, S. S., Mitchell, D. J., Lim, M., Rothbard, J. B., and Steinman, L. (1988). *J. Neuroimmunol.* **19**, 21–32.

Sobel, R. A., Tuohy, V. K., Lu, Z., Laursen, R. A., and Lees, M. B. (1990). *J. Neuropath. Exp. Neurol.* **49**, 468–479.

Soos, J. M., Schiffenbauer, J., Wegrzyn, L., and Johnson, H. M. (1993). *J. Immunol.* **150**, 192A (Abstr. 1091).

Steinman, L., Schwartz, G., Waldor, M., O'Hearn, M., Lim, M., and Sriram, S. (1984). *In EAE: A Good Model for MS* (E. C. Alvord, M. W. Kies, and A. Suckling, Eds.), pp. 393–397. Alan R. Liss, New York.

Suckling, A. J., Kirby, J. A., Wilson, N. R., and Rumsby, M. G. (1984) *In EAE: A Good Model for MS* (E. C. Alvord, M. W. Kies and A. Suckling, Eds.), pp. 7–12. Alan R. Liss, New York.

Tuohy, V. K., Lu, Z., Sobel, R. A., Laursen, R. A., and Lees, M. B. (1988). *J. Immunol.* **141**, 1126–1130.

Tuohy, V. K., Lu, Z., Sobel, R. A., Laursen, R. A., and Lees, M. B. (1989). *J. Immunol.* **142**, 1523–1527.

Whitham, R. H., Jones, R. E., Hashim, G. A., Hoy, C. M., Wang, R.-Y., Vandenbark, A., and Offner, H. (1991). *J. Immunol.* **147**, 3803–3808.

Zamvil, S. S., and Steinman, L. (1990). *Ann. Rev. Immunol.* **8**, 579–621.

Zamvil, S., Nelson, P., Mitchell, D., Knobler, R., Fritz, R., and Steinman, L. (1985). *J. Exp. Med.* **162**, 2107–2124.

Zamvil, S. S., Mitchell, D. J., Moore, A. C., Kitamura, K., Steinman, L., and Rothbard, J. (1986). *Nature* **324**, 258–260.

Chapter 2

Rat Experimental Autoimmune Encephalomyelitis

Ahmad Al-Sabbagh and Howard L. Weiner

Center for Neurologic Diseases, Brigham and Womens Hospital and Harvard Medical School, Boston, Massachusetts 02115

I. History and Introduction

Several spontaneously occurring organ-specific autoimmune diseases in man have experimental models that can be induced in laboratory animals by immunization with specific antigen(s) from the target organ. Experimental autoimmune encephalomyelitis (EAE) has been the most widely used model for the human disease, multiple sclerosis (MS) since Rivers and Schwentker first produced EAE in monkeys in 1935. Since then there has been steady progress in producing EAE in different animal species, including rabbits, guinea pigs, rats, and mice. In 1949 Lumsden unsuccessfully attempted to induce EAE in the albino rat. In 1953, Lipton and Freund were the first to successfully induce EAE in rats of the Sherman strain by the intracutaneous injection of central nervous system (CNS) tissue, together with killed and dried tubercle bacilli suspended in an emulsifying agent in paraffin oil. The use of *Mycobacterium tuberculosis* (Mt) to enhance sensitization and the route of injection were crucial to establishing the EAE model in rats (Freund, 1932). Subsequently, the Lewis strain of rats became standard for EAE studies as well as other animal autoimmune models. Lewis rats were produced from animals selected and inbred at Wistar institute by Margaret Reed Lewis in 1956.

II. Animals and Housing

Lewis rats are albino and are generally used at 7–10 weeks of age (between 175–350 g). Animals may be housed in a conventional or a virus-antibody-free (VAF) facility. [VAF refers to negative, enzyme-linked immunosorbent (ELISA) assays for serum antiviral antibodies.] Animals are housed in a large plastic cage with a stainless steel top (four to five per cage, depending on size and weight) containing bedding, water, and food pellets. Each cage carries an individual card holder with information established by the committee of the animal resource center, including the investigator's name, permit number, the date of birth and date of arrival of animals, species, strain, and sex. In a conventional care facility, there is no need to autoclave material used for housing animals. As a general practice, gloves and masks are worn, but there are no dressing requirements for entering the animal room. In a virus-free facility, rats arrive from a virus-antibody-free colony. They are kept in special microaislator cages which have a cage cover with a special replaceable filter to prevent cross-contamination of cages. Gowns, gloves, head covers, shoe covers, and masks are required to enter the VAF room. All cages, food, water, and accessories must be autoclaved before the rats are housed, and there must be a hood in which cages can be uncovered to minimize cross-contamination. Other precautions exist, depending on the regulations of each facility.

III. Genetic Background

EAE in Lewis rats is generally induced by injecting guinea pig myelin basic protein (GP-MBP) and is determined by a single dominant gene which is linked to the $Ag-B^1$ histocompatibility locus (Gasser et al., 1973) and to the $Ag-B^1/AgB^3$ histocompatibility locus in the (Lewis × brown Norway) F_1 rat. The gene for EAE susceptibility has been designated Ir-EAE (Williams and Moore, 1973). The Ir-EAE gene is also involved in cell-mediated immunity to GP-MBP. Six inbred strains possessing the $Ag-B^1$ histocompatibility allele are susceptible to EAE. The brown Norway (BN) strain is much less susceptible to EAE then Lewis rats. However, EAE can be produced in BN rats by immunization with rat spinal cord and carbonyl iron particulate adjuvants (Levine and Sowinski, 1975; Happ et al., 1988). T-cell lines and clones selected with GP-MBP in vitro have been shown to preferentially utilize the $V\beta8.2$ allele of the T-cell receptor (TCR; Burns et al., 1989). Some genetically resistant rats (PVG strain) which resist active induction of EAE are susceptible to and can generate EAE effector T-cell lines (Ben-Nun et al., 1982a).

IV. Disease Induction

EAE may be actively induced by immunization with myelin basic protein or proteolipid apoprotein (PLP), or by specific peptides encompassing the encephalitogenic regions. MBP and PLP are the major protein components of CNS myelin. For disease induction, the protein or peptide must be emulsified (water in oil solution) in Freund's complete adjuvant (CFA), or adsorbed on the surface of particulates such as carbon, kaolin, or talc (Levine *et al.*, 1972). The emulsified adjuvant acts as a slow-releasing repository of emulsified antigen at the injection site and creates a granulomatous reaction that stimulates mononuclear cells to induce a CD4+ T-cell response (Freund, 1953). Freund's complete adjuvant holds an established place in the laboratory as a means of attaining high levels of antibody against protein antigens and inducing cell-mediated responses. It is made by adding various mycobacterial species to a simple water in oil emulsion. There are different strains of mycobacteria that are effective in such mixtures, including *M. tuberculosis* (human and bovine strains), *M. avium*, *M. phlei* (soprophytic strains), *M. sinegmatis*, and *M. kansasii* (atypical strains). Unlike murine EAE, the use of pertussis toxin or pertussis organisms is not required to induce acute EAE in Lewis rats. Pertussis is required, however, for the induction of hyperacute EAE, which is an animal model of acute hemorrhagic necrotizing leukoencephalopathy in humans (Levine and Saltzman, 1989; Levine, 1969). The encephalitogenic determinant of MBP varies among species. In Lewis rats, the encephalitogenic determinant of guinea pig MBP is 68–86, with the minimal epitope being 75–84 or 72–84 (Chou *et al.*, 1977; McFarlin *et al.*, 1973; Kardys and Hashim, 1981; Mannie *et al.*, 1985). Guinea pig MBP is the antigen most commonly used to induce EAE in Lewis rats. There is a hierarchy of encephalitogenicity of MBP from different species, with guinea pig MBP being the most encephalitogenic; it is worth noting that the response to rat (self-MBP) MBP is lower than to guinea pig MBP (Happ *et al.*, 1988; Miller *et al.*, 1992).

For immunization, guinea pig MBP is dissolved in phosphate-buffered saline at a concentration of 0.5 mg–1 mg. *Mycobacterium tuberculosis* H37Ra is dissolved in incomplete Freund's adjuvant (IFA) at a concentration of 2 mg/ml. GP-MBP and Mt are emulsified in equal volumes (1:1 v/v) and once the emulsion is formed, the appearance of the mixture is white and thick. If the emulsion is not complete and is liquid in texture so that it separates easily, it will interfere with the induction of EAE. The emulsion can be prepared in either glass or plastic syringes, and a stainless steel or a plastic three-way stopcock used. Plastic syringes and the three-way valve are preferable. Each rat receives 0.1 ml of emulsion, injected subcutaneously in either one or two footpads in which 0.1 ml of emulsion contains 0.025 mg or 0.05 mg of GP-

MBP and 0.1 mg of Mt H37Ra. There are some variations in which the GP-MBP is at a concentration of 0.5 mg/ml and the amount of MT (H37Ra) is increased to 4 mg/ml. In this case, 0.1 ml of emulsion will contain 0.025 mg GP-MBP and 0.2 mg of MT (H37Ra). Signs of clinical disease appear beginning from day 9 to day 12.

EAE may also be induced in Lewis rats by injection of bovine proteolipid apoprotein (Yamamura et $al.$, 1986) PLP is dissolved in water at a concentration of 2 mg/ml and emulsified in an equal volume of complete Freund's adjuvant containing 4 mg/ml of Mt (H37Ra) strain. Each rat is immunized with a total of 0.1 ml of emulsion containing 0.1 mg of PLP and 0.2 mg of Mt divided equally into the hind footpads. Clinical EAE develops approximately 18 days after injection, with demyelination being a more prominent feature than with MBP-induced EAE.

Although EAE is a cell-mediated autoimmune disease that is not transferrable by antibodies, antimyelin antibodies against myelin oligodendrocyte glycoprotein can enhance the severity of EAE and be associated with demyelination (Schluesener et $al.$, 1987; Linington et $al.$, 1988).

Adoptive transfer of EAE is often used to study immunoregulatory events in the EAE model in Lewis rats. For adoptive transfer, lymph node cells are removed from MBP/CFA immunized animals 10–14 days after immunization and cultured in $vitro$ with either MBP for 3–4 days or a T-cell mitogen such as concanavalin A (ConA) for 2–3 days prior to transfer. Clinical signs of EAE usually appear 4–7 days after transfer (Hinrichs, 1984; Miller et $al.$, 1993). Briefly, inguinal, popliteal, and paraaortic lymph nodes are aseptically removed on days 10–14 postimmunization. The nodes are ground through a wire mesh screen to form a single-cell suspension and washed several times with Hank's balanced salt solution (HBSS) and resuspended in complete RPMI 1640 medium containing 5% heat-inactivated fetal calf serum or 1% autologous rat serum, 2 mM L-glutamine, 1% penicillin (100 u/ml) plus streptomycin (100 μg/ml), 1% MEM nonessential amino acids, 1% sodium pyruvate, 1% HEPES, and 2×10^{-5} 2 mercaptoethanol. Cells are adjusted to a density of 2×10^{6} and incubated for 3–4 days at 37.5° C with 5% CO_2 and GP-MBP or ConA, at a final concentration of 10–50 μg/ml MBP or 1.5–2.5 μg/ml ConA, in 75 cm^2 culture flasks (40 ml of medium) or in a petri dish (10 ml of medium). Following incubation, cells are collected, washed three times in HBSS, and counted, with a determination of viability by standard trypan blue exclusion. Viable cells are adjusted to 4–5 $\times$ 10^7/ml in HBSS prior to injection either intravenously or intraperitoneally in a volume of 1–2 ml. If spleen cells are used, red blood cells are removed by lysis with 0.2% ammonium chloride solution for 3 min followed by washing three times with HBSS. T-cell lines or clones can also transfer passive EAE in rats and there are different techniques for the preparation of encephalitogenic T-cell lines or clones (Ben-Nun *et al.*, 1982b). The characteristics of the encephalitogenic cells are CD4+TCR Vβ8.2Vα2 (Offner *et al.*, 1989). It is important to know that the number of T-cell lines or clones needed to transfer EAE is much smaller than that for primed lymph nodes described earlier.

Chronic relapsing EAE (CR-EAE) can be induced in rats (Feuer *et al.*, 1985; Brod *et al.*, 1991). There are two forms of CR-EAE; one form has a latent period of 2–3 months between the time of immunization with isogenic spinal cord in CFA and the first clinical sign of EAE (Raine, 1983). In the other form, a first attack occurs 2 weeks after immunization, followed by recovery and onset of relapse between 8 and 12 weeks postimmunization (Lassmann *et al.*, 1979). In general, Lewis rats immunized with GP-MBP in CFA suffer a single (monophasic) episode of paralysis from which they recover spontaneously and become refractory to induction of further episodes of paralysis by immunization with GP-MBP in CFA. CR-EAE can be induced in Lewis rats by immunization with guinea pig spinal cord homogenate (GP-SCH) in CFA into the footpad. Lewis rats are immunized in each hind footpad with 0.1 ml of emulsion containing GP-SCH in phosphate-buffered saline (PBS) (290 mg/ml) plus an equal volume of CFA containing 11 mg/ml of *Mycobacterium tuberculosis* (H37Ra) according to Feuer *et al.*, (1985). Clinical EAE is first observed on days 9–12 postimmunization.

Approximately 1 week after the acute attack, a second attack occurs. An interesting feature of hindlimb paralysis in the chronic variant of EAE is that initially flaccid paralysis of the classic type occurs but with time spasticity of hindlimbs can develop. Ascending paralysis is observed not only during acute monophasic EAE, but also during the onset of relapses, in which the initial behavioral impairment is recapitulated.

Lewis rats that have recovered from EAE are resistant to subsequent attempts at induction. Such resistance may be associated with postrecovery suppressor or regulatory cells that secrete suppressive cytokines such as transforming growth factor-β (TGF-β) and interleukin-4 (IL-4) (Karpus and Swanborg, 1991; Khoury *et al.*, 1992).

V. Quantitation

The most common clinical impairment is flaccid paralysis of the hindlimbs, which in rats occurs more often than forelimb paralysis. The ascending (caudal to cranial) progression of paralysis during EAE has long been recognized as the clinical hallmark of the disease. In species with long tails such as rats, the ascending progression can be easily monitored. The first neurological sign is a decreased tendency of the tail to curl around the examiner's finger, followed by a limp tip or half length of the tail, and then complete atony. Clinical signs of EAE usually appear by days 9–12 postimmunization.

Animals may be scored according to the following clinical scale: 0, no clinical signs; 1+, loss of tail tone (flaccid tail); 2+, tail weakness plus hindlimb paresis (ataxia); 3+, moderate hindlimb paralysis; 4+, total hindlimb paralysis (paraplegia), often accompanied by urinary incontinence and fecal impaction; 5+, death. Some groups score 3+ as total hindlimb paralysis and 4+ as tetraplegia.

The histological hallmark of acute EAE in the Lewis rat is a perivascular infiltrate of mononuclear cells (Sobel et al., 1984). Demyelination is only seen in chronic disease. The infiltrate may also include polymorphonuclear neutrophilic leukocytes. For histologic analysis, animals are sacrificed on day 16 after immunization, and their brains removed and fixed in either 10% formalin or a solution of 3% formaldehyde, 60% ethanol, and 4% acetic acid. Tissue sections are then dehydrated and embedded in paraffin. Transverse (7–10 μm) sections are stained with hematoxylin and eosin and duplicate slides for each animal are assessed for perivascular mononuclear infiltrates and scored as follows: 1+, 1–10 lesions; 2+, 11–30 lesions; 3+, more than 30 lesions. In Lewis rats, because the spinal cord is more predominantly affected, spinal cord histology is preferred by some investigators.

In our studies of chronic EAE (Brod et al., 1991), demyelination was determined in two ways. First, demyelination foci were assigned for each anatomical level on a subjective scale of 0 (no demyelination) to 4 (multifocal, large areas of demyelination). Second, areas of demyelination were measured directly in each section using a Bioquant system image analyzer attached to a computer. Microscopic fields with demyelinated foci in the white matter were selected from coded luxol fast blue hematoxylin–eosin-stained paraffin sections. Images were projected from fields magnified to 468 times on a monitor and areas of demyelination were outlined on a digitizer pad. Vessel lumina, inflammatory cell aggregates in which cells were too close to determine if demyelination was present, and clusters of inflammatory cells within the Virchow–Robin spaces were excluded from measurement. All histological analysis should be performed by a person blind to the protocols.

VI. Expert Experience

Animals from a conventional care facility have an earlier onset of disease (days 9–10) and more severe clinical signs of EAE than those from a VAF facility (disease onset, 11–13 days). Occasionally animals may show clinical signs different from those previously mentioned. For example, some animals will develop only front limb paralysis with no decreased tail tone or hind leg paralysis. At times, animals develop an axial rotatory movement, in which any attempt to examine the rat results in a vigorous rotation with a twisted neck. Also during the clinical course of EAE, many paraplegic rats develop a black ring around the eyes that lasts until the end of the recovery stage. This sign does not appear in every rat within a group. Rarely, after a full recovery from EAE, some rats have a spontaneous relapse that can last from a few days to a week. Viral infection and parasitic infestation may affect the induction as well as the clinical course of EAE and *in vitro* immunologic assays. Bad batches of Mt will decrease the incidence and severity of EAE and not all batches of Mt work equally well and must be individually tested. EAE can be induced by injection of whole CNS tissue or purified antigens such as MBP and PLP emulsified in CFA into other sites beside the hind footpads, for example, into the base of the tail, flanks, nuchal area, and into the back. This gives the researcher the advantage of being able to use larger volumes of emulsions and larger areas of inoculation.

References

Ben-Nun, A., Wekerle, H., and Cohen, I. R. (1982a). *Eur. J. Immunol.* **11**, 195–201.

Ben-Nun, A., Eisenstein, S., and Cohen, I. R. (1982b). *J. Immunol.* **129**, 918–919.

Brod, S. A., Al-Sabbagh, A., Sobel, R. A., Hafler, D. A., and Weiner, H. L. (1991). *Ann. Neurol.* **29**, 615–622.

Burns, F. R., Li, X., Shen, N., Offner, H., Chou, Y., Vanderbark, A. A., and Heverkatz, E. (1989). *J. Exp. Med.* **169**, 27–34.

Chou, C. H. J., Chou, F. C. H., Kowalski, T. J., Shapira, R., and Kibler, R. F. J. (1977). *Neurochemistry* **28**, 115–119.

Feuer, C., Prentice, D. E., and Cammisuli, L. (1985). *J. Neuroimmunol.* **10**, 159–165.

Freund, J. (1932). *Science* **75**, 418–420.

Gasser, D. L., Newlin, C. M., Palm, J., and Gonatas, N. K. (1973). *Science* **181**, 872–873.

Happ, P. M., Wertstein, P., Dietzchold, B., and Heber-Katz, E. J. (1988). *Immunology* **141**, 1489–1494.

Hinrichs, D. T. (1984). *In* "Immunoregulatory Processes in Experimental Allergic Encephalomyelitis and Multiple Sclerosis" (A. A. Vandenbark, and J. C. M. Rans, Eds.). Research Monographs in Immunology, Vol. 7, pp. 63–98. Elsevier, Amsterdam.

Kardys, J., and Hashim, G. (1981). *J. Immunol.* **127**, 862–867.

Karpus, W., and Swanborg, R. (1991). *J. Immunol.* **146**, 1163–1168.

Khoury, S. J., Hancock, W. W., and Weiner, H. L. (1992). *J. Exp. Med.* **176**, 1355–1364.

Lassman, H., and Wisniewski, H. M. (1979). *Arch. Neurol.* **36**, 490–496.

Levine, S. (1969). "Relationship of Experimental Allergic Encephalomyelitis to Human Disease" *In* (L. P. Rowland, Ed.) *Immunological Disorder of the Nervous System*. Proceedings of the Association for Research in Nervous and Mental Diseases. Vol. 49. pp. 33–49. Williams and Wilkins. Baltimore.

Levine, S., and Saltzman, A. (1989). *J. Neurol.* **48**, 255–162.

Levine, S., and Sowinski, R. (1975). *J. Immunol.* **114**, 2, Part 1, 297–629.

Levine, S., Sowinski, R., Gruenewald. R., and Kies, M. W. (1972). *Immunology* **23**, 609–614.

Linington, C., Bradl, M., Lassmann, H., Brunner, C., and Vass, K. (1988). *Am. J. Pathol.* **130**, 443–454.

Lipton, M. M., and Freund, J. (1953). *J. Immunol.* **71**, 98–109.

Lumsden, C. E. (1949). *Brain* **72**, 198–226.

McFarlin, D. E., Blank, S. E., Kibler, R. F., McKneally, S., and R. Shapira. (1973). *Science* **179**, 478–480.

Mannie, M. D., Paterson, P. Y., U'Prichard, D. C., and Flouret, G. (1985). *Proc. Natl. Acad. Sci.* **82**, 5515–5519.

Miller, A., Lider, O., Al-Sabbagh, A., and Weiner, H. L. (1992). *J. Neuroimmunol.* **39**, 245–250.

Miller, A., Zhang, Z. J., Sobel, R. A., Al-Sabbagh, A., and Weiner, H. L. (1993). *J. Neuroimmunol.* **46**, 73–82.

Offner, H., Hashim, G. A., Celnik, B., Galang, A., Li, X., Burns, F. R., Shen, N., Hever-Katz, E., and Vandenbark, A. A. (1989). *J. Exp. Med.* **170**, 355–362.

Raine, C. S. (1983). *Lab. Invest.* **48(3)**, 275–284.

Rivers, T. M., and Schwentker, F. F. (1935). *J. Exp. Med.* **61**, 689–702.

Schluesener, H. J., Sobel, R. A., Livingston, C., and Weiner, H. L. (1987). *J. Immunol.* **139**, 4016–4021.

Sobel, R., Blanchette, B., Bhan, A., and Colvin, R. (1984). *J. Immunol.* **132**, 2393–2401.

Williams, R. M., and Moore, M. J. (1973). *J. Exp. Med.* **138**, 775–781.

Yamamura, T., Namikawa, T., Endo, M., Kumishita, T., and Tabira, T. (1986). *J. Neuroimmunol.* **12**, 143–153.

Chapter 3

Theiler's Virus-Induced Demyelinating Disease

Stephen D. Miller,[1] William J. Karpus,[1] Jonathan G. Pope,[1] Mauro C. Dal Canto,[2] and Roger W. Melvold[1]

Departments of [1]Microbiology-Immunology and [2]Pathology, Northwestern University Medical School, Chicago, Illinois 60611

I. History and Relevance of the Model

Theiler's murine encephalomyelitis viruses (TMEV) are members of the cardiovirus group of the Picornaviridae, and along with the other cardio-viruses—mengovirus and encephalomyocarditis virus—are natural pathogens in mice (Pevear *et al.*, 1987, 1988). TMEV is composed of three capsid proteins (VP1, VP2, and VP3) which surround a single-stranded, plus-sense RNA genome associated with a fourth structural protein, VP4. TMEV was first isolated in 1937 from a spontaneous case of paralysis in the mouse colony of Dr. Max Theiler (Theiler, 1937). TMEV has since been shown to infect both wild and colony-bred mice. There are two subgroups of TMEV. One group includes GD VII and FA viruses, which grow to high titers, are highly virulent, and induce fatal encephalitis. The second group, known as the Theiler's original (TO) subgroup, includes the Daniels (DA) and BeAn 8386 strains that have low virulence, grow to relatively low titers, and produce persistent infection of central nervous system (CNS) white matter with extensive demyelination (Lipton, 1980). A natural encounter with the TO strains initially leads to enteric infections in mice, with a small percentage of susceptible strains developing a subsequent infection of the central nervous system, which can lead to a chronic, progressive, demyelinating disease characterized by spastic hindlimb paralysis (Theiler, 1937; Theiler and Gard, 1940; Feltz *et al.*, 1953). The demyelination is linked to persistent TMEV infection of the CNS, and is characterized histologically by CNS, perivascular, mononuclear cell infiltrates, and primary demyelination (Lipton, 1975; Dal Canto and Lipton, 1975; Lipton *et al.*, 1984).

Mechanistic, histopathologic, genetic, and clinical similarities between this chronic, virally induced murine disease and human multiple sclerosis (MS) make TMEV-induced demyelinating disease an excellent experimental model for MS (Dal Canto, 1990). Demyelination in both MS (Waksman, 1989; Hafler and Weiner, 1987) and TMEV-induced demyelinating disease (Clatch *et al.*, 1985, 1986, 1987a,b; Peterson *et al.*, 1992; Welsh *et al.*, 1987; Borrow *et al.*, 1992; Gerety *et al.*, 1993b) is clearly immune mediated and thought to be due primarily to the activity of inflammatory responses mediated via production of proinflammatory cytokines produced by antigen-specific $CD4^+$ T cells. The pathological lesions are very similar, with inflammation and demyelination being Closely linked in Theiler's virus infection (Lipton, 1975; Dal Canto and Lipton, 1975; Lehrich *et al.*, 1976; Lipton and Dal Canto, 1979b), as they are in acute MS lesions (Prineas, 1975). In addition, the cellular nature of the mononuclear infiltrates in both diseases consists primarily of monocytes, macrophages, and T lymphocytes (Traugott *et al.*, 1983; Clatch *et al.*, 1990). Both diseases are under multigenic control; susceptibility is associated with both major histocompatibility complex (MHC) genes and non-MHC genes, including T-cell receptor β-chain genes (Spielman and Nathanson, 1982; Gonatas *et al.*, 1986; Ho *et al.*, 1982; Clatch *et al.*, 1985, 1987b; Rodriguez and David, 1985; Rodriguez *et al.*, 1986b; Melvold *et al.*, 1987, 1990). Finally both MS and TMEV infection of mice lead to chronic and/or relapsing paralytic symptoms.

Consistent with TMEV-induced demyelinating disease as a model of MS, it is highly relevant that chronic demyelination following TMEV infection is induced in the apparent absence of autoimmune antimyelin responses (Miller *et al.*, 1987, 1990). Similarly, there is no convincing evidence that antimyelin responses play a major, or even a secondary, effector role in MS (Ota *et al.*, 1990; Waksman and Reynolds, 1984). However, epidemiologic studies strongly favor a viral etiology for MS (Nathanson and Miller, 1978; Kurtzke and Hyllested, 1986), although the causative agent(s) remains unidentified. Thus, elucidation of the immunopathologic mechanisms underlying chronic demyelination following TMEV infection of susceptible mouse strains could lead to a better understanding of the etiology of chronic demyelination and to the development of therapeutic applications for human demyelinating diseases, including MS.

II. The Animals

Inbred mouse strains differ in their susceptibility to development of TMEV-induced demyelination (Lipton and Dal Canto, 1979a; Clatch et al., 1987a). Table I shows a list of mouse strains which are highly susceptible, intermediately susceptible, or highly resistant to the development of Theiler's virus-induced demyelinating disease.

III. Genetics of Susceptibility or Resistance

The genetic basis for a differential susceptibility to development of Theiler's virus-induced demyelinating disease is multigenic and complex (Lipton and Melvold, 1984), and was recently reviewed by Blankenhorn and Stranford (1993). Both MHC (Lipton and Melvold, 1984; Rodriguez and David, 1985; Patick et al., 1990) and non-MHC (Melvold et al., 1987, 1990; McAllister et al., 1990; Bureau et al., 1992) genes are involved, and the loci found to have predominant effects in one comparison (e.g., resistant C57BL/6 vs susceptible DBA/2 mice) may differ from those in another comparison (e.g., resistant BALB/c vs susceptible SJL mice). In addition, resistance may be the dominant trait in some hybrids between susceptible and resistant strains, while susceptibility may be dominant in other hybrids.

Table I
Strain Differences in Susceptibility to TMEV-induced Demyelination

Highly susceptible	Intermediately susceptible	Highly resistant
SJL	C3H	BALB/c[a]
DBA/1[b]	CBA	C57BL/6
DBA/2	AKR	C57BL/10[a]
SWR	A	C57L
PL	C57BR	129/J[b]
P[b]		
NZW[b]		

[a] Although these strains are generally cited as resistant, substrain variation has been observed (R. W. Melvold, unpublished).
[b] R. W. Melvold, unpublished observations.

Several specific loci involved in differential susceptibility have been mapped (Table II), including two known or likely to be involved in T-cell regulation—the class I MHC locus *H-2D*, and the *Tmevd-1* locus, which is located in or among the loci encoding the β-chain of the T-cell receptor. The role of the *Tmevd-2* locus, located near the *Car-2* locus at the telomeric end of chromosome 3, is unknown. The strong association of a class I MHC gene (*H-2D*) in determining the presence or absence of an MHC class II-restricted, TMEV-specific delayed-type hypersensitivity (DTH) response, which is associated with development of disease (see later discussion), has been interpreted as reflecting either the role of a $CD8^+$ cytotoxic T lymphocyte (CTL) in clearing the virus (Rodriguez *et al.*, 1986b; Rossi *et al.*, 1991; Lindsley *et al.*, 1991), or the role of a $CD8^+$ regulatory cell controlling development of TMEV-specific DTH reactivity (Olsberg *et al.*, 1993). One other genetic trait, sex, has been shown to contribute to differential susceptibility between some strain combinations, in which males have a higher incidence of disease than females (Kappel *et al.*, 1990). Additional relevant loci remain to be mapped.

The resistance of some strains to the development of demyelination after infection with TMEV is not always intrinsic and absolute. Several reports indicate that immunopotentiating agents, applied prior to infection, permit development of demyelination in normally resistant animals. Rodriguez *et al.* (1990) reported that a high incidence of demyelinating lesions occurred in C57BL/10 mice exposed to 300 R of γ-irradiation 1 day prior to infection. Olsberg *et al.* (1993) reported that low doses of cyclophosphamide (20 mg/kg) 2 days prior to infection resulted in a 75–80% disease incidence in normally resistant $B6D2F_1$ hybrids. However, resistance could be restored in the cyclophosphamide-treated animals by adoptive transfer of spleen cells from syngeneic, noncyclophosphamide-treated donors. Comparable results have been

Table II

Genetic Loci Associated with Susceptibility to TMEV-Induced Demyelination

Locus	Chromosome	References
H-2D	17	Clatch *et al.* (1985)
		Rodriguez *et al.* (1986b)
		Clatch *et al.* (1987b)
Tmed-1	6	Melvold *et al.* (1987)
	(3 ± 3 cm from *TcR*β constant gene)	Kappel *et al.* (1991)
Tmevd-2	3	Melvold *et al.* (1990)
	(4 ± 4 cm from *Car-2*)	

found in B6D2F$_1$ hybrids receiving low-dose (50–200 rads) γ-irradiation. As with cyclophosphamide-treated B6D2F$_1$ animals, the irradiation-induced susceptibility can be reversed by adoptive transfer of spleen cells from syngeneic, unirradiated donors (Pelka *et al.*, 1993). Low-dose irradiation of a resistant BALB/c substrain (BALB/cByJ) also results in a disease incidence comparable to that seen in a susceptible substrain (BALB/cAnNCr) (Nicholson, *et al.*, 1994). Taken together, these results suggest the presence of a radiation-sensitive, cyclophosphamide-sensitive cell which confers and maintains protection against development of demyelination in certain resistant strains.

It is thus apparent that many genetically resistant strains are not absolutely so, but rather carry a "latent susceptibility" which can be expressed when "normal" regulatory mechanisms are perturbed. Not all resistant strains, however, can be converted to the susceptible phenotype. C57BL/6 mice, in our hands, remain resistant despite pretreatment with irradiation, cyclophosphamide, or both. It is likely that the basis for resistance in this strain is different from that in the "latently susceptible" C57BL/10, B6D2F$_1$, or BALB/c strains.

IV. The Disease

A. Virus Production and Purification

1. Infecting Stock

BHK-21 cells (American Type Culture Collection) are grown in complete Dulbecco's Modified Eagle's Medium (DMEM) (high glucose, GIBCO, Grand Island, New York), containing 7.5% donor calf serum (GIBCO), 0.295% tryptose phosphate broth (Difco, Detroit, Michigan), 1.0% gentamicin (Sigma Chemical Co., St. Louis, Missouri), and 0.5% penicillin/streptomycin solution (GIBCO), in two 175-cm^2 tissue culture flasks at 37°C and 5% CO_2 until confluent. The medium is aspirated off, the cells are washed once with sterile phosphate-buffered saline (PBS), and approximately 2.25 ml of sterile 1X trypsin (GIBCO) added to the monolayers. When the cells begin to detach, 5 ml of complete DMEM are added to each disrupted monolayer and the cell suspension is pipetted against the side of the flask to break up remaining clumps, creating a single-cell suspension. The contents of the two flasks are suspended in 1 liter of complete DMEM; 25 ml of the suspension are distributed into each of 40 glass petri plates (150 mm × 20 mm), which are incubated at 37°C and 5% CO_2 until confluent. Approximately 3 days later the BHK-21 monolayer will be confluent, at which point the medium is aspirated off and replaced with 25 ml DMEM, containing 0.1% sterile bovine serum albumin (BSA, Sigma), 0.5% penicillin–streptomycin solution, and 4 ml thawed TMEV, BeAn 8386 strain. The plates are incubated at 33°C and 5% CO_2 until all the cells are lysed (floating). The lysate is then harvested from the glass plates with the aid of a rubber policeman and clarified by three cycles of alternate centrifugation (3000 rpm in a table-top centrifuge for 15 min) and sonication. Finally, the virus-containing supernatant is collected, aliquoted into 2-ml samples, and frozen at −70°C. It is advisable to determine the titer of the infecting virus stock by standard plaquing on BHK-21 cells.

2. Purification of TMEV

To obtain purified TMEV for immunological studies, the above protocol is followed through the point of harvesting the cell lysate from the glass petri plates. The pH of the lysate is adjusted using concentrated HCl such that the solution appears slightly orange. At this stage of the procedure, the cell lysates are either frozen at −20°C until needed, or used directly for the next step in purification (freezing appears to maximize the virus yield). The bottles of viral lysate are thawed in a 37°C shaking water bath, taking care that the bottles do not become too warm. To each bottle of viral lysate, 14.5 g NaCl and 30 g polyethylene glycol (PEG) (MW = 8000) are added and the solution is stirred overnight at 4°C. The precipitated lysate is divided into two 250-ml Nalgene centrifuge bottles and centrifuged at 6800 rpm in a Sorvall HB-4 swinging bucket rotor for 45 min at 4°C to collect the precipitate. The supernatant is discarded and each pellet immediately resuspended in 9 ml hypertonic TNE buffer (0.02 M Tris base, 0.5 M NaCl, 0.002 M EDTA). The contents of each bottle are sonicated as necessary to separate the virus from the cellular membranes and to break up cellular DNA. Following sonication, the pooled lysates are warmed and incubated with 1 ml 10% sodium dodecy/ sulfate (SDS) for each 9 ml lysate for 30 min at 37°C. The lysate is clarified by centrifugation (15 min, 3000 rpm at room temperature) to remove any large membranous debris. The pellet is discarded and the supernatants are overlaid onto 22 ml of a 35% sucrose solution in 14 × 89 mm Beckman Ultra-Clear centrifuge tubes. The virus is pelleted through the sucrose cushion by centrifugation in a SW28 rotor at 20,000 rpm for 20 hr at room temperature.

The following day the supernatant is poured off, each SW28 pellet is resuspended in 2 ml hypertonic TNE buffer, and sonicated on ice as necessary to remove clumps. To break up the remaining membrane fractions, the virus solution is treated with 0.1 ml 10% SDS for every 1 ml solution and incubated for at least 10 min at 37°C. Using a two-chambered gradient maker (Hoefer Scientific, San Francisco California), linear sucrose gradients are poured directly into SW41 Ultra-Clear centrifuge tubes by placing 4.5 ml of 20% sucrose in the left chamber and 4.5 ml 70% sucrose in the right chamber and mixing with air in the right chamber while the gradient pours down the wall of the centrifuge tube. Each gradient should take 5–10 min to pour properly. The SDS-treated virus solution is clarified as described previously; 2–3 ml of the resulting supernatant are overlaid onto each of the 20–70% sucrose gradients; and these are centrifuged at 35,000 rpm for 3 hr at room temperature. After centrifugation, a blue band is visible by UV or halogen light, approximately 1–2 cm from the bottom of the tube. The virus-containing blue bands are collected by puncturing the side of the tube using a syringe fitted with a 21-gauge needle and pooled into a new test tube. Pooled virus bands are divided equally into SW50.1 Ultra-Clear centrifuge tubes (maximum volume of virus solution per tube is 1.5 ml) and 2.2 ml Cs_2SO_4 (1 g/ml in hypotonic TNE buffer; pH = 7.0; RI = 1.384; filtered) is added. These are topped off with hypotonic TNE buffer (0.02 M Tris base, 0.15 M NaCl, 0.002 M EDTA), thoroughly mixed, and centrifuged at 40,000 rpm for 22 hr at 5°C.

The next day the virus is collected by puncturing the side of the tube using a 23-gauge needle and syringe, and pulling a white particulate band, visible 1 cm from the bottom of the tube. To pellet the resulting virus, 2–3 ml per tube of the pooled white virus bands are added to SW41 centrifuge tubes, which are filled to the top with hypotonic TNE buffer, mixed well, and centrifuged at 35,000 rpm for at least 3 hr at 5°C.

In the final purification step, the supernatant from the SW41 tubes is discarded, the virus pellet is resuspended in 0.2 ml PBS, and incubated for 1–24 hr at 4°C. At this point, better yields of virus are obtained by sonicating the resulting suspension to deaggregate the virus and to remove any virus nonspecifically adhering to the centrifuge tube. The mixture is gently vortexed and subsequently clarified in a microcentrifuge for 1 min. This supernatant is saved. The SW41 tubes are rinsed with PBS; the rinse is used to resuspend the pellet in the microcentrifuge tube which is centrifuged again and this supernatant is combined with the first supernatant. To quantitate the virus yield, appropriate dilutions of virus are made (e.g., 1:50, 1:100, 1:200) and each A_{280} measured is multiplied by its dilution factor. The average of the resulting numbers is used to determine the amount of virus by the following equation: (average $A_{280} \times 10/35$) = mg virus (including RNA). Purity is assessed by SDS–PAGE.

B. Disease Induction

Six to eight-week-old mice are anesthetized with methoxyflurane (Pitman-Moore, Washington Crossing, New Jersey) and inoculated in the right cerebral hemisphere with 2.9×10^6 plaque-forming units (PFU) of BeAn strain TMEV infecting stock (produced as described above) in 30 μl, using a 27-gauge needle with a guard to ensure penetration to a depth of no more than

3.5 mm. The mice are returned to their cages 1–2 min later when they regain consciousness. Control mice are inoculated in the same manner with 30 μl DMEM. Mice are marked for individual evaluation of clinical and histological disease.

C. Clinical Course of the Disease

The clinical presentation of TMEV-induced disease in a susceptible strain, such as SJL/J, differs when different strains of the virus are used for infection. Thus, when the brain-derived DA strain of virus is used, mice first develop a flaccid paralysis similar to that produced by polio virus (Lipton, 1975). This phase is generally self-limited and mice recover in approximately 2 weeks. Two to 3 weeks after infection, mice develop a spastic paresis of the hindlimbs, which, in SJL/J mice, has a chronic course resulting in severe paralysis (Lipton, 1975).

In contrast, infection of SJL/J mice with the tissue culture-adapted BeAn 8386 strain does not produce clinical evidence of a first phase of polio-like disease. Clinical signs develop slowly with no major changes in gait from day to day. Mice begin to show signs of clinical disease 35–40 days postinfection and develop a chronic, progressive paralysis with no recovery or remitting episodes. Mice are monitored for disease progression two to three times per week beginning 10 days before the predicted onset of disease and continuing for 100–200 days postinfection. With the onset of spastic paralysis, mice are monitored once a day, and with onset of total hindlimb paralysis, they are monitored twice a day. Each mouse is assigned a numerical score based on the severity of impairment: 0, asymptomatic, 1, abnormal waddling gait; 2, spastic paralysis; 3, hindlimb paralysis. The clinical course of disease is plotted as the mean clinical severity score for the experimental group versus time (in days) postinfection.

D. Pathological Course of the Disease

The pathology that follows infection with the DA or BeAn 8386 strains differs significantly. The major difference is in the degree of gray matter involvement in both brain and spinal cord. Whereas the DA strain produces a clear-cut, polio-like phase in both organs, BeAn-infected mice develop only a mild degree of gray matter inflammation, with only occasional foci of neuronophagia, which are abundant in DA-infected animals (Lipton, 1975; Lipton and Dal Canto, 1979b). Interestingly, the polio-like phase in DA-infected mice heals to the point that, at 6–8 weeks postinfection, there are no significant qualitative differences between the anterior horns in DA and BeAn infection. Counts of motor neurons in the two infections have not been performed.

The timing and appearance of white-matter lesions in the chronic phase of the disease also differ in DA- and BeAn-infected animals. Lesions in BeAn-infected animals develop more slowly than those in DA-infected mice. Pathological lesions in DA-infected animals are fully developed 2–3 weeks after TMEV inoculation, whereas lesions in BeAn-infected animals first appear at around 2 weeks postinfection, but do not become fully developed until 3–4 weeks after inoculation, concomitant with the appearance of clinical signs (Lipton, 1975; Lipton and Dal Canto, 1979b). Thus, up to 2 weeks of subclinical pathology of the spinal cord may occur following BeAn infection.

The initial pathological lesion in TMEV-induced demyelination is the development of lymphocytic infiltrates in meninges and along venules in the spinal cord parenchyma. This phase is followed soon by myelin breakdown in strict spatial relationship with such infiltrates (Figure 1) (Dal Canto and Lipton, 1975). Macrophages with myelin debris are always present in these

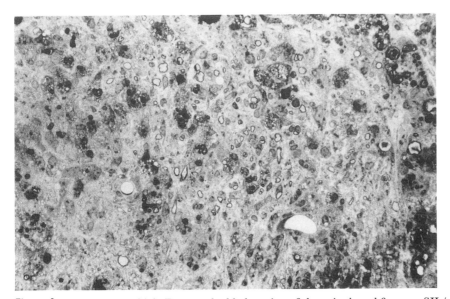

Figure 1   One micron-thick, Epon-embedded section of the spinal cord from an SJL/J mouse 140 days postinfection with BeAn virus stained with toluidine blue. The anterior column of the spinal cord shows an area of extensive demyelination. Several macrophages are still present in the subarachnoid space on the right-hand side of the picture. Other macrophages are scattered in the demyelinated white matter. A few scattered remyelinated axons, characterized by thin myelin sheaths, are seen. ×250.

areas. In addition, and particularly in SJL/J mice chronically infected with the BeAn strain, a considerable degree of axonal compromise may follow, which in some animals may become quite severe (M. C. Dal Canto, unpublished observations). As lesions become chronic, gliosis sets in; macrophages decrease in number; and the whole area becomes a gliotic plaque, in which naked axons can still be recognized.

Ultrastructurally, two main mechanisms of myelin breakdown can be recognized. One is characterized by vesicular dissolution of myelin in the presence of an intact axon. Myelin is thus reduced to a delicate network of thin lamellar loops representing the disrupted sheath. Activated monocytes often are seen in close contact with this form of myelin dissolution (Dal Canto and Lipton, 1975). The second mechanism is that of "myelin stripping," which consists of the penetration of monocyte processes into the myelin sheath, followed by progressive stripping of myelin lamellae, eventually leading to a naked axon (Dal Canto and Lipton, 1975). In both types of myelin destruction, therefore, the monocyte/macrophage appears to be the necessary element for carrying out the damage, a feature consistent with the hypothesis of bystander myelin injury (Dal Canto and Lipton, 1975; Dal Canto and Rabinowitz, 1982; Clatch *et al.*, 1985).

Ultrastructural immunohistochemical studies have attempted to determine the identity of the main cellular reservoir for this infection. The neuron and its processes are infected initially, followed by other cell types, including astrocytes, oligodendrocytes, and especially macrophages (Dal Canto and Lipton, 1982). The timing of oligodendrocyte infection relative to the onset of demyelination is not clear. It appears that oligodendrocytes are not initially infected, as detected by immunohistochemical techniques (Dal Canto and Lipton, 1982). However, at later times oligodendrocytes may become infected (Rodriguez *et al.*, 1983), but the contribution of this primary oligo-dendroglial infection to the overall demyelinating process is not clear. There is little doubt that the macrophage harbors most of the infectious virus during the chronic phase of the infection. By ultrastructural immunohistochemistry, macrophages are the most frequently and the most heavily stained cells in chronically infected spinal cords, and viral antigen appears associated with cytoskeletal elements, a feature generally associated with active viral synthesis (Dal Canto and Lipton, 1982). This was proven by macrophage isolation studies (Clatch *et al.*, 1990).

E. Immune Reactivities—Specificity, Transfer, and Regulation

There is an abundance of direct and indirect evidence favoring an immune-mediated basis for TMEV-induced demyelinating disease. A dramatic reduction in the extent of mononuclear cell infiltration and prevention of demyelination is observed in mice nonspecifically immunosuppressed by treatment with cyclophosphamide and/or antithymocyte serum (Lipton and Dal Cánto, 1976, 1977; Roos *et al.*, 1982). Treatment of mice with monoclonal anti-Ia antibodies (directed against MHC class II gene products) results in reversal of chronic paralysis, and reduced inflammation and demyelination when given concomitant with or after the establishment of persistent infection (Friedmann *et al.*, 1987; Rodriguez *et al.*, 1986a). The mononuclear cell nature of the inflammatory infiltrate associated with the CNS demyelinating lesions and linkage of strain susceptibility to both *H-2* and *TcR* genes are suggestive of a T-cell-mediated pathogenic process. In contrast, disease susceptibility does *not* correlate with a number of other parameters, including: (1) splenic TMEV-specific T-cell proliferative (Tprlf) responses—both susceptible and resistant strains generate TMEV-specific T-cell proliferation (Clatch *et al.*, 1985, 1986, 1987a,b); (2) serum anti-TMEV antibody titers (either total or neutralizing antibody)—both susceptible and resistant strains synthesize high titers of TMEV-specific antibody (Clatch *et al.*, 1985, 1986, 1987a,b); and (3) the amount of TMEV plaqued from the CNS (Clatch *et al.*, 1985, 1987a,b).

The failure of adult, thymectomized, irradiated, bone marrow-reconstituted, susceptible SJL/J mice to develop clinical or histological signs of TMEV-induced demyelinating disease following infection with the BeAn strain of virus (Gerety *et al.*, 1993b) indicates that the pathologic process is T-cell dependent. In addition, transfer of TMEV-specific T-cell blasts (either polyclonally activated from lymph node cells of TMEV-primed mice or long-term T-cell lines) results in an increase in the incidence and severity of disease in syngeneic recipients infected intracerebrally with a suboptimal dose of TMEV, but not in uninfected recipients (Gerety *et al.*, 1993b).

In vivo monoclonal antibody depletion experiments have yielded disparate results regarding the nature of the effector T cells responsible for demyelination. Welsh *et al.* (1987) found that CBA mice depleted of total T cells or CD4$^+$ cells after infection with the BeAn strain of TMEV, but prior to the onset of clinical signs of demyelination, exhibited a reduced disease incidence of approximately 50%. Similarly, studies with SJL/J mice in our laboratory have shown that monoclonal antibody depletion of CD4$^+$ cells, beginning 10–14 days after infection with the BeAn strain of TMEV, resulted in a decreased incidence of demyelinating disease as well as a slower onset of disease in those mice which eventually became clinically affected (Gerety *et al.*, 1993b). In addition, essentially all of the activated [i.e., interleukin-2 (IL-2) receptor-bearing] lymphocytes infiltrating the CNS are CD4$^+$ as determined by flow cytometry (Pope *et al.*, submitted for publication). In contrast, the incidence and onset of clinical disease in BeAn-infected CBA and SJL/J mice treated with a monoclonal anti-Lyt 2 antibody to deplete CD8$^+$ T cells parallel that of control mice (Borrow *et al.*, 1992; Gerety *et al.*,

1993b). However, demyelination induced by the DA strain of TMEV has been reported to be inhibited by depletion of CD8[+], but not CD4[+] T cells (Rodriguez and Sriram, 1988). The varied effects of monoclonal antibody depletion of T cell subsets on clinical and histologic disease thus may relate to the strain of virus employed.

Support for a CD4[+] T-cell-mediated (CMl) pathogenesis of TMEV-induced demyelinating disease derives from studies showing that susceptibility strongly correlates with the development of chronic, high levels of TMEV-specific DTH (Clatch et al., 1985, 1986, 1987a,b). DTH in BeAn-infected susceptible SJL/J mice develops within 10–14 days postinfection, preceding the onset of clinical signs, and remains at high levels for at least 6 months postinfection (Clatch et al., 1986). TMEV-specific DTH in SJL mice is mediated by L3T4[+] (CD4[+]) Lyt 2[-] (CD8[-]) T cells and is restricted by I-A^s determinants (Clatch et al., 1986). DTH and Tprlf responses in susceptible SJL/J mice, whether infected with the viable BeAn strain of TMEV or peripherally immunized with UV-inactivated BeAn emulsified in CFA, cross-react to a significant extent with the closely related encephalomyocarditis virus, but only marginally with the MEF1 strain of poliovirus, a more distantly related picornavirus.

In addition, extensive cross-reactivity at the polyclonal T-cell level is observed between members of the serologically related subgroups of TMEV [i.e., the relatively avirulent, demyelinating TO subgroup of TMEV (BeAn and VL strains) and the highly neurovirulent GDVII subgroup (GDVII strain); Miller et al., 1987]. Thus, functional T-cell cross-reactivity among members of the picornavirus family, as reflected by DTH and Tprlf assays, correlates with the degree of sequence homology among the capsid proteins of the picornavirus strains. VP2 contains the immunodominant T-cell determinant(s) in TMEV-infected SJL/J mice, as 80–90% of the DTH response is directed against this virion protein (Gerety et al., 1991). In contrast, resistant C57BL/6 mice generally respond equivalently to VP1, VP2, and VP3. These results suggest that susceptibility or resistance to TMEV-induced demyelinating disease may be influenced by the T-cell repertoire. More recent studies have mapped the SJL/J T cell epitope to a 17-amino-acid peptide on VP2 (VP2$_{70-86}$) (Gerety et al., 1993a). Systemic transfer of an SJL/J-derived, VP2$_{74-86}$-specific T-helper cell line (Th1), sTV1, exacerbates the incidence and severity of disease in mice infected intracerebrally with suboptimal amounts of TMEV, demonstrating the immunopathologic potential of CD4[+] T-cell responses to the dominant epitope (Gerety et al., 1993b).

Autoimmune T-cell reactivity against the major myelin proteins, myelin basic protein (MBP) and proteolipid protein (PLP) does not appear to be involved in the induction of the demyelination process following TMEV infection. Demyelination cannot be transferred from TMEV-infected donors to normal, non-TMEV-infected recipients with either serum or lymphoid cells (Barbano and Dal Canto, 1984). Neuroantigen-specific T-cell responses are not detected in SJL/J mice at any time following intracerebral inoculation with TMEV, including time points prior to the onset of clinical signs of disease (day + 23), shortly after the onset of disease (day +69), and 8–12 weeks after the onset of disease (day +127) (Miller *et al.*, 1987). T cells from TMEV-infected mice also do not respond to the peptide fragments of MBP (amino acids 91–104) and PLP (139–151) known to be encephalitogenic in SJL/J mice (Miller *et al.*, 1990). The lack of neuroantigen reactivity in TMEV-infected mice, as measured by functional T-cell analyses, is paralleled by the absence of significant amino acid homology between the TMEV capsid proteins (VP1, VP2, or VP3) and MBP or PLP (Miller *et al.*, 1987).

In addition, induction of tolerance in SJL/J mice via the i.v. injection of syngeneic splenocytes coupled with mouse spinal cord homogenate (MSCH) (a heterogeneous mixture of myelin and nonmyelin antigens) failed to affect the development of clinical and histological signs of TMEV-induced demyelinating disease and the accompanying virus-specific CMI and antibody responses induced by TMEV infection (Miller *et al.*, 1990). However, this tolerogenic regimen is extremely effective in reducing the incidence of clinical and histological signs of MSCH-induced relapsing experimental autoimmune encephalomyelitis and the accompanying neuroantigen-specific DTH responses (Miller *et al.*, 1990; Kennedy *et al.*, 1988). In contrast, induction of tolerance using intact TMEV virions coupled to syngeneic splenocytes, which specifically anergizes virus-specific Th1 responses (Peterson *et al.*, 1993), results in a dramatic reduction in the incidence and severity of demyelinating lesions and clinical disease in SJL/J mice subsequently infected with TMEV (Kapus *et al.*, submitted for publication).

Collectively, these results strongly indicate that chronic demyelination can occur in the apparent absence of neuroantigen-specific autoimmune responses, which is consistent with the hypothesis that virus-specific DTH is the major effector mechanism of CNS demyelination following TMEV infection (Clatch *et al.*, 1986). According to this hypothesis, intracerebral infection leads to an initial viremia followed by a persistent, low-level CNS infection which can last for virtually the lifetime of the animal (Lipton *et al.*, 1984). As a consequence of this infectious process, MHC class II-restricted, TMEV-specific Th1 cells clonally expand, either in the periphery or locally within the CNS. Subsequent release of proinflammatory cytokines interferon-γ and lymphotoxin/TNF-β) by the tumor-necrosing factor-β T helper (Th1) cells in the CNS leads to the recruitment and activation of monocytes and macrophages which cause myelin destruction by a terminal nonspecific *bystander* mechanism (Dal Canto and Lipton, 1975). This hypothesis is also consistent with the characteristic mononuclear cell infiltrates associated with destructive demyelinating lesions (Dal Canto and Lipton, 1975; Lehrich *et al.*, 1976) and would account for the chronic replenishing of host monocytes or macrophages in which TMEV is known to persist primarily (Clatch *et al.*, 1990). Recent isolation of an SJL/J-derived cloned TMEV-specific Th1 line (sTV1), which can increase the incidence and severity of demyelinating disease upon transfer to recipient mice infected with a suboptimal dose of TMEV (Gerety *et al.*, 1993b), lends strong support to a major effector role for DTH reactivity in the pathogenesis of demyelinating lesions. A major role for TMEV-specific Th1 activity is also supported by the finding that anti-TMEV antibody response in susceptible mice is dominated by immunoglobulin G2a [IgG2a, known to be under the regulatory control of Th1 cells (Mosmann and Coffman, 1989)], whereas Th2-regulated IgG1 anti-TMEV responses dominate in TMEV-resistant strains (Peterson *et al.*, 1992).

V. Lessons

As detailed previously TMEV-induced demyelinating disease is an extremely relevant model of MS owing to close mechanistic, pathologic, genetic, and clinical similarities. An important feature of the pathogenesis of the disease is the surprising finding that a member of a normally highly cytocidal family of picornaviruses can persist exclusively in the CNS for virtually the lifetime of the murine host (Lipton *et al.*, 1984). Because of its small size, low tissue titers, and failure to produce any characteristic inclusions, it can only be detected by immunohistochemical staining or *in situ* hybridization (Dal Canto and Lipton, 1982; Cash *et al.*, 1985; Brahic *et al.*, 1984). Most important, it appears that chronic demyelination in TMEV-infected mice is immune-mediated, but induced in the apparent absence of autoimmune responses against myelin proteins. These latter points are highly relevant in light of epidemiological studies favoring a viral etiology in MS yet a failure to clearly associate a specific CNS virus infection with MS, as well as a lack of convincing evidence that antimyelin T-cell responses correlate with the clinical course of MS.

References

Barbano, R. L., and Dal Canto, M. C. (1984). *J. Neurol. Sci.* **66**, 283–293.

Blankenhorn, E. P., and Stranford, S. A. (1993). *Reg. Immunol.*, **4**, 331–343.

Borrow, P., Tonks, P., Welsh, C. J. R., and Nash, A. A. (1992). *J. Gen. Virol.* **73**, 1861–1865.

Brahic, M., Haase, A. T., and Cash, E. (1984). *Proc. Natl. Acad. Sci. USA* **81**, 5445–5448.

Bureau, J. F., Montagutelli, X., Lefebvre, S., Guenet, J. L., Pla, M., and Brahic, M. (1992). *J. Virol.* **66**, 4698–4704.

Cash, E., Chamorro, M., and Brahic, M. (1985). *Virology* **144**, 290–294.

Clatch, R. J., Melvold, R. W., Miller, S. D., and Lipton, H. L. (1985). *J. Immunol.* **135**, 1408–1414.

Clatch, R. J., Lipton, H. L., and Miller, S. D. (1986). *J. Immunol.* **136**, 920–927.

Clatch, R. J., Lipton, H. L., and Miller, S. D. (1987a). *Microb. Pathogen.* **3**, 327–337.

Clatch, R. J., Melvold, R. W., Dal Canto, M. C., Miller, S. D., and Lipton, H. L. (1987b). *J. Neuroimmunol.* **15**, 121–135.

Clatch, R. J., Miller, S. D., Metzner, R., Dal Canto, M. C., and Lipton, H. L. (1990). *Virology* **176**, 244–254.

Dal Canto, M. C. (1990). *In* "Handbook of Multiple Sclerosis" (S. D. Cook, Ed.), pp. 63–100. Marcel Dekker, New York/Basel.

Dal Canto, M. C., and Lipton, H. L. (1975). *Lab. Invest.* **33**, 626–637.

Dal Canto, M. C., and Lipton, H. L. (1982). *Am. J. Pathol.* **106**, 20–29.

Dal Canto, M. C., and Rabinowitz, S. G. (1982). *Ann. Neurol.* **11**, 109–127.

Feltz, E. T., Mandel, B., and Racker, E. (1953). *J. Exp. Med.* **98**, 427–436.

Friedmann, A., Frankel, G., Lorch, Y., and Steinman, L. (1987). *J. Virol.* **61**, 898–903.

Gerety, S. J., Clatch, R. J., Lipton, H. L., Goswami, R. G., Rundell, M. K., and Miller, S. D. (1991). *J. Immunol.* **146**, 2401–2408.

Gerety, S. J., Karpus, W. J., Cubbon, A. R., Goswami, R. G., Rundell, M. K., Peterson, J. D., and Miller, S. D. (1994a). *J. Immunol.* **152**, 908–918

Gerety, S. J., Rundell, M. K., Dal Canto, M. C., and Miller, S. D. (1994b). *J. Immunol.*, **152**, 919–929.

Gonatas, N. K., Greene, M. I., and Waksman, B. H. (1986). *Immunol. Today* **7**, 121–126.

Hafler, D. A., and Weiner, H. L. (1987). *Immunol. Rev.* **100**, 307–332.

Ho, H. Z., Tiwari, J. L., Haile, R. W. Terasaki, P. I., and Morton, N. E. (1982). *Immunogenetics* **15**, 509–517.

Kappel, C. A., Melvold, R. W., and Kim, B. S. (1990). *J. Neuroimmunol.* **29**, 15–19.

Kappel, C. A., Dal Canto, M. C., Melvold, R. W., and Kim, B. S. (1991). *J. Immunol.* **147**, 4322–4326.

Kennedy, M. K., Dal Canto, M. C., Trotter, J. L., and Miller, S. D. (1988). *J. Immunol.* **141**, 2986–2993.

Kurtzke, J. F., and Hyllested, K. (1986). *Neurology* **36**, 307–328.

Lehrich, J. R., Arnason, B. G. W., and Hochberg, F. (1976). *J. Neurol. Sci.* **29**, 149–160.

Lindsley, M. D., Thiemann, R., and Rodriguez, M. (1991). *J. Virol.* **65**, 6612–6620.

Lipton, H. L. (1975). *Infect. Immun.* **11**, 1147–1155.

Lipton, H. L. (1980). *J. Gen. Virol.* **46**, 169–177.

Lipton, H. L., and Dal Canto, M. C. (1976). *Science* **192**, 62–64.

Lipton, H. L., and Dal Canto, M. C. (1977). *Infect. Immun.* **15**, 903–909.

Lipton, H. L., and Dal Canto, M. C. (1979a). *Infect. Immun.* **26**, 369–374.

Lipton, H. L., and Dal Canto, M. C. (1979b) *Ann. Neurol.* **6**, 25–28.

Lipton, H. L., and Melvoid, R. (1984). *J. Immunol.* **132**, 1821–1825.

Lipton, H. L., Kratochvil, J., Sethi, P., and Dal Canto, M. C. (1984). *Neurology* **34**, 1117–1119.

McAllister, A., Tangy, F., Aubert, C., and Brahic, M. (1990). *J. Virol.* **64**, 4252–4257.

Melvold, R. W., Jokinen, D. M., Knobler, R. L., and Lipton, H. L. (1987). *J. Immunol.* **138**, 1429–1433.

Melvold, R. W., Jokinen, D. M., Miller, S. D., Dal Canto, M. C., and Lipton, H. L. (1990). *J. Virol.* **64**, 686–690.

Miller, S. D., Clatch, R. J., Pevear, D. C., Trotter, J. L., and Lipton, H. L. (1987). *J. Immunol.* **138**, 3776–3784.

Miller, S. D., Gerety, S. J., Kennedy, M. K., Peterson, J. D., Trotter, J. L., Tuohy, V. K., Waltenbaugh, C., Dal Canto, M. C., and Lipton, H. L. (1990). *J. Neuroimmunol.* **26**, 9–23.

Mosmann, T. R., and Coffman, R. L. (1989). *Ann. Rev. Immunol.* **7**, 145–174.

Nathanson, N., and Miller, A. (1978). *Am. J. Epidemiol.* **107**, 451.

Nicholson, S. M., Peterson, J. D., Miller, S. D., Dal Canto, M. C., and Melvold, R. W. (1994) *J. Neuroimmunol.* in press.

Olsberg, C., Pelka, A., Miller, S. D., Waltenbaugh, C., Creighton, T. M., Dal Canto, M. C., Lipton, H. L., and Melvold, R. (1993). *Reg. Immunol.*, **5**, 1–10.

Ota, K., Matsui, M., Milford, E. L., Mackin, G. A., Weiner, H. L., and Hafler, D. A. (1990). *Nature* **346**, 183–187.

Patick, A. K., Pease, L. R., David, C. S., and Rodriguez, M. (1990). *J. Virol.* **64**, 5570–5576.

Pelka, A., Olsberg, C., Miller, S., Waltenbaugh, C., Creighton, T. M., Dal Canto, M. C., and Melvold, R. (1993). *Cell. Immunol.* **152**, 440–455.

Peterson, J. D., Waltenbaugh, C., and Miller, S. D. (1992). *Immunology* **75**, 652–658.

Peterson, J. D., Karpus, W. J., Clatch, R. J., and Miller, S. D. (1993). *Eur. J. Immunol.*, **23**, 46–55.

Pevear, D. C., Calenoff, M., Rozhon, E., and Lipton, H. L. (1987). *J. Virol.* **61**, 1507–1516.

Pevear, D. C., Borkowski, J., Luo, M., and Lipton, H. (1988). *Ann. N.Y. Acad. Sci.* **540**, 652–653.

Prineas, J. (1975). *Hum. Pathol.* **6**, 531–554.

Rodirguez, M., and David, C. S. (1985). *J. Immunol.* **135**, 2145–2148.

Rodriguez, M., and Sriram, S. (1988). *J. Immunol.* **140**, 2950–2955.

Rodriguez, M., Leibowitz, J. L., and Lampert, P. W. (1983). *Ann. Neurol.* **13**, 426–433.

Rodriguez, M., Lafuse, W. P., Leibowitz, J., and David, C. S. (1986a). *Neurology* **36**, 964–970.

Rodriguez, M., Leibowitz, J., and David, C. S. (1986b). *J. Exp. Med.* **163**, 620–631.

Rodriguez, M., Patick, A. K., and Pease, L. R. (1990). *J. Neuroimmunol.* **26**, 189–199.

Rodriguez, M., and Sriram, S. (1988). *J. Immunol.* **140**, 2950–2955.

Roos, R. P., Firestone, S., Wollmann, R., Variakojis, D., and Arnason, B. G. (1982). *J. Neuroimmunol.* **2**, 223–234.

Rossi, C. P., McAllister, A., Fiette, L., and Brahic, M. (1991). *Cell. Immunol.* **138**, 341–348.

Spielman, R. S., and Nathanson, N. (1982). *Epidemiol. Rev.* **4**, 45–65.

Theiler, M. (1937). *J. Exp. Med.* **65**, 705–719.

Theiler, M., and Gard, S. (1940). *J. Exp. Med.* **72**, 49–67.

Traugott, U., Reinherz, E. L., and Raine, C. S. (1983). *Science* **219**, 308–310.

Waksman, B. H. (1989). *Curr. Opin. Immunol.* **1**, 733–739.

Waksman, B. H., and Reynolds, W. E. (1984). *Proc. Soc. Exp. Biol. Med.* **175**, 282–294.

Welsh, C. J., Tonks, P., Nash, A. A., and Blakemore, W. F. (1987). *J. Gen. Virol.* **68**, 1659–1667.

Chapter 4

Experimental Autoimmune Neuritis

Christopher Linington and Hartmut Wekerle

Max-Planck-Institute of Psychiatry, D 82152 Martinsried, Germany

I. Introduction

The origins of experimental autoimmune neuritis (EAN) date back to the mid-1950s (Waksman and Adams, 1955), when it was already clear that "autoallergic" diseases of the central nervous system (CNS) could be induced in experimental animals not only by immunization with brain homogenate, but also by various CNS protein extracts (Waksman *et al.*, 1954). Waksman and Adams extended these studies to examine the pathological response following immunization with peripheral nerve tissue in adjuvant. In this paradigm, "autoallergic" disease was also tissue specific, but the inflammatory response was restricted exclusively to the peripheral nervous system (PNS) (Waksman and Adams, 1955). Detailed analysis of this disease model, EAN, revealed that it shared many characteristics with experimental autoimmune encephalomyelitis (EAE); for example, the disease was passively transferred to naive recipients by lymphocytes (Aström and Waksman, 1962), but not serum. Moreover, the methodology that allowed the isolation of encephalitogenic, myelin basic protein (MBP)-specific T-cell lines could be promptly used to isolate neuritogenic T lines specific for the P2 protein of peripheral nerve myelin—the immunodominant autoantigen responsible for the induction of EAN (Linington *et al.*, 1984). However, EAN has never reached the popularity of EAE as a model for T-cell-mediated autoimmunity. Yet in combination with EAE, EAN has proved an invaluable adjunct to determining the specificity of T-cell migration through the nervous system, the molecular properties of autoimmunogenic proteins, and the development of potential therapies for autoimmune-mediated diseases of the nervous system.

II. Isolation and Composition of Peripheral Nerve Myelin

The autoantigens used to induce EAN are all derived from the components of the PNS myelin sheath. In the PNS, myelin is formed and maintained by Schwann cells (SCs) each of which enwraps a single axonal segment to form a spiral of compact multilamellar myelin. Myelinating SCs maintain a strict one-to-one relationship with their axonal segment and can synthesize a sheath containing up to 100 layers of compacted membrane and one or more millimeters in length. This is in contrast to myelin formation within the CNS, in which the myelinated internodal length is generally shorter, but where the myelinating cell, the oligodendrocyte, myelinates several independent axonal segments. The function of myelin in both the CNS and PNS is to increase the velocity of nerve conduction by inducing saltatory conduction between the nodes of Ranvier.

Myelin is a lipid-rich membrane which contains only 22–28% protein by dry weight. Moreover, the protein composition of the isolated membrane is very simple, three protein components—the P0 glycoprotein, myelin basic protein, and the P2 protein—accounting for at least 80% of the total protein content of the membrane. Details of the composition of PNS myelin are reviewed in Norton and Cammer (1984). The high lipid content of myelin simplifies its purification by density-gradient centrifugation and thereafter only simple chromatographic techniques are required to purify the major protein components. The best sources of PNS myelin for the induction of EAN are bovine nerve roots and peripheral nerves, which can be obtained from most slaughterhouses. The tissue should be transported to the laboratory on ice as quickly as possible, adhering connective and adipose tissue should be removed, and the nerves chopped into small pieces and stored at −80°C.

EAN can be induced by using either PNS tissue homogenates, purified myelin, or isolated myelin proteins emulsified in complete Freund's adjuvant (CFA). In our experience, purified myelin provides an immunogen that is easier to work with and that provides more consistent results than crude tissue homogenates. High yields of myelin from peripheral nerve are obtained by first grinding the tissue to a fine powder. In this step the connective tissue structures within the nerve are thoroughly broken up, which facilitates subsequent homogenization. The concentration of myelin relative to other membrane fractions in the nerve (axonal, fibroblast, and Schwann cell microsomal fractions) is very high; therefore we routinely use the abbreviated purification scheme illustrated in Figure 2.

The purity of the isolated and washed myelin membranes is best assessed by SDS-PAGE. The major protein, the P0 glycoprotein, accounts for >50% of the total membrane protein in all species studied while MBP and the P2 protein make up the bulk of the remaining membrane protein. The concentration of MBP and P2, however, vary considerably among different species. In bovine PNS myelin, the P2 protein is approximately 20% of the total membrane protein, whereas in the rat, P2 protein accounts for > 0.1% of PNS myelin protein (Figure 1).

All three of these proteins seem to be able to induce a neuritogenic autoimmune response under certain conditions. Although MBP is a component of both CNS and PNS myelin, MBP-specific T cells preferentially attack the CNS. Why they commonly spare the PNS is not understood. It should also be noted that although the P2 protein is specific for PNS myelin in the rat, it is also expressed in the rabbit, bovine, and human CNS. Schemes for purification of the P2 and P0 proteins from PNS myelin are given in Figures 3 and 4. MBP is more easily purified from CNS tissue or purified CNS myelin (Eylar *et al.*, 1979). In addition to these major proteins, PNS myelin contains many quantitatively minor proteins and glycoproteins the immunological properties of which are poorly defined.

III. Basic Features of EAN

EAN is readily inducible in many mammalian species by immunization with either peripheral nerve tissue, PNS myelin, purified PNS myelin antigens, or even synthetic peptides representing PNS protein sequences. The two PNS myelin proteins known to induce EAN are the P2 protein (Uyemura *et al.*, 1982; Olee *et al.*, 1988; Rostami *et al.*, 1990; Hahn *et al.*, 1991), and the P0 glycoprotein (Carlo *et al.*, 1975; Milner *et al.*, 1987; Linington *et al.*, 1992).

Actively induced EAN is normally a monophasic disease that develops 10 to 14 days after immunization. The classic clinical signs of the disease are an ascending paraparesis and paralysis that typically first affects tail tone and then gradually ascends rostrally, involving the hindlimbs. Clinical signs of disease then normally resolve over a period of 1–2 weeks, although in severe cases tetraplegia and death can occur. The histopathological changes associated with EAN may vary markedly among different species, and are dependent on the autoantigens and immunization protocols used. There are, however, several common features shared by all major variants of EAN. As a

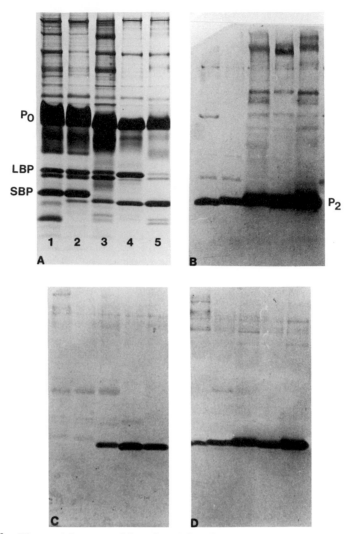

Figure 1 The protein composition of peripheral nerve myelin isolated from several mammalian species. Lane 1, mouse; lane 2, rat; lane 3, human; lane 4, rabbit; lane 5 cow. Fifty-microgram samples of PNS myelin protein were separated by SDS-polyacylamide gel electrophoresis and either stained directly with Coomassie blue (A), or electroblotted onto cellulose nitrate membranes, and P2 protein detected using either a polyclonal rabbit anti-P2 antisera (B), or mouse monoclonal antibodies (MAb) generated using purified bovine P2 protein (C and D). In contrast to the P0 glycoprotein, which is the major protein component of PNS myelin in all five species, the concentrations of P2 protein and MBP vary dramatically. The samples have been applied to the gel so that the concentration of MBP in PNS myelin is clearly seen to decrease from mouse to cow, whereas the concentration of P2 protein increases. This is also seen in B to D in which the P2 protein is specifically stained. Also note that the two mouse MAbs detect a heterogenity in the mouse antibody response to bovine P2. The MAb used in C binds to an epitope common to the cow, rabbit, and human proteins, but which is absent in the mouse protein. In contrast, the MAb used in D reacts with the P2 protein of all five species. (Illustration by courtesy of Dr. T. V. Waehneldt.)

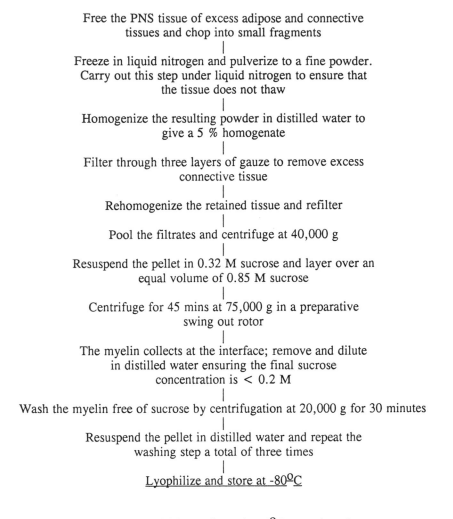

Free the PNS tissue of excess adipose and connective
tissues and chop into small fragments
|
Freeze in liquid nitrogen and pulverize to a fine powder.
Carry out this step under liquid nitrogen to ensure that
the tissue does not thaw
|
Homogenize the resulting powder in distilled water to
give a 5 % homogenate
|
Filter through three layers of gauze to remove excess
connective tissue
|
Rehomogenize the retained tissue and refilter
|
Pool the filtrates and centrifuge at 40,000 g
|
Resuspend the pellet in 0.32 M sucrose and layer over an
equal volume of 0.85 M sucrose
|
Centrifuge for 45 mins at 75,000 g in a preparative
swing out rotor
|
The myelin collects at the interface; remove and dilute
in distilled water ensuring the final sucrose
concentration is < 0.2 M
|
Wash the myelin free of sucrose by centrifugation at 20,000 g for 30 minutes
|
Resuspend the pellet in distilled water and repeat the
washing step a total of three times
|
Lyophilize and store at -80°C

All steps should be performed at 4°C or on ice, the
solutions required must be adjusted to pH 7.4 prior to use.

Figure 2   Purification of peripheral nerve myelin.

rule, the onset of clinical disease is associated with mononuclear infiltration of PNS tissue and endoneurial edema. This is then followed by varying degrees of focal demyelination and axonal degeneration. The cellular infiltrates are mainly composed of $CD4^+$ T lymphocytes and blood-derived monocytes or macrophages. In fact, macrophages are thought to be the major effector

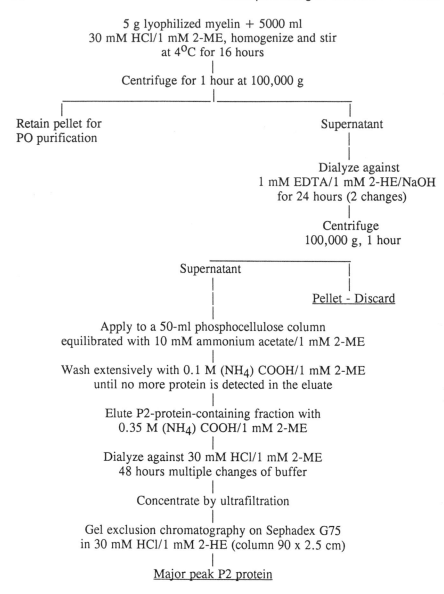

5 g lyophilized myelin + 5000 ml
30 mM HCl/1 mM 2-ME, homogenize and stir
at 4°C for 16 hours
|
Centrifuge for 1 hour at 100,000 g

Retain pellet for   Supernatant
PO purification |

Dialyze against
1 mM EDTA/1 mM 2-HE/NaOH
for 24 hours (2 changes)
|
Centrifuge
100,000 g, 1 hour

Supernatant |
| |
| Pellet - Discard
|
Apply to a 50-ml phosphocellulose column
equilibrated with 10 mM ammonium acetate/1 mM 2-ME
|
Wash extensively with 0.1 M (NH₄) COOH/1 mM 2-ME
until no more protein is detected in the eluate
|
Elute P2-protein-containing fraction with
0.35 M (NH₄) COOH/1 mM 2-ME
|
Dialyze against 30 mM HCl/1 mM 2-ME
48 hours multiple changes of buffer
|
Concentrate by ultrafiltration
|
Gel exclusion chromatography on Sephadex G75
in 30 mM HCl/1 mM 2-HE (column 90 x 2.5 cm)
|
Major peak P2 protein

The P2 protein containing fractions should be briefly
dialyzed against distilled water, lyophilized and
stored at -80°C.

Figure 3   Purification of bovine P2 protein.

This is a modification of the method described by Kitamura et al. (1976) starting from the acid-insoluble extract of PNS myelin obtained during the isolation of P2 protein

Acid insoluble fraction of PNS myelin
|
Dissolve in acidified chloroform-methanol (2:1 v/v)
using 50 ml/g of the starting material,
lyophilized PNS myelin
|
Centrifuge to remove any insoluble material
|
Add a few drops of 1 M NaOH, final pH 7.5 - 8.0
Stir for 45 minutes
|
Collect the precipitate by centrifugation
|
Wash with 50 ml chloroform-methanol (2:1 v/v)
for 10 minutes, three times
|
Wash once in methanol (100 ml)
|
Wash twice with water
|
Lyophilize
|
Dissolve at 60°C in
100 mM Tris/HCl, pH 8.0/10 mM dithiothreitol (DTT)
containing 10% SDS (approx. 15 mg/ml)
|
Gel exclusion chromatography on Sephacryl S-300
in 100 mM Tris/HCl/10 mM DTT/2% SDS pH 8.0
(column 90 x 2.5 cm)
|
Pool appropriate fractions, lyophilize, then extract with acetone-water (4:1 v/v), methanol and finally water to remove SDS and salts before final lyophilization.

For further variations on this method see Mezei and Verpoorte (1981) and Milner et al. (1987) for the generation of a neuritogenic PO/lysophosphatidyl choline complex.

Figure 4   Purification of bovine P0 glycoprotein.

cell within the EAN lesion. They not only phagocytose myelin debris, but also actively mediate demyelination by stripping sheets of membrane from the myelin sheath. However, it should be noted that demyelination in EAN may be mediated by more than one mechanism. In addition to direct macrophage-mediated mechanisms of primary demyelination, severe edema and associated ischemic changes in the nerve lead to axonal degeneration, resulting in a secondary loss of myelin (Powell et al., 1983).

The extent of primary demyelination in acute models of EAN depends upon the intensity of the inflammatory response within the nerve. In actively induced EAN, this can be modulated by varying the dose and composition of immunogen, or in T-cell-mediated models of adoptively transferred EAN, by injecting different doses of neuritogenic T cells. Low doses of immunogen or T cells result in a mild clinical disease in which the lesions are confined to the nerve roots. In this situation, focal demyelination is observed and the axonal pathology is minimal. Increasing the dose of immunogen, or T cells, induces a progressively more severe clinical disease which in extreme cases has a fatal outcome. In animals with severe EAN, the entire PNS can be affected; inflammation of the peripheral nerves is intense, and axonal degeneration and secondary demyelination are the major pathological features. A consequence of this axonal loss is a profound neurophysiological deficit that may persist for many weeks following onset of disease.

In addition to the classic monophasic models of EAN, chronic relapsing variants of EAN (CREAN) have been induced in a variety of species. CREAN is seen in some monkeys, rabbits, guinea pigs, and, more rarely, in the Lewis rat following immunization with PNS tissue (Wisniewski et al., 1974; Pollard et al., 1975). The incidence of CREAN appears to be age dependent; the frequency of this variant of EAN is increased in adolescent guinea pigs, while adult animals generally develop an acute monophasic disease (Suzumura et al., 1985). In addition, the original immunization protocols can be varied to produce CREAN in appropriate strains of experimental animals. For example, treatment with cyclosporin A initially prevents the development of EAN in rats and guinea pigs (King et al., 1983), but withdrawal of the drug results in relapses (King et al., 1983; McCombe et al., 1990). Finally, relapsing–remitting courses of EAN can be simulated by the repeated transfer of neuritogenic T-cell lines (Lassmann et al., 1991).

A. T-Cell-Mediated Models of EAN

The pathogenic agents mediating EAN are T lymphocytes that recognize PNS myelin proteins, in particular the P2 and P0 proteins. This has been formally proven in the Lewis rat by the adoptive transfer of homogeneous T-cell lines specific for either the P2 or P0 PNS myelin proteins (Linington *et al.*, 1984; Rostami *et al.*, 1985; Linington *et al.*, 1992). This autoaggressive T-cell response is the *minimal* requirement to initiate EAN. After activation *in vivo*, P2- or P0-specific T cells mediate the whole spectrum of histopathological and clinical changes seen in acute EAN induced by using PNS tissue in adjuvant (Izumo *et al.*, 1985; Linington *et al.*, 1992).

The P2 protein was the first PNS myelin protein identified as a neuritogenic autoantigen (Brostoff *et al.*, 1972). Subsequently, the Lewis rat was found to provide a highly reproducible model of EAN using purified bovine P2 protein in Freund's complete adjuvant as the immunogen (Kadlubowski *et al.*, 1979). The central role of the P2 protein-specific, T-cell response in the immunopathogenesis of EAN was proven by the adoptive transfer of P2-specific T-cell lines into syngeneic rats (Linington *et al.*, 1984; Rostami *et al.*, 1985; Linington *et al.*, 1986). Intravenous injection of as few as 5×10^4 P2-specific T cells can induce definite though mild clinical signs of EAN in the Lewis rat 4–5 days after cell transfer (Linington *et al.*, 1984). As stated previously, the intensity of the clinical and histological signs of T-cell mediated EAN is directly related to the number of antigen-specific T cells transferred. Low numbers of T cells result in the formation of focal perivascular infiltrates of mononuclear cells, predominantly CD4+ T cells and macrophages (Izumo *et al.*, 1985) which are associated with local edema, and a plasma protein exudate that indicates an increased permeability of the endothelial blood–nerve barrier (BNB). These pathological changes are also often accompanied by focal primary demyelination (Izumo *et al.*, 1985). This inflammatory response within the nerve and the extent of demyelination increase as the number of neuritogenic T cells transferred is increased. However, the transfer of large numbers of P2-specific T cells induces massive axonal degeneration, resulting in secondary rather than primary demyelination (Izumo *et al.*, 1985). Axonal degeneration in this model of EAN often extends into the dorsal columns of the spinal cord and this is also observed in a relapsing model of EAN produced by the repeated transfers of P2-specific T cells (Lassmann *et al.*, 1991).

The P2 protein is, however, not the only neuritogenic myelin component. Active immunization with P0 glycoprotein in adjuvant induces EAN in the Lewis rat with a similar efficiency, pathology, and time course (Milner *et al.*, 1987). This is remarkable because these two proteins differ completely with respect to their physiochemical properties, concentration, function, and cellular localization. The P2 protein is a small, basic protein that accounts for less than 0.1% of the total PNS myelin protein in the rat (Milek *et al.*, 1981). The function of P2 is uncertain but it is structurally related to a number of lipid binding proteins (Bergfors *et al.*, 1987; Jones *et al.*, 1988) and may be involved in lipid transport. This proposal is supported by the localization of P2 protein within the cytoplasmic domains of the PNS myelin sheath.

In contrast to P2, which is clearly inaccessible to antibody present in the extracellular fluid, P0 is a transmembrane glycoprotein with clearly defined extracellular, transmembrane, and cytoplasmic domains (Lemke, 1988). Thus in principle, immunization with P0 glycoprotein can trigger both cellular and humoral autoimmune responses that may contribute to the development of EAN. Recent transfer experiments showed that P0-specific T-cell lines produce a form of EAN indistinguishable from that induced by either P2-specific T cells, or active immunization with PNS tissue (Linington *et al.*, 1992). Thus a T-cell-mediated effector mechanism seems to predominate in the pathogenesis of EAN in general.

The autoimmune T-cell response to both P2 and P0 has been analyzed in great detail in the Lewis rat and the neuritogenic T-cell epitopes identified for both proteins. The P2 protein contains a single immunodominant neuritogenic determinant located within residues 61–72 of the protein's amino acid sequence. EAN can be induced by either active immunization with synthetic peptides corresponding to this sequence, or by the passive transfer of P2 61–72 peptide-specific T-cell lines (Olee *et al.*, 1989). The P2 sequence(s) recognized by neuritogenic T cells in the brown Norway rat are, however, located in different regions (Linington *et al.*, 1986).

It is well established that in several EAE models, the diversity of *TcR* genes used by the encephalitogenic anti-MBP T-cell response is extremely limited. In the Lewis rat (Burns *et al.*, 1989; Chluba *et al.*, 1989), and in PL/J or B10.PL mice (Acha-Orbea *et al.*, 1988; Urban *et al.*, 1988), almost all encephalitogenic T cells use the *Vβ8.2* gene, often together with *Vα2*, and a narrow selection of *J* genes. *TcR* gene use in EAN is less clear. Polymerase chain reaction (PRC) studies of one group have indicated biased use of *Vβ8.2* in neuritogenic anti-P2 T cells of the Lewis rat as well (Clark *et al.*, 1992). Using a *Vβ8.2*-specific MAb (Torres-Nagel *et al.*, 1993), we were neither able to confirm preferential selection of *Vβ8.2* in a panel of P2-specific T-cell lines, nor did we observe accumulation of *Vβ8.2$^+$* T cells in EAN infiltrates (Gold *et al.*, submitted).

In contrast to P2, in the Lewis rat the T-cell response against the P0 protein appears to be focused on at least two distinct epitopes. Peptide mapping and T-cell transfer studies identified one epitope located within the amino acid residues 56–71 of the extracellular IgG-like domain of P0, and a second within residues 180–199 of the cytoplasmic, carboxyl terminal sequence (Linington *et al.*, 1992). The immunological properties of these two domains of P0 are very different. The cytoplasmic epitope is clearly immunodominant and EAN-inducing T-cell lines specific for this epitope can be selected from the T-cell repertoire of rats immunized with PNS tissue homogenate. This is not the case for the epitope identified within the extracellular epitope of P0. No T-cell response to this epitope was observed following immunization with either PNS tissue, myelin, or purified P0 protein, indicating that the epitope remains cryptic when the intact protein is processed and presented to T cells in the peripheral immune system.

This situation is reminiscent of the T-cell response to the immunodominant encephalitogenic autoantigen responsible for EAE, MBP. In the Lewis rat, the dominant epitope is located within sequence 70–88. A second, cryptic epitope, however, is contained in the abutting sequence, 87–99 (Sun et al., 1992b; Offner et al., 1992). The presence of cryptic, but nevertheless pathogenic T-cell epitopes in the P0 glycoprotein suggests that the processing pathways responsible for the degradation of myelin proteins and their binding to MHC products differ considerably between antigen-presenting cells (APCs) within nervous system and lymphoid tissue. This observation is of critical importance to any clinical study attempting to characterize autoaggressive T-cell responses of patients with a putative autoimmune disease using APCs obtained from the peripheral blood. As in our experimental studies, APCs from human target organs may process cellular autoantigens in other ways, as would APCs present in the blood.

The finding that PNS myelin components with such different functions, localization, and structure as the P0 glycoprotein and P2 protein initiate similar T-cell-mediated EAN suggests that other neuritogenic PNS autoantigens will be identified.

B. Autoantibody-Mediated EAN

The original models of EAN, which were based on the immunization of experimental animals with PNS tissue homogenates, established the cellular nature of the neuritogenic autoimmune response. However, at the same time, other studies indicated the presence of humoral demyelinating factors. In some situations, serum from animals with EAN induced demyelination either in vivo following direct intraneural injection, or in vitro when added to myelinating organotypic cultures (Saida et al., 1978, 1979a, b, c). Furthermore, plasmapheresis significantly reduced the clinical score of animals with EAN, again indicating a role for circulating antibody to peripheral nerve antigens in the pathogenesis of the disease (Gross et al., 1983; Harvey et al., 1988).

It is now clear that humoral autoantibodies to myelin can play a (secondary) role in the pathogenesis of EAN. Circulating autoantibodies that recognize surface determinants of myelin, in particular galactosyl cerebroside (GC), will enhance T-cell-mediated demyelination by both complement and antibody-dependent cell-mediated cytotoxicity (ADCC) effector mechanisms and will further amplify the inflammatory response by the local production of complement-derived proinflammatory factors (Hughes and Powell, 1984).

These autoantibodies are, however, unable to trigger demyelination without prior disruption of the endothelial BNB. In both actively induced and passively transferred EAN, this is achieved in the course of the local T-cell-induced inflammatory response. In addition, the neuritogenic T-cell response recruits effector cells, primarily macrophages, into the lesions, which can then mediate an ADCC response directed against the myelin sheath.

The only myelin autoantigen for which there is clear evidence for a demyelinating autoantibody response is GC. Rabbits mount a high titer antibody response to GC following immunization with either myelin or GC absorbed to bovine serum albumin. These antisera mediate demyelination *in vitro*, an activity that can be abolished by absorption with GC (Joffe *et al.*, 1963; Niedieck *et al.*, 1965; Dubois-Dalcq *et al.*, 1970; Fry *et al.*, 1974; Gregson *et al.*, 1974; Saida *et al.*, 1979b). This demyelinating antibody response recognizes epitopes involving the galactose head group of the glycolipid. This is remarkable because the antibody does not bind to simple micellar dispersions of the purified lipid. In these complexes, the galactose head group is firmly hydrogen bonded within the micelles' hydrophobic or hydrophilic interface, and the target epitopes are not accessible to the antibody.

This is not the case in either mixed micelles containing phospholipids and cholesterol in addition to GC, or in the myelin membrane. In this situation, the galactose head group is accessible to antibody, as shown by the binding of anti-GC antibody to myelin and its ability to mediate demyelination (Dubois-Dalcq *et al.*, 1970; Fry *et al.*, 1974). Tissue culture showed that anti-GC antibody can interact with myelinating membranes in several ways. In the absence of complement, binding of anti-GC antibody to the myelin surface results in the separation of compacted myelin lamellae, that is, myelin swelling. Myelin destruction *in vitro*, however, depends on complement and is very rapid.

The ability of GC to induce an EAN in the rabbit (Saida *et al.*, 1979c) suggests that a purely antibody-mediated model of EAN can be induced by active immunization. However, disease incidence is not 100% and rabbits can remyelinate the PNS despite the continued presence of high titers of demyelinating anti-GC antibody in the peripheral blood (Stoll *et al.*, 1986). These observations suggest that other factors in addition to the anti-GC antibody response are involved in the pathogenesis of GC-induced models of EAN. The usefulness of GC as a model autoantigen is also limited by its markedly varied effect in different species. Rabbits and guinea pigs are generally high responders, while mice and rats are poor responders. However, active immunization protocols are now being replaced by murine monoclonal anti-GC antibodies, which can be used to investigate the role of autoantibody in the pathogenesis of disease.

C. Effector Phase of EAN

The primary targets of autoaggressive, neuritogenic T cells within the PNS are any cell type that is able to properly present local (auto-)antigen. First is a population of pericytes that constitutively express MHC class II products and that may function as resident APCs within the PNS. In addition, tissue culture studies showed that nonmyelinating Schwann cells can be induced to express MHC class II products by interferon-γ and could therefore act as facultative APCs in the PNS (Wekerle *et al.*, 1986; Kingston *et al.*, 1989; Zhang *et al.*, 1990).

The antigen-specific interaction between T cell and APC is the essential first step for triggering a variety of cellular functions in both cell types. One key result of this encounter is the local production of proinflammatory cytokines. These cytokines may determine the nature of the subsequent inflammatory response either by acting directly on local cells, or recruiting additional effector cells from the peripheral blood.

The earliest changes affect the vascular endothelium. As in any inflammatory response, cytokines profoundly modulate the expression of cell adhesion molecules (CAM) on the vascular surface of the endothelium (Shimizu *et al.*, 1992; Butcher, 1992). Some CAMs are newly induced on the vascular endothelium during the course of the inflammatory response; the expression of others may be enhanced or even downmodulated. Vascular permeability is also increased both by the direct effects of cytokines on endothelial cells (Brett *et al.*, 1989), indirectly via cytokine-induced mast cell degranulation (Brosnan *et al.*, 1985), or as a consequence of massive T-cell diapedesis (Claudio *et al.*, 1990). Among the many cytokines that are involved in the early response phase, interferon-γ appears to play a central role. It is known to affect vascular permeability and the expression of MHC molecules and cell adhesion molecules on PNS elements, and it activates infiltrating monocytes. Thus systemic injection of recombinant interferon-γ enhances the clinical and histopathological signs of T-cell-mediated EAN, while treatment with antibodies against this cytokine can suppress the development of disease (Hartung *et al.*, 1990).

The pathological changes of EAN are usually initiated by vasogenic edema. This is the result of increased endothelial permeability to serum proteins. Edema is associated with perivascular influx of small numbers of blood-borne CD4+ T cells and also some monocytes. These events are initiated about 72 hr after intravenous injection of activated P2-specific T cells. They precede the onset of clinical disease by 12–24 hr (Linington *et al.*, 1986). In full-blown EAN, the BNB seems to break down completely, allowing rapid immigration and accumulation of numerous inflammatory cells, predominantly macrophages, but extravascularization of erythrocytes can also be observed (Izumo *et al.*, 1985; Heininger *et al.*, 1986). Endoneurial fluid pressure and endoneurial edema also increase rapidly. These pathological changes within the nerve are associated with rapid deterioration of nerve conduction and eventually a complete block of conduction 4–5 days after T-cell transfer (Heininger *et al.*, 1986). These electrophysiological changes initially reflect paranodal demyelination, but in severe inflammatory lesions, conduction failure is due to the overwhelming destruction of axons (Hahn *et al.*, 1991).

There is good evidence that macrophages are responsible for many of the pathological effects in the EAN lesion. Activated macrophages secrete a large number of cytotoxic agents, including proteases, lipases, glycosidases, reactive oxygen metabolites, and toxic cytokines (Hartung *et al.*, 1988a,b). These factors may act on endothelium to produce leakage of the BNB; they may damage Schwann cells to deregulate the local milieu and cause myelin degeneration; or they may directly affect axons. Depletion of the macrophage population (e.g., by quartz treatment) or inhibition of their biological activities suppresses the development of clinical disease, demonstrating their importance in the pathogenesis of disease (Craggs *et al.*, 1984; Hartung *et al.*, 1988; Heininger *et al.*, 1988; Schabet *et al.*, 1991). The endoneurial pressure that rises as a consequence of edema may in itself trigger local ischemia and axonal degeneration (Powell *et al.*, 1991).

The interaction of macrophages with myelin in EAN lesions appears to be selective. Macrophages first attach to apparently normal myelin sheaths and then strip the myelin lamellae from the axon. The molecular basis of this interaction is unknown; however, antibody-independent activation of the alternative complement pathway by the P0 protein on myelin or myelin debris (Koski *et al.*, 1985) may deposit C3i on the membrane surface, providing a ligand for a macrophage CR3 receptor.

Finally, myelin-specific, neuritogenic T cells may directly contribute to demyelination by acting as cytotoxic killer cells. Direct lysis of MHC class II-induced rat Schwann cells by syngeneic P2-specific, neuritogenic T-cell lines has been demonstrated *in vitro*, but its significance *in vivo* is uncertain (Wekerle *et al.*, 1989).

IV. Immunopathogenesis of EAN—A Model for Therapeutic Studies

EAN models in which disease is initiated by the passive transfer of well-defined T cells have opened new approaches to studying the pathophysiology of acute inflammatory, demyelinating PNS disease in the presence or absence of antimyelin antibody response. As reviewed earlier, the initial step in T-cell-mediated EAN is the activation of PNS autoantigen reactive CD4+ T cells within the peripheral immune repertoire. Migration of activated, autoreactive T cells through the BNB is followed by an antigen-specific interaction with local MHC class II-positive APCs. This then triggers the local inflammatory responses that are responsible for clinical EAN. All these stages in the development of EAN may be amenable to therapeutic intervention.

In principle, immunotherapy of EAN follows the principles established for treatment of EAE and other tissue-specific autoimmune diseases (Hohlfeld, 1989; Adorini *et al.*, 1990; Wekerle and Hohfeld, 1992). Most of the new immunotherapies aim at the neutralization of the specific pathogens, the autoaggressive T cells. The strategies may attempt to eliminate these T cells, to push them to a paralytic state of nonreactivity, or to prevent them from interacting with their (antigen-presenting) target cells.

T-Cell tolerance to the neuritogenic P2 protein has been induced by pre-treatment of rats with soluble P2 in the absence of adjuvant (Brosnan *et al.*, 1984). Suppression of EAE inducibility by oral administration of MBP has been spectacularly successful (Bitar and Whitacre, 1988; Higgins and Weiner, 1988). We know of no reports of this treatment in EAN, but trust that this gap will be filled.

Monoclonal antibodies (MAb) to T-cell differentiation antigens have become invaluable tools to eliminate or functionally inhibit the autoaggressive CD4$^+$ T-cell population. Unfortunately, anti-CD4 MAb treatment works best when given prophylactically (Holmdahl *et al.*, 1985). These MAbs have only a moderate effect once clinical disease is established. In some cases, MAbs against T-cell membrane antigens may even produce quite erratic results. Anti-CD5 MAbs may prevent induction of EAE (Sun *et al.*, 1992a), but in EAN such treatment paradoxically enhanced the clinical severity of EAN and caused relapses (Strigard *et al.*, 1989).

A more promising approach uses an antibody that recognizes the rat *TcR*. This antibody not only inhibits the development of T-cell-mediated EAN, but also reverses the development of actively induced EAN when given therapeutically (Jung *et al.*, 1992). Immunotherapy or rat EAN with *TcR V* gene-specific MAbs has become a reality with the development of new reagents (Torres-Nagel *et al.*, 1993). At present, it is not clear at all whether the neuritogenic T-cell response is dominated by the use of the *Vβ8.2* gene, as is the encephalitogenic reaction. Finally, attempts to prevent EAN induction by vaccination with attenuated P2-specific T-cell lines have been unsuccessful (Jung *et al.*, 1991).

References

Acha-Orbea, H., Mitchell, D. J., Timmermann, L., Wraith, D. C., Tausch, G. S., Waldor, M. K., Zamvil, S. S., McDevitt, H. O., and Steinman, L. (1988). *Cell* **54**, 263–273.
Adam, A. M., Atkinson, P. F., Hall, S. M., et al. (1989). *Neuropathol. Appl. Neurobiol.* **15**, 249–256.
Adorini, L., Barnaba, V., Bona, C., Celada, F., Lanzavecchia, A., Sercarz, E., Suciu-Foca, N., and Wekerle, H. (1990). *Immunol. Today* **11**, 383–386.
Aström, K.-E., and Waksman, B. H. (1962). *J. Pathol. Bacteriol.* **83**, 89–107.
Bergfors, T., Sedzik, J., Unge, T., et al. (1987). *J. Mol. Biol.* **198**, 357–362.
Bitar, D., and Whitacre, C. C. (1988). *Cell. Immunol.* **112**, 364–370.

Brett, J., Gerlach, H., Nawroth, P., Steinberg, S., Godman, G., and Stern, D. M. (1989). *J. Exp. Med.* **169**, 1977–1991.

Brosnan, C. F., Craggs, R. I., King, R. H. M., and Thomas, P. K. (1984). *Acta Neuropathol.* **64**, 153–160.

Brosnan, C. F., Lyman, W. D., Tansey, F. A., and Carter, T. H. (1985). *J. Neuropathol. Exp. Neurol.* **44**, 196–203.

Brostoff, S. W., Burnett, P., Lampert, P. W., and Eylar, E. H. (1972). *Nature* **235**, 210–212.

Butcher, E. C. (1992). *Cell* **67**, 1033–1036.

Burns, F. R., Li, X., Shen, H., Offner, H., Chou, Y. K., Vandenbark, A. A., and Heber-Katz, E. (1989). *J. Exp. Med.* **169**, 27–40.

Carlo, D. J., Karkhanis, Y. D., Bailey, P. J., Wisniewski, H. M., and Brostoff, S. W. (1975). *Brain Res.* **88**, 580–584.

Chluba, J., Steeg, C., Becker, A., Wekerle, H., and Epplen, J. T. (1989). *Eur. J. Immunol.* **19**, 279–284.

Clark, L., Heber-Katz, E., and Rostami, A. (1992). *Ann. Neurol.* **31**, 587–592.

Claudio, L., Kress, Y., Factor, J., and Brosnan, C. F. (1990). *Am. J. Pathol.* **137**, 1033–1045.

Craggs, R. I., King, R. H. M., and Thomas, P. K. (1984). *Acta Neuropathol.* **62**, 316–323.

Cunningham, J. M., Powers, J. M., and Brostoff, S. W. (1983). *Brain Res.* **258**, 285–289.

Dubois Dalcq, M., Neidieck, B., and Buyse, M. (1970). *Pathol. Eur.* **5**, 331–337.

Eylar, E. H., Kniskern, P. J., and Jackson, J. J. (1979). *Methods Enzymol.* **32B**, 323–341.

Fry, J. M., Weissbarth, S., Lehrer, G. M., and Bornstein, M. B. (1974). *Science* **183**, 540–542.

Gregson, N. A., Kennedy, M., and Leibowitz, S. (1974). *Immunology* **26**, 743–750.

Gross, M. L. P., Craggs, R. I., King, R. H. M., and Thomas, P. K. (1983). *J. Neurol. Sci.* **61**, 149–160.

Hahn, A. F., Feasby, T. E., Wilkie, L., and Lovgren, D. (1991). *Acta Neuropathol.* **82**, 60–65.

Hartung, H.-P., Schäfer, B., Heininger, K., Stoll, G., and Toyka, K. V. (1988a). *Brain* **111**, 1039–1059.

Hartung, H.-P., Heininger, K., Schaefer, B., et al. (1988b). *Ann. N.Y. Acad. Sci.* **540**, 122–161.

Hartung, H.-P., Schäfer, B., Van der Meide, P. H., Fierz, W., Heininger, K., and Toyka, K. V. (1990). *Ann. Neurol.* **27**, 247–257.

Harvey, G. K., Schindhelm, K., Anthony, J. H., and Pollard, J. D. (1988). *J. Neurol. Sci.* **88**, 207–218.

Heininger, K., Stoll, G., Linington, C., Toyka, K. V., and Wekerle, H. (1986). *Ann. Neurol.* **19**, 44–49.

Heininger, K., Schäfer, B., Hartung, H.-P., Fierz, W., Linington, C., and Toyka, K. V. (1988). *Ann. Neurol.* **23**, 326–331.

Higgins, P. J., and Weiner, H. L. (1988). *J. Immunol.* **140**, 440–445.

Hohlfeld, R. (1989). *Ann. Neurol.* **25**, 531–538.

Holmdahl, R., Olsson, T., Moran, T., and Klareskog, L. (1985). *Scand. J. Immunol.* **22**, 257–269.

Hughes, R. A. C., and Powell, H. C. (1984). *J. Neuropathol. Exp. Neurol.* **43**, 154–161.

Izumo, S., Linington, C., Wekerle, H., and Meyermann, R. (1985). *Lab. Invest.* **53**, 209–218.

Joffe, S. J., Rapport, M. M., and Graf, L. (1963). *Nature* **197**, 60–62.

Jones, T. A., Bergfors, T., Sedzik, J., and Unge, T. (1988). *EMBO J.* **7**, 1597–1604.

Jung, S., Schluesener, H. J., Toyka, K. V., and Hartung, H.-P. (1991). *J. Neuroimmunol.* **35**, 1–11.

Jung, S., Krämer, S., Schluesener, H. J., Hünig, T., Toyka, K. V., and Hartung, H.-P. (1992). *J. Immunol.* **148**, 3768–3775.

Kadlubowski, M., and Hughes, R. A. C. (1979). *Nature* **277**, 140–141.

Kadlubowski, M., Hughes, R. A. C., and Gregson, N. A. (1980). *Brain Res.* **184**, 439–454.

King, R. H. M., Craggs, R. I., Gross, M. L. P., Tompkins, C., and Thomas, P. K. (1983). *Acta Neuropathol.* **59**, 262–268.

Kingston, A. E., Bergsteinsdottir, K., Jessen, K. R., Van der Meide, P. H., Colston, M. J., and Mirsky, R. (1989). *Eur. J. Immunol.* **19**, 177–183.

Kitamura, K., Suzuki, M., and Uyemura, K. (1976). *Biochim. Biophys. Acta* **455**, 806–816.

Koski, C. L., Vanguri, P., and Shin, M. L. (1985). *J. Immunol.* **134**, 1810–1814.

Laemmli, U. K. (1970). *Nature* **227**, 668–685.

Lassmann, H., Fierz, W., Neuchrist, C., and Meyermann, R. (1991). *Brain* **114**, 429–442.

Lemke, G. (1988). *Neuron* **1**, 535–543.

Linington, C., Izumo, S., Suzuki, M., Uyemura, K., Meyermann, R., and Wekerle, H. (1984). *J. Immunol.* **133**, 1946–1950.

Linington, C., Mann, A., Izumo, S., Uyemura, K., Suzuki, M., Meyermann, R., and Wekerle, H. (1986). *J. Immunol.* **137**, 3826–3831.

Linington, C., Lassmann, H., Oxawa, K., Kosin, S., and Mongan, L. (1992). *Eur. J. Immunol.* **22**, 1813–1817.

Mezei, C., and Verpoorte, J. A. (1981). *J. Neurochem.* **37**, 550–557.

McCombe, P. A., van der Kreek, S. A., and Pender, M. P. (1990). *J. Neuroimmunol.* **28**, 131–140.

Milek, D. J., Sarvas, H. O., Greenfiled, S., Weise, M. J., and Brostoff, W. W. (1981). *Brain Res.* **208**, 387–396.

Milner, P., Lovelidge, C. A., Taylor, W. A., and Hughes, R. A. C. (1987). *J. Neurol. Sci.* **79**, 275–285.

Niedieck, B., Kuwert, E., Palacios, O., and Crees, O. (1965). *Ann. N.Y. Acad. Sci.* **122**, 266–276.

Norton, W. T., and Cammer, W. (1984). *In* "Myelin" (P. Morrell, Ed.), pp. 147–179. Plenum Press, New York.

Offner, H., Vainiene, M., Gold, D. P., Celnik, B., Wang, R., Hashim, G. A., and Vandenbark, A. A. (1992). *J. Immunol.* **149**, 1706–1711.

Olee, T., Powers, J. M., and Brostoff, S. W. (1988). *J. Neuroimmunol.* **19**, 167–174.

Olee, T., Weise, M. J., Powers, J. M., and Brostoff, S. W. (1989). *J. Neuroimmunol.* **21**, 235–240.

Pollard, J. D., King, R. H. M., and Thomas, P. K. (1975). *J. Neurol. Sci.* **24**, 365–383.

Powell, H. C., Braheny, S. L., Myers, R. R., Rodriguez, M., and Lampert, P. W. (1983). *Lab. Invest.* **48**, 332–338.

Powell, H. C., Olee, T., Brostoff, S. W., and Mizisin, A. P. (1991). *J. Neuropathol. Exp. Neurol.* **50**, 658–674.

Rostami, A., Burns, J., Brown, M. J., Rosen, J., Zweiman, B., Lisak, R. P., and Pleasure, D. (1985). *Cell. Immunol.* **91**, 354–361.

Rostami, A., Gregorian, S. K., Brown, M. J., and Pleasure, D. E. (1990). *J. Neuroimmunol.* **30**, 145–151.

Saida, T., Saida, K., Silberberg, D. H., and Brown, M. J. (1978). *Nature* **272**, 639–641.

Saida, T., Saida K., and Silberberg, D. H. (1979a). *Acta Neuropathol. (Berlin)* **48**, 19–25.

Saida, K., Saida, T., Brown, M. J., and Silberberg, D. H. (1979b). *Am. J. Pathol.* **95**, 99–116.

Saida, T., Saida, K., Dorfman, S. H., Silberberg, D. H., Sumner, A. J., Manning, M. C., Lisak, R. P., and Brown, M. J. (1979c). *Science* **204**, 1103–1106.

Schabet, M., Whitaker, J. N., Schott, K., Stevens, A., Zürn, A., Bühler, R., and Wiethölter, H. (1991). *J. Neuroimmunol.* **31**, 265–272.

Shimizu, Y., Newman, W., Tanaka, Y., and Shaw, S. (1992). *Immunol. Today* **13**, 106–113.

Stoll, G., Reiners, K., Schwendemann, G., et al. (1986). *Ann. Neurol.* **19**, 189–192.

Strigard, K., Larsson, P., Holmdahl, R., Klareskog, L., and Olsson, T. (1989). *J. Neuroimmunol.* **23**, 11–18.

Sun, D., Branum, K., and Sun, Q. (1992a). *Cell. Immunol.* **145**, 263–271.

Sun, D., Gold, D. P., Smith, L., Brostoff, S., and Coleclough, C. (1992b). *Eur. J. Immunol.* **22**, 591–594.

Suzumura, A., Sobue, G., Sugimura, K., Matsuoka, Y., and Sobue, I. (1985). *Acta Neurol. Scand.* **71**, 364–372.

Torres-Nagel, N. E., Gold, D. P., and Hünig, T. (1993). *Immunogenetics* **37**, 305–308.

Urban, J. L., Kumar, V., Kono, D. H., Gomez, C., Horvath, S. J., Clayton, J., Ando, D. G., Sercarz, E. E., and Hood, L. (1988). *Cell* **54**, 577–592.

Uyemura, K., Suzuki, M., Kitamura, K., Horie, K., Ogawa, Y., Matsuyama, H., Nozaki, S., and Muramatsu, I. (1982). *J. Neurochem.* **39**, 895–898.

Waksman, B. H., and Adams, R. D. (1955). *J. Exp. Med.* **102**, 213–235.

Waksman, B. H., Porter, H., Lees, M. B., Adams, R. D., and Folch, J. (1954). *J. Exp. Med.* **100**, 451–471.

Wekerle, H., and Hohlfeld, R. (1992). *In* "The Autoimmune Diseases II" (N. R. Rose and I. R. Mackay, Eds.), pp. 387–407. Academic Press, Orlando.

Wekerle, H., Schwab, M., Linington, C., and Meyermann, R. (1986). *Eur. J. Immunol.* **16**, 1551–1555.

Wekerle, H., Pette, M., Fujita, K., Nomura, K., and Meyermann, R. (1989). *Prog. Immunol.* **7**, 813–820.

Wisniewski, H. M., Brostoff, S. W., Carter, H., and Eylar, E. H. (1974). *Arch. Neurol.* **30**, 347–358.

Zhang, Y., Porter, S., and Wekerle, H. (1990). *Am. J. Pathol.* **136**, 111–122.

Chapter 5

Experimental Autoimmune Uveoretinitis—Rat and Mouse

Rachel R. Caspi

Laboratory of Immunology, National Eye Institute, National Institutes of Health, Bethesda, Maryland 20892

I. Introduction

Experimental autoimmune uveoretinitis (EAU) is a prototypic T-cell-mediated autoimmune disease that targets the neural retina and related tissues (Caspi, 1989; Gery *et al.*, 1985). A unique advantage of the EAU model is that it permits direct visual inspection of disease development and progression, thanks to the natural transparency of the ocular media. The model is used to represent a number of human eye diseases of a putative autoimmune nature, and to study basic mechanisms in tolerance and autoimmunity to organ-specific antigens residing in immunologically privileged sites. EAU models exist in a number of rodent species as well as in primates. Only the rat and mouse models are covered in this chapter. EAU models in the guinea pig, the rabbit, and the monkey have been reviewed elsewhere (Caspi, 1989; Faure, 1980; Gery *et al.*, 1986a).

EAU can be induced against a number of purified protein antigens extracted from the retina. The vast majority of studies have been done using heterologous, usually bovine, antigens; for obvious reasons, autologous rat or mouse retinal proteins cannot be obtained in sufficient quantities. As a rule, uveitogenic retinal proteins are evolutionarily well-conserved molecules, whose homologs can be found as far down the phylogenetic scale as the invertebrates (Applebury and Hargrave, 1986; Borst *et al.*, 1989; Mirshahi *et al.*, 1985). The better-known (but not the only) retinal uveitogens are:

1. The retinal-soluble antigen (S-Ag, arrestin). This 48-kDa intracellular photoreceptor protein is involved in the phototransduction cascade. It binds to photoactivated-phosphorylated rhodopsin, thereby apparently preventing the transducin-mediated activation of phosphodiesterase (Pfister *et al.*, 1985).

2. Interphotoreceptor retinoid-binding protein (IRBP). This 148-kDa protein is found in the interphotoreceptor matrix, and is thought to transport vitamin A derivatives between the photoreceptor and the retinal pigment epithelium (RPE). IRBP is composed of four homologous domains, which are thought to have arisen by gene duplication (Borst *et al.*, 1989).

3. Rhodopsin, and its illuminated form, opsin. This 40-kDa intracellular protein is the rod visual pigment (Applebury and Hargrave, 1986). Pathogenicity of this protein appears to be conformation-dependent, as rhodopsin is more pathogenic than opsin (Schalken *et al.*, 1988).

Immunization with microgram quantities of a uveitogenic protein or peptide in complete Freund's adjuvant (CFA) can induce disease that within a period of days or weeks results in disruption of the retinal architecture and complete destruction of the photoreceptor cell layer (Figure 1). EAU induced in mice and in rats with the different uveitogens appears to share essential immunological mechanisms and histological features. However, there are species-specific and strain-specific differences in the course of disease, in susceptibility to the different uveitogenic proteins, and in the pathogenic epitopes recognized (Caspi, 1989, 1993; Caspi *et al.*, 1988a; Gery *et al.*, 1985, 1986a). Cellular mechanisms have been better worked out in the rat, which is an older and more established model, whereas immunogenetic studies are

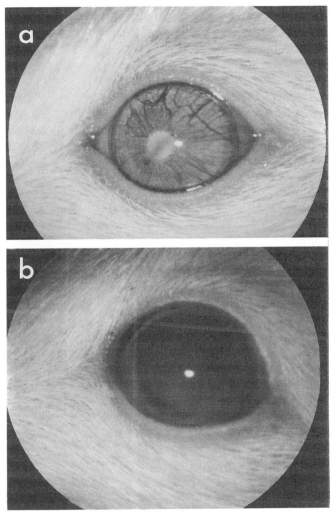

Figure 1   Clinical appearance of EAU in the Lewis rat by anterior chamber examination. (a) Normal eye; translucent appearance; pupil and iris blood vessels are clearly visible and the vessels are not congested. (b) Uveitic eye; the eye appears larger due to swelling and proptosis; red reflex is absent and pupil is obscured

more appropriately done in mice. Physical size of the animal and of the target organ may constitute another consideration. The choice of model will therefore depend on the specific needs of the study.

II. Rat EAU

A. History

The model of EAU initially developed in 1963 by Aronson *et al.* in the guinea pig using homologous uveal tissue was adapted to the rat in 1973 by Wacker and Kalsow using whole retinal extracts, and subsequently refined in 1981 by de Kozak and Faure using the retinal S-Ag. Major milestones in the further development of the rat model included the demonstration that essentially identical disease manifestations could be induced using different retinal proteins, that the disease was T-cell-mediated and transferable with long-term $CD4^+$ T-cell lines specific to retinal antigens, and finally the characterization of the pathogenic epitopes of the various uveitogenic proteins (reviewed in Caspi, 1989; Faure, 1980; Gery *et al.*, 1986a).

B. Animals

The most popular strain for EAU studies is the Lewis rat, which develops characteristically severe uveitis and has served as a "standard" against which responses of other strains are compared. Both males and females appear to be equally susceptible. There are no controlled studies of age dependency of susceptibility. We have used animals between 6 weeks and 6 months of age, without observing clear-cut differences in disease development (R. R. Caspi, unpublished). No special preparation of Lewis rats (such as irradiation or pretreatment with cyclophosphamide (CY) to downregulate natural resistance mechanisms) is necessary prior to the uveitogenic challenge, be it by active immunization or by adoptive transfer; however, such treatments can help to enhance the disease.

C. Genetic Background—MHC and Non-MHC Genes

The strain dependence of susceptibility in rats has been studied by a number of investigators. It appears that both major histocompatibility complex (MHC) and non-MHC genes play a role; however, owing to the limited availability of congenic and MHC-recombinant rat strains, their relative effects have not been well separated. In the case of most strains, poor susceptibility to disease can be enhanced by treatment with pertussis organisms or with pertussis toxin concurrently with immunization. It is thought that this treatment can overcome some non-MHC mechanisms of resistance, whereas resistance due to nonrecognition of pathogenic epitopes is not affected (Caspi, 1993; Hirose *et al.*, 1991). Obviously, the latter situation will be more frequently encountered when synthetic peptides representing single epitopes are used for immunization. Table I summarizes the susceptibility of some common inbred rat strains to EAU induced with the native S-Ag or IRBP.

D. Disease Induction

1. Immunization, Pathogenic Epitopes

Lewis rats are susceptible to all three major uveitogenic proteins: S-Ag, IRBP, and rhodopsin. The usual dose is 30 to 50 μg of S-Ag or IRBP, or 50 to 100 μg of rhodopsin emulsified in complete Freund's adjuvant that has been supplemented with additional *Mycobacterium tuberculosis* (usually 2.5 mg/ml). A suspension of heat-killed pertussis bacteria (10^{10} organisms/animal) may be injected at the time of immunization as additional adjuvant to maximize the disease. If pertussis is used, the dose of antigen should be reduced. Although footpad injections of antigen emulsified in CFA have been the traditional uveitogenic regimen, neither use of CFA nor the footpad route of immunization are mandatory. Subcutaneous (s.c.) immunization in the thighs and base of the tail with an emulsion of S-Ag or IRBP in CFA was as good as or better for induction of disease than the footpad route (Mozayeni and Caspi, unpublished). Complications resulting from use of CFA include crippling arthritis, particularly in the case of footpad immunization, and severe granulomatous inflammation of the injection site that can sometimes lead to

Table I

Susceptibility of Some Inbred Rat Strains to EAU

Strain	MHC	Susceptibility	Antigen	References
Lewis	RTl[l]	High	S-Ag, IRBP	Caspi *et al.* (1992b); Gery *et al.* (1985)
LeR	RTl[l]	Low[a]	S-Ag	Gery *et al.* (1986a)
F344	RTl[lvl]	Low	S-Ag, IRBP peptide	Caspi *et al.* (1992b); Gery *et al.* (1985)
CAR	RTl[l]	High	S-Ag	Caspi *et al.* (1992b); Gery *et al.* (1985)
BN	RTl[n]	Low[b]	S-Ag	Gery *et al.* (1986a)
PVG	RTl[c]	High	S-Ag	de Kozak *et al.* (1981)
WKAH	RTl[k]	Low	S-Ag	Hirose *et al.* (1991)
AVN	RTl[a]	Low	S-Ag	Gery *et al.* (1986a)
MAXX	RTl[n]	Low[b]	S-Ag	Gery *et al.* (1986a)

[a] Resistance of this strain may vary in different colonies (Caspi *et al.*, 1992b).

[b] Resistance is not overcome by pertussis treatment.

tissue necrosis. In such cases the animal(s) should be promptly euthanized. Hunter's adjuvant was recently shown to be as effective as CFA for EAU induction in rats, without the undesirable granulomatous and arthritogenic side effects that accompany immunization with CFA (Roberge *et al.*, 1992).

A number of pathogenic epitopes of S-Ag, IRBP, and opsin have been defined for the Lewis rat ($RT1B^l$), but information concerning epitopes pathogenic for other rat haplotypes is sparse. Table II lists the currently known epitopes that were found to be consistently pathogenic in the Lewis strain. As a rule of thumb, the peptides which are pathogenic at low doses are considered to contain a major pathogenic epitope. Frequently such peptides show immunological cross-reactivity with the native protein at the cellular level, indicating that they are recognized in the context of the whole molecule. However, some pathogenic epitopes may fail to elicit lymphocyte proliferation (de Smet *et al.*, 1993; Gregerson *et al.*, 1989; Kotake *et al.*, 1990a), so that this criterion is not applicable in all cases.

2. Adoptive Transfer

The full histopathological picture of EAU can be induced by adoptive transfer of immune lymph node cells or long-term CD4+, MHC class II-restricted T-cell lines in the absence of detectable titers of serum antibodies (Caspi *et al.*, 1986; Mochizuki *et al.*, 1985). The cells must be activated with antigen or mitogen just prior to transfer in order to efficiently mediate disease, suggesting that activation-dependent functions (lymphokine production, expression of adhesion molecules, etc.) are important. The minimum number of cells required to transfer the disease depends on their source and specificity. For example, as many as 50×10^6 activated (unselected) lymph node cells specific to bovine S-Ag may be needed for a successful transfer, dropping to 5×10^6 cells for a T-lymphocyte line of the same specificity, to as few as 2×10^4 cells after reselection of that line with the major pathogenic epitope of human S-Ag, peptide 35 (Beraud *et al.*, 1992; Caspi *et al.*, 1986; Mochizuki *et al.*, 1985). This suggests that only a minority of the cells carried in T-cell lines derived to the whole S-Ag protein recognize epitope(s) that are pathogenic. It is not necessary to transfer the cells intravenously; except when transferring limiting numbers of cells, the intraperitoneal (i.p.) route gives very satisfactory results.

The method currently used in our laboratory to generate uveitogenic rat T-cell lines consists of stimulating the draining lymph node cells (collected approximately 11 days after immunization) with the antigen for 48 hr, after which the proliferating blast cells are enriched by density centrifugation over Ficoll, and the CD4+ cells are isolated by panning. The cells are subsequently maintained on a weekly cycle of 2 days of stimulation with antigen in the presence of antigen-presenting cells (APC), followed by 5 days of expan-

Table II
Retinal Protein-Derived Peptides That Are Pathogenic for Lewis Rats

Source	Nickname (if any)	Position[a]	a.a. sequence[b]	Minimum dose[c]	References
Bovine S-Ag	Peptide N	281–302 (287–297)	VPLLANNRERRGIAL DGKIKHE	50 μg	Donoso et al. (1988); Singh et al. (1988)
	Peptide M	303–320 (303–317)	DTNLASSTIIKEGIDK TV	50 μg	Donoso et al. (1987)
	—	333–352 (339–352)	LTVSGLLGELTSSE VATEVP	0.5 μg	Merryman et al. (1991)
	—	343–362 (352–364[d])	TSSEVATEVPFRLM HPQPED(PD[d])	0.5 μg[e]	Gregerson et al. (1990)
Human S-Ag	Human N	286–305 (289–300)	LLANNRERRGIALDG KIKHE	100 μg	Donoso et al. (1988)
	Human M	306–325 (306–317)	DTNLASSTIIKEGIDR TVLG	100 μg	Donoso et al. (1988)
	Peptide 1	1–20	MAASGKTSKSEPN HVIFKKI	100 μg[f]	de Smet et al. (1993)
	Peptide 6	51–70	VDPDLVKGKKVYVT LTCAFR	100 μg[f]	de Smet et al. (1993)
	Peptide 19	181–200	VQHAPLEMGPQPRA EATWQF	25 μg	de Smet et al. (1993)
	Peptide 20	191–210	QPRAEATWQFFMSD KPLHLA	100 μg[f]	de Smet et al. (1993)
	Peptide 26	251–270	VVLYSSDYYVKPVA MEEAQE	100 μg[f]	de Smet et al. (1993)
	Peptide 29	281–300	TLTLLPLLANNRERR GIAL	100 μg[f]	de Smet et al. (1993)
	Peptide 31	301–320	GKIKHEDTNLASSTII KEGI	100 μg[f]	de Smet et al. (1993)
	Peptide 35	341–360 (343–356)	GFLGELTSSEVATE VPFRLM	5 μg	de Smet et al. (1993); Merryman et al. (1991)
	Peptide 36	351–370 (356–366)	VATEVPFRLMHPQP EDPAKE	50 μg	de Smet et al. (1993); Gregerson et al. (1990)
Bovine IRBP	R23	1091–1115	PNNSVSELWTLSQL EGERYGSKKSM	100 nM (280 μg)	Kotake et al. (1991a)
	R4	1158–1180	HVDDTDLYLTIPTAR SVGAADGS	67 μg	Sanui et al. (1988)
	R14	1169–1191 (1182–1190)	PTARSVGAADGSS WEGVGVVPDV	0.1 nM (0.2 μg)	Kotake et al. (1991b); Sanui et al. (1989)
	—	271–283[g]	SQTWEGSGVLPCV	1.5 nM (2 μg)	Kotake et al. (1990b)
	—	880–892[g]	GEAWDLAGVEPDI	150 nM (200 μg)	Kotake et al. (1990b)
Human IRBP	HIRBP 715	521–540 (527–534)	YLLTSHRTATAAEEF AFLMQ[h]	0.1 μg	Donoso et al. (1989)
	HIRBP 778	531–550	AAEEFAFLMQSLGW ATLVGE[i]	50 μg[f]	Donoso et al. (1989)

(continued)

Table II—*Continued*

Source	Nickname (if any)	Position[a]	a.a. sequence[b]	Minimum dose[c]	References
	HIRBP 730	821–840	KDLYILMSHTSGSA AEAFAH	50 μg[f]	Donoso *et al.* (1989)
	HIRBP 745	1121–1140	SKKSMVILTSTVTAG TAEEF	50 μg[f]	Donoso *et al.* (1989)
	HIRBP 808	1131–1150	TVTAGTAEEFTYIMK RLGRA[j]	50 μg[f]	Donoso *et al.* (1989)
	HIRBP 720	621–640	ALVEGTGHLLEAHY ARPEVV	50 μg[f]	Donoso *et al.* (1989)
	HIRBP 722	661–680	DLESLASQLTADLQ EVSGDH	50 μg[f]	Donoso *et al.* (1989)
	HIRBP 724	701–720	PAVPSPEELTYLIEA LFKTE	50 μg[f]	Donoso *et al.* (1989)
	HIRBP 804	1051–1070	EHIWKKIMHTDAM IIDMRFN	50 μg[f]	Donoso *et al.* (1989)
Bovine rhodopsin	—	61–75	VTVQHKKLRTPLNYI	100 μg[f,k]	Adamus *et al.* (1992)
	—	230–252	VKEAAAQQQESATT QKAEKEVTR	100 μg[f,k]	Adamus *et al.* (1992)
	—	324–348	GKNPLGDDEASTTV SKTETSQVAPA	100 μg[f,k]	Adamus *et al.* (1992)

[a] In parenthesis: position of minimal sequence (if known).
[b] The minimal pathogenic sequence (if known) is underlined.
[c] Pathogenicity was tested in most cases using pertussis vaccine as additional adjuvant (1–2×10^10 heat-killed organisms per rat).
[d] Two additional amino acids (sequence: PD) at the C-terminal are required to elicit pathogenicity when the short peptide is used, possibly to stabilize the peptide-MHC class II complex, but are not considered to be part of the pathogenic epitope.
[e] Pertussis was not used.
[f] Lower doses were not tested.
[g] Structural repeats of 1182–1190 within the IRBP molecule (Borst *et al.*, 1989).
[h] An additional epitope may be encoded by the N terminus (sequence; YLLTSHRTATAA).
[i] Overlaps 521–540, but pathogenic epitope appears to be different.
[j] Overlaps 1121–1140.
[k] Animals were preinjected with 20 mg/kg of cyclophosphamide 3 days before immunization. Pertussis adjuvant was not used.

sion and then rest in interleukin-2 (IL-2)-containing medium. Highly pathogenic, phenotypically homogeneous T-cell lines are generated by this method after only three stimulation cycles. While we and others (D. Gregerson, personal communication) have found it difficult to clone uveitogenic rat T cells, the line cells (particularly when they are specific to defined pathogenic peptides) can be generated in large numbers and maintain their pathogenicity for many stimulation cycles. Pathogenic T-cell lines express T-cell receptor (TCR) genes of the *Vβ8* family. Some data suggest that a pathogenic clonotype in S-Ag-induced EAU may be *Vβ8.2*, and a pathogenic clonotype in IRBP-induced EAU may be *Vβ8.3* (Egwuagu *et al.*, 1992; Gregerson *et al.*, 1991; Merryman *et al.*, 1991).

3. Course of Disease

The course of disease in the Lewis rat is typically acute and of short duration. The time of onset will vary according to the severity of the developing disease, the antigen, and mode of induction. For example, immunization with 30 μg of S-Ag in CFA usually results in onset around day 14; a similar dose of IRBP in CFA results in onset around day 12. If pertussis is used as additional adjuvant, the time of onset will be earlier by 2 to 3 days, and will usually be more uniform than without pertussis. Onset of EAU induced by adoptive transfer is usually on days 4–7, that is, about a week shorter than for active immunization. Development of the disease can be very rapid, and within 24 hr clinical manifestations can reach a score of 2 or 3 (see later discussion for scoring method). The active EAU in the Lewis rat lasts 1–2 weeks, and the disease does not relapse. This might be due in part to typically massive destruction of photoreceptors and depletion of the source of autoantigen. Another reason might be development of active suppression, and a number of reports suggest that active suppression might have a role in curtailing uveitis in the Lewis rat model (see later discussion). The rapid onset and acute course of EAU in the Lewis rat makes it difficult to evaluate therapeutic intervention during active disease. A workaround for looking at efferent-stage disease is to begin intervention 7 days after immunization, when immune lymphocytes are already present, or to use an adoptive transfer system. Alternative rat models of EAU in strains that exhibit a more protracted clinical course have been described, but have not gained wide acceptance (de Kozak *et al.*, 1981; Stanford *et al.*, 1987).

E. Quantitation

1. Clinical

Onset of disease in an albino strain such as the Lewis rat can be recognized and its development followed simply by inspecting the eyes with the aid of a good flashlight (Figure 2). The normal eye appears translucent and reflects the light (red reflex). The first sign of uveitis is engorgement of blood vessels in the iris and an irregular pupil that cannot contract in response to light (caused by the iris adhering to the lens). Leukocyte infiltration and deposition of fibrin is first seen as dulling of the red reflex, progressing to

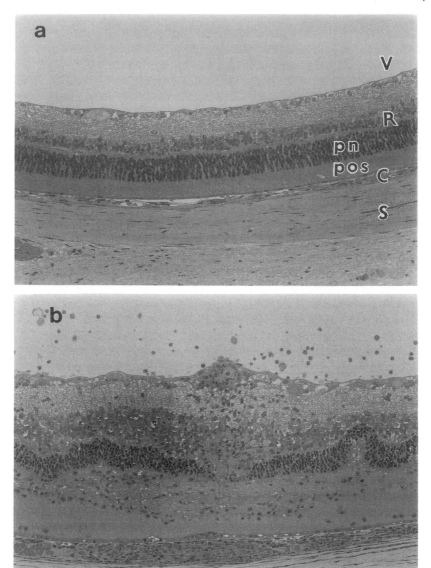

Figure 2 Histopathology of EAU in the Lewis rat. (a) Normal retina. V, vitreous; R, retina; pn, photoreceptor nuclei; pos, photoreceptor outer segments; C, choroid; S, sclera. Note ordered retinal layers. (b) Uveitic retina. Note disorganized retinal architecture, massive inflammatory cell infiltration, serous retinal detachment, and photoreceptor cell damage (grade 3 disease).

complete opacification of the anterior chamber. The eye swells and can protrude from its socket (proptosis). In very severe cases, hemorrhages in the anterior chamber and even perforation of the cornea can occur. In the latter case, the animal should be euthanized. We grade clinical EAU on a scale of 0 (no disease) to 4 (severe disease), as follows (each higher grade includes criteria for the preceding one):

0.5 (trace) Dilated iris blood vessels

1 Engorged iris vessels, abnormal pupil contraction

2 Hazy anterior chamber, decreased red reflex

3 Moderately opaque anterior chamber, but pupil still visible; dull red reflex

4 Opaque anterior chamber and obscured pupil, absence of red reflex, proptosis

2. Histopathology

EAU is defined primarily as a posterior segment disease, because the target antigens reside in the retina. Therefore, although clinical follow-up by anterior chamber inflammation is important and yields valuable information, the final readout should be done by histopathology. In addition, the appearance of the anterior chamber does not always parallel the extent of retinal damage (see Section IV,7). We grade EAU by histopathology on an arbitrary scale of 0 to 4, in half-point increments, as follows (Caspi *et al.*, 1993):

0.5 (trace) Mild inflammatory cell infiltration of the retina, with or without photoreceptor damage, in less than one-fourth of the retinal section area

1 Mild inflammation and/or photoreceptor outer segment damage in at least one-fourth of the retinal section area

2 Mild to moderate inflammation and/or lesion extending to the outer nuclear layer in at least one-fourth of the retinal section area

3 Moderate to marked inflammation and/or lesion extending to the inner nuclear layer in at least one-fourth of the retinal section area

4 Severe inflammation and/or full thickness retinal damage in at least one-fourth of the retinal section area

The grading is conveniently done on methacrylate-embedded tissue sections, 4 to 6 microns thick, stained by hematoxylin and eosin. To arrive at the final grading, several sections cut through the pupillary–optic nerve plane should be examined for each eye. It should be remembered that in this type of visual scoring, there is always an element of subjectivity. Therefore, it is important that the results be read in a masked fashion, preferably always by the same person.

F. Resistance to Disease: Natural and Acquired

Some rat strains are genetically resistant to EAU, such as the F344 and the brown Norway strains. The basis for resistance of most strains is unknown, but in many cases low susceptibility correlates with low numbers of mast cells in the eye (Caspi, 1993; Li *et al.*, 1992; Mochizuki *et al.*, 1984). Frequently, resistance can be successfully overcome by administering *Bordetella pertussis* organisms or pertussis toxin (10^{10} organisms or 1 μg) at the time of immunization (Gery *et al.*, 1986a). It is thought that resistance which cannot be overcome by pertussis treatment is due to lack of recognition of pathogenic epitopes (Hirose *et al.*, 1991). Others have used low-dose CY to enhance the uveitogenic response (Adamus *et al.*, 1992).

Acquired resistance to EAU in the susceptible Lewis strain can be induced by a number of experimental manipulations, most of which (1–4) appear to be due to an active suppressor cell response:

1. Injection of T-suppressor cells (Caspi *et al.*, 1988b).
2. Induction of anti-idiotypic responses by "vaccination" with uveitogenic T-helper cells or selected antigenic peptides (Beraud *et al.*, 1992; de Kozak, 1990).
3. Priming with antigen administered through the anterior chamber of the eye, resulting in a response known as anterior chamber-associated immune deviation (ACAID) (Mizuno *et al.*, 1989).
4. Feeding of antigen (oral tolerance) (Nussenblatt *et al.*, 1990; Thurau *et al.*, 1991).
5. Immunization under cover of treatment with T-cell targeting agents, such as cyclosporin A or FK506 (Fujino *et al.*, 1988; Kawashima *et al.*, 1990).
6. Intravenous administration of soluble antigen or antigen coupled to syngeneic splenocytes (Dua *et al.*, 1992; Sasamoto *et al.*, 1992).

III. Mouse EAU

A. History

Successful induction of EAU in mice was first reported in 1988 by Caspi *et al.* (1988a). Numerous attempts to induce EAU in mice with S-Ag yielded disappointing results, until findings by Gery *et al.* in 1986, who showed that IRBP is a potent uveitogen in rats (Gery *et al.* 1986b), prompted us to evaluate this protein as a uveitogen in mice. IRBP turned out to be a much better uveitogen for mice than S-Ag and made possible the development of a workable mouse EAU model which has since been used in many studies.

B. Animals

As in rats, age and sex do not appear to have a major influence on susceptibility to disease. As a species, mice appear to be less susceptible to EAU than
rats. In fact, "susceptible" mouse strains require an immunization regimen
of an intensity similar to that used to induce EAU in "resistant" strains of
rats. Initially, EAU in mice was induced after pretreatment with CY with a
split-dose immunization protocol that employed heat-killed pertussis as additional adjuvant (Caspi *et al.*, 1988a). However, optimization of the immunization protocol has shown that severe disease can be induced in susceptible
mice with a single immunization of IRBP in CFA plus pertussis toxin (Caspi
et al., 1990). Generally, CY pretreatment should not be required, except under suboptimal conditions of immunization.

C. Genetic Background—MHC and Non-MHC Genes

There are distinct differences in EAU susceptibility among mouse strains
(Caspi *et al.*, 1992a). EAU expression in mice requires both a susceptible
MHC haplotype and a "permissive" genetic background, for example, B10.
When tested on the permissive B10 background, the highly susceptible hap-
lotypes are $H\text{-}2^r$ and $H\text{-}2^k$. $H\text{-}2^b$ appears to have intermediate susceptibility,
and $H\text{-}2^d$ is poorly susceptible. Primary MHC control of susceptibility appears
to depend on the I-A subregion, at least as determined for strains expressing
the $I\text{-}A^k$. In contrast, expression of the $I\text{-}E^k$ appeared to have a protective
effect. Secondary control of susceptibility is exerted by the genetic background. In strains having a "nonpermissive" genetic background (e.g., A or
AKR), EAU is reduced or abrogated, despite the presence of a susceptible
I-A type. Table III lists the currently known susceptible and resistant mouse
strains.

D. Disease Induction

1. Immunization, Pathogenic Epitopes

As mentioned above, IRBP is a good uveitogen for mice, whereas S-Ag is a
relatively poor uveitogen. Data concerning uveitogenicity of rhodopsin in
mice are not available. Use of a sufficient dose of pertussis toxin as additional
adjuvant is mandatory for disease development. With 0.5 to 1 μg of pertussis
toxin given i.p., IRBP doses of 50–100 μg in CFA should normally cause
severe disease in susceptible strains such as the B10.A and B10.RIII. An
alternative induction protocol has been published that relies on multiple
immunizations with S-Ag using *Klebsiella* lipopolysaccharide as the sole adju-

Table III
Susceptibility of Different Mouse Strains to IRBP-EAU

Strain	H-2	Susceptibility[a]
B10.A	a^b	High
A/J	a	Medium
C57bl/6	b	Medium
C57bl/10	b	Medium
Balb/c	d	Low
B10.D2	d	Low to medium
B10.M	f	Low
A.CA	f	Low
B10.BR	k	High
AKR/J	k	Low
B10.Q	q	Low
DBA.1	q	Low
B10.Rlll	r	High
LP.Rlll	r	Medium
A.SW	s	Low
B10.S	s	Low
B10.PL	u	Low
B10.SM	v	Low
NZW	z	Low

[a] Mice were immunized by the split-dose method with 100 μg IRBP in CFA in the footpads and were given 1 μg of pertussis toxin i.p. Eyes were harvested at 5 weeks.
[b] $H\text{-}2^a$ mice are $I\text{-}A^k$.

vant (Iwase *et al.*, 1990), but has not gained popularity. As with rats, the s.c. immunization route is as good as or better for inducing disease than the footpad route, and appears less distressful to the animals. The epitopes of the IRBP molecule pathogenic for the $H\text{-}2^b$, $H\text{-}2^r$, and $H\text{-}2^k$ haplotypes are being studied. The sequences SGIPYVISYLHPGSTVSHVD (aa 161–180 of human IRBP) and HPGNTILHVDTIYNRPSNTT (aa 171–190) contain a major and a minor pathogenic epitope, respectively, for the $H\text{-}2^r$ haplotype (Silver *et al.*, 1994; Caspi *et al.*, 1994b; Silver *et al.*, submitted). Preliminary data indicate that the sequence LRHNPGGPSSAVPLLLSYFQ (aa 461–480 of human IRBP) contains a minor pathogenic epitope for $H\text{-}2^b$ (Silver *et al.*, 1993). Data obtained with fusion proteins representing different repeated domains of bovine IRBP indicate that the first and last domains may contain epitopes pathogenic for $H\text{-}2^k$ (P. Silver *et al.*, unpublished).

2. Adoptive Transfer

Uveitogenic T-cell lines in mice have only recently become available. We have generated long-term IRBP-specific and peptide-specific T-cell lines from draining lymph node cells and from uveitic eyes of IRBP-immunized mice by using a method similar to the one described for generation of rat T-cell lines, by alternating cycles of stimulation with antigen and APC, followed by expansion in IL-2-containing medium. One B10.A T-cell line specific to whole bovine IRBP is still pathogenic at 1×10^5 cells/mouse after 18 antigen stimulation cycles, and appears to elaborate an unrestricted lymphokine profile. This line is composed of TCR α/β bearing cells. Interestingly, over time, *Vβ8.2* and *Vβ6*-bearing cells gradually became the dominant TCR types (Rizzo *et al.*, 1993). In contrast, we have found it difficult to consistently transfer EAU in mice with primary cultures of IRBP-primed lymph node cells.

3. Course of Disease

The severity and clinical course of EAU in mice varies, depending on the strain and the immunization regimen. In the susceptible B10.A strain, it is possible to control the course of disease by adjusting the respective doses of antigen and pertussis toxin, so that the whole spectrum of disease, from chronic to hyperacute, can be obtained (Caspi *et al.*, 1990). High-intensity immunization results in an acute form of disease with an early onset (ca. day 14) and diffuse photoreceptor damage, whereas lower antigen and pertussis toxin doses will result in milder disease with progressively later onset. In the milder form of disease, pathology is typically focal and a large portion of the photoreceptor cell layer may be spared. This type of disease tends to take on a chronic form, or may remit and be followed by a relapse after a brief disease-free period (Applebury and Hargrave, 1986). The number of relapses that can occur has not been determined.

E. Quantitation

1. Clinical

In the susceptible mouse strains (B10 background), strong pigmentation of the eyes and the typically mild involvement of the anterior chamber usually precludes detection of disease by anterior chamber inspection, as is done in rats. However, in pigmented strains it is possible to observe changes in the fundus of the eye under a binocular microscope after dilating the pupil with a clinical ophthalmic dilating solution (Tropicamide, 1%) (Figure 3). The nature, number, and severity of the lesions are used as criteria for clinical scoring on a scale of 0 (no change) to 4 (severe disease) (Whitcup *et al.*, 1993):

0.5 (trace) Few (1–2) very small, peripheral focal lesions; minimal vasculitis/vitritis.
1 Mild vasculitis; <5 small focal lesions; max. 1 linear lesion

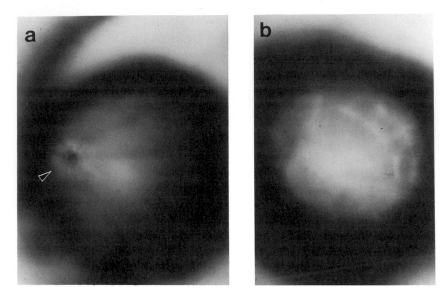

Figure 3 Clinical appearance of EAU in the B10.A mouse by fundoscopic exam. (a) Normal eye; note blood vessels radiating from the optic nerve head (arrowhead). (b) Uveitic eye.; note retinal detachment obscuring the optic nerve head and numerous white linear lesions.

2 Multiple (>5) chorioretinal lesions and/or infiltrations; severe vasculitis (large size, thick wall infiltrations); few linear lesions (<5)

3 Pattern of linear lesions; large confluent lesions; subretinal neovascularization; retinal hemorrhages; papilledema

4 Large retinal detachment; retinal atrophy

2. Histopathology

The final readout should be confirmed by histopathology. Histological grading is done on methacrylate-embedded tissue sections, 4 to 6 microns thick, stained by hematoxylin and eosin (Figure 4). Disease is scored on a scale of 0 to 4 in half-point increments, on the basis of the type, number and severity of lesions, and the extent of inflammation (Caspi *et al.*, 1988a).

0.5 Mild inflammatory cell infiltration. No tissue damage

1 Infiltration; retinal folds and focal retinal detachments; few small granulomas in choroid and retina, perivasculitis.

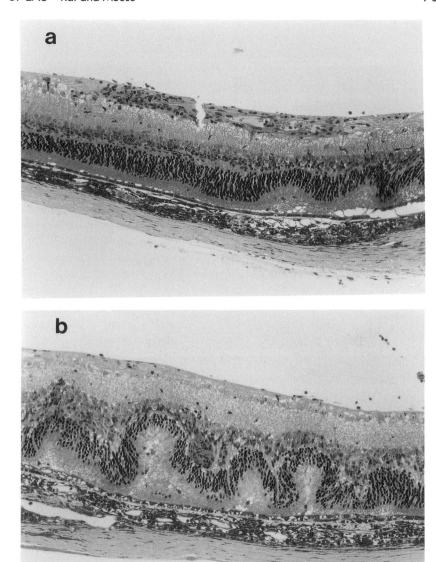

Figure 4　Histopathology of EAU in the B10.A mouse. (a) Mild disease of the chronic type (grade 1); note well-preserved photoreceptor cell layer. (b) Severe disease of the acute type; note diffuse photoreceptor damage (grade 3).

2 Moderate infiltration; retinal folds, detachments and focal photoreceptor cell damage; small- to medium-sized granulomas, perivasculitis and
vasculitis

3 Medium to heavy infiltration; extensive retinal folding with detachments, moderate photoreceptor cell damage; medium-sized granulomatous
lesions; subretinal neovascularization

4 Heavy infiltration; diffuse retinal detachment with serous exudate and
subretinal bleeding; extensive photoreceptor cell damage; large granulomatous lesions; subretinal neovascularization

To arrive at the final grading, several sections cut through the pupillary–
optic nerve plane should be examined for each eye. This is particularly important when disease scores are low and changes are focal because lesions
may be visible in only some of the sections. It should be remembered that in
this type of visual scoring, there is always an element of subjectivity. Therefore, it is important that the results be read in a masked fashion, preferably
always by the same person.

F. Resistance to Disease: Natural and Acquired

As already mentioned, even the most susceptible mouse strains are about as
susceptible to EAU as resistant strains of rats. Pertussis toxin is needed to
overcome this low natural propensity of mice to develop EAU. Even in susceptible mouse haplotypes, a "nonpermissive" background can largely or completely prevent the expression of disease, despite the presence of a highly
susceptible *H-2* haplotype and despite the fact that pertussis toxin is routinely included in the immunization protocol. Factors which may determine
"permissiveness' or "nonpermissiveness" of a particular genetic background
are largely unknown at present, but one determining factor could be regulation of the systemic interferon-γ (IFNγ) responses. Treatment with a
monoclonal antibody to IFNγ upregulates EAU in some strains, and can
even alter the response pattern from resistance to susceptibility (Caspi *et al.*,
1992b). Irrespective of whether it is MHC or non-MHC-related, resistance
to EAU is not absolute (at least when using the whole multiepitope IRBP or
S-Ag protein for immunization) and can be partly overcome by a more intense immunization protocol. A case in point: immunization by the s.c. route
in the thighs and base of tail tends to cause stronger EAU than footpad
immunization with the same dose of antigen (s.c. immunization employs a
larger volume of CFA, resulting in a higher dose of mycobacteria, and more
injection sites). DBA/1 mice, which completely failed to develop EAU after
footpad immunization with 100 μg of IRBP (Caspi *et al.*, 1988a), did develop
mild EAU when the same dose was delivered by the s.c. route (Caspi *et al.*,
1992b).

IV. Expert Experience

A. Choice of Strain

Some common laboratory mouse strains have congenital retinal degeneration (recessive *rd* gene) which manifests itself as partial to complete loss of the photoreceptor cell layer. Such strains are obviously unsuitable for uveitis studies. Strains that carry the *rd* gene include SJL, PL/J, CBA/J, SWR/J, C3H, and others (Robison *et al.*, 1983).

B. Animal Husbandry and Health

Even in mice and rats with a normal retina, prolonged exposure to strong light can cause photoreceptor degeneration, which will confound experimental results (Robison *et al.*, 1983). Albinos are more susceptible than pigmented strains. It is therefore important not to leave incoming animals in strong light on the facility loading dock for many hours, and to adjust lighting conditions in the animal rooms. The experimental animals must be in good health. Although not strictly required, it is recommended that animals be purchased and maintained under specific pathogen-free conditions. Abnormal uveitogenic responses are seen in animals harboring an active infection. EAU in mice can be experimentally regulated by manipulating systemic IFNγ levels (Caspi *et al.*, 1992b; and Caspi *et al.*, 1994a). It is therefore a plausible hypothesis that, in infected animals, the development of immunity to the uveitogenic protein is being influenced by systemic levels of lymphokines produced as part of the host defense mechanisms.

C. Pitfalls of Surgical Anesthesia

Anesthetized animals sleep with their eyes open and do not blink. Therefore, if animals are going to be asleep for more than a few minutes, it is necessary to place an ointment on the eyes to prevent drying of the cornea. Drying of the eyes will inevitably result in exposure keratitis, which will cause corneal opacification and will make follow-up of clinical disease difficult or impossible. Also, it is important not to expose the eyes of anesthetized animals that had their pupils dilated to light for any longer than necessary because strong light can damage the photoreceptor cells.

D. Collection of Blood

Drawing blood from the retroorbital plexus is not recommended, for obvious reasons.

E. Handling of Eye Specimens for Histology

Enucleation in rats should be performed by carefully dissecting the globe from the periocular tissues and the optic nerve without excessive squeezing, to avoid maceration of delicate ocular tissues that become even more fragile when inflamed. In mice, the eye should be made to protrude by applying pressure on the skull, and plucked free of the tissue with a curved forceps. Eyes should be collected within 15 min of euthanasia, because autolysis sets in very rapidly and will preclude correct evaluation of the results. It is important to prefix the eyes in 4% buffered glutaraldehyde for 1 hr, after which the eyes are transferred to 10% buffered formalin at least overnight. This brief fixation in 4% glutaraldehyde prevents artifactual detachment of the retina from the choroid. However, leaving the eyes in glutaraldehyde for too long will cause excessive hardening of the lens, which will make sectioning difficult.

F. Maintenance of T-Cell Lines

Uveitogenic rat and mouse T-cell lines tend to lose their antigenic specificity if maintained constantly in fetal bovine serum (FBS). Syngeneic rat or mouse serum (1 to 1.5%) should be used during the stage of antigen stimulation, otherwise proliferation of FBS-specific cells may result, causing high backgrounds *in vitro* and loss of pathogenicity *in vivo*. The rat/mouse serum should be fresh or fresh-frozen to maintain maximum nutritional quality, and does not need to be heat inactivated (although inactivation may help to guard against mycoplasma). We have tested commercially available mouse serum (PelFreeze) as culture supplement, and found it to be inadequate and even toxic.

G. Evaluation of Clinical Disease

a. Rats. The extent of anterior chamber disease does not always parallel the extent of retinal damage. Retinal damage in the absence of overt anterior chamber inflammation tends to occur in rats adoptively transferred with some S-Ag-specific lines (Caspi *et al.*, 1986). Conversely, it is not unusual to find considerable anterior chamber inflammation without any tissue damage in the posterior pole of the eye. In particular, immunization with the R16 peptide of IRBP or adoptive transfer of cells specific to this epitope tends to give this picture. Eyes should never be harvested too early after onset (a frequent temptation is to collect the eyes at the peak of clinical disease) because anterior inflammation precedes posterior disease and there may be little if any photoreceptor damage at that point. A good time to collect the eyes is 1 week after clinical onset.

b. Mice. Appropriate optics and good coaxial illumination through the objective lens are needed because of the smallness and extreme curvature of the mouse eye. The pupil is first dilated with an ophthalmic dilating solution. It takes several minutes for the drops to take effect. The evaluation technique is as follows: grasp enough skin on the back of the scalp to draw the eyelids up and prevent the mouse from blinking, and place a drop of sterile saline and a microscope coverslip on the cornea to equalize refraction. Manipulate the head of the mouse under the microscope (while keeping the coverslip level) to inspect as far up the sides of the retina as possible because the linear lesions are frequently seen there. With some practice, fundoscopy can be performed on nonanesthetized animals, but if disease is borderline or severity scores are to be assigned, it advisable to lightly anesthetize the mouse prior to fundoscopy to facilitate a more thorough inspection.

V. Lessons

The EAU models in animals are used to represent human posterior uveitic diseases of a putative autoimmune nature, such as sympathetic ophthalmia, birdshot retinochoroidopathy, Behcet's disease, and others (Nussenblatt and Palestine, 1989). While none of the animal models mimics the full spectrum of the human disease, each has distinguishing characteristics that are reminiscent of different aspects of clinical uveitis. Although the putative retinal antigens involved in human uveitis are still unknown, the fact that a number of retinal proteins provoke essentially the same disease in a number of species suggests that similar mechanisms might operate in the human disease. Clinically, the EAU model has served as an invaluable tool to evaluate novel immunotherapeutic and conventional therapeutic strategies. So far, the success of a given modality to downregulate EAU in animals has served as a good predictor of its clinical usefulness. Basic questions are being asked concerning the genetic control of susceptibility vs resistance to ocular autoimmunity, the cellular and molecular mechanisms that contribute to maintenance or breakdown of tolerance to organ-specific antigens, and the immunological events that constitute the autoimmune amplification cascade which culminates in the expression of disease (Caspi, 1993; Caspi and Nussenblatt, 1993). Thus, EAU is useful as a tool for clinical as well as for basic studies of ocular and organ-specific autoimmunity.

References

Adamus, G., Schmied, J. L., Hargrave, P. A., Arendt, A., and Moticka, E. J. (1992). Induction of experimental autoimmune uveitis with rhodopsin synthetic peptides in Lewis rats. *Curr. Eye Res.* **11**, 657–667.

Applebury, M. L., and Hargrave, P. A. (1986). Molecular biology of the visual pigments. *Vision Res.* **26**, 1881–1895.

Aronson, S. B., Hogan, M. J., and Zweigart, P. (1963a). Homoimmune uveitis in the guinea-pig. I. General concepts of auto- and homoimmunity, methods and manifestations. *Arch. Ophthalmol.* **69**, 105–109.

Aronson, S. B., Hogan, M. J., and Zweigart, P. (1963b). Homoimmune uveitis in the guinea-pig. II. Clinical manifestations. *Arch. Ophthalmol.* **69**, 203–207.

Aronson, S. B., Hogan, M. J., and Zweigart, P. (1963c). Homoimmune uveitis in the guinea-pig. III. Histopathologic manifestations of the disease. *Arch. Ophthalmol.* **69**, 208–219.

Beraud, E., Kotake, S., Caspi, R. R., Oddo, S. M., Chan, C. C., Gery, I., and Nussenblatt, R. B. (1992). Control of experimental autoimmune uveoretinitis by low dose T cell vaccination. *Cell. Immunol.* **140**, 112–122.

Borst, D. E., Redmond, T. M., Elser, J. E., Gonda, M. A., Wiggert, B., Chader, G. J., and Nickerson, J. M. (1989). Interphotoreceptor retinoid-binding protein. Gene characterization, protein repeat structure, and its evolution. *J. Biol. Chem.* **264**, 1115–1123.

Caspi, R. R. (1989). Basic mechanisms in immune-mediated uveitic disease. *In* "Immunology of Eye Disease" (S. L. Lightman, Ed.), Chap. 5, pp. 61–86. Kluwer Academic Publishers, Lancaster, UK.

Caspi, R. R. (1993). Immunogenetic aspects of clinical and experimental uveitis. *Reg. Immunol.* **4**, 321–330.

Caspi, R. R., Roberge, F. G., McAllister, C. G., el Saied, M., Kuwabara, T., Gery, I., Hanna, E., and Nussenblatt, R. B. (1986). T cell lines mediating experimental autoimmune uveoretinitis (EAU) in the rat. *J. Immunol.* **136**, 928–933.

Caspi, R. R., Roberge, F. G., Chan, C. C., Wiggert, B., Chader, G. J., Rozenszajn, L. A., Lando, Z., and Nussenblatt, R. B. (1988a). A new model of autoimmune disease. Experimental autoimmune uveoretinitis induced in mice with two different retinal antigens. *J. Immunol.* **140**, 1490–1495.

Caspi, R. R., Kuwabara, T., and Nussenblatt, R. B. (1988b). Characterization of a suppressor cell line which downgrades experimental autoimmune uveoretinitis in the rat. *J. Immunol.* **140**, 2579–2584.

Caspi, R. R., Chan, C. C., Leake, W. C., Higuchi, M., Wiggert, B., and Chader, G. J. (1990). Experimental autoimmune uveoretinitis in mice. Induction by a single eliciting event and dependence on quantitative parameters of immunization. *J. Autoimmun.* **3**, 237–246.

Caspi, R. R., Fujino, Y., Najafian, F., Grover, S., Hansen, C. B., and Wilder, R. L. (1993). Recruitment of antigen-nonspecific cells plays a pivotal role in the pathogenesis of a T cell-mediated organ-specific autoimmune disease, experimental autoimmune uveoretinitis. *J. Neuroimmunol.*, **47**, 177–178.

Caspi, R. R., Grubbs, B. G., Chan, C. C., Chader, G. J., and Wiggert, B. (1992a). Genetic control of susceptibility to experimental autoimmune uveoretinitis in the mouse model: Concomitant regulation by MHC and non-MHC genes. *J. Immunol.* **148**, 2384–2389.

Caspi, R. R., Chan, C.-C., Fujino, Y., Oddo, S., Najafian, F., Bahmanyar, S., Heremans, H., Wilder, R. L., and Wiggert, B. (1992b). Genetic factors in susceptibility and resistance to experimental autoimmune uveoretinitis. *Curr. Eye Res.* **11**(Suppl.), 81–86.

Caspi, R. R., Parsa, C., Chan, C. C., Grubbs, B. G., Bahmanyar, S., Heremans, H., Billiau, A., and Wiggert, B. (1994a). Endogenous systemic Interferon-gamma has a protective role against ocular autoimmunity in mice. *J. Immunol.* **152**, 890–899.

Caspi, R. R., Silver, P. B., Chan, C. C., Wiggert, B., Redmond, T. M., and Donoso, L. A. (1994b). Immunogenetics of experimental autoimmune uveoretinitis (EAU). *Regional Immunol.* (suppl.), (in press).

Caspi, R. R., and Nussenblatt, R. B. (1994). Natural and therapeutic control of ocular autoimmunity—Rodent and man. *In* "Autoimmunity: Physiology and Disease" (A. Coutinho and M. Kazatchkine, Eds.), pp. 377–405. Wiley-Liss, Inc.

de Kozak, Y. (1990). Regulation of retinal autoimmunity via the idiotypic network. *Curr. Eye Res.* **9**(Suppl.), 193–200.

de Kozak, Y., Sakai, J., Thillaye, B., and Faure, J. P. (1981). S antigen-induced experimental autoimmune uveo-retinitis in rats. *Curr. Eye Res.* **1**, 327–337.

de Smet, M. D., Bitar, G., Roberge, F. G., Gery, I., and Nussenblatt, R. (1993). Human S-Antigen: Presence of multiple immunogenic and immunopathogenic sites in the Lewis rat. *J. Autoimmun.*, in press.

Donoso, L. A., Merryman, C. F., Sery, T. W., Shinohara, T., Dietzschold, B., Smith, A., and Kalsow, C. M. (1987). S-antigen: Characterization of a pathogenic epitope which mediates experimental autoimmune uveitis and pinealitis in Lewis rats. *Curr. Eye Res.* **6**, 1151–1159.

Donoso, L. A., Yamaki, K., Merryman, C. F., Shinohara, T., Yue, S., and Sery, T. W. (1988). Human S-antigen: Characterization of uveitopathogenic sites. *Curr. Eye Res.* **7**, 1077–1085.

Donoso, L. A., Merryman, C. F., Sery, T., Sanders, R., Vrabec, T., and Fong, S. L. (1989). Human interstitial retinoid binding protein. A potent uveitopathogenic agent for the induction of experimental autoimmune uveitis. *J. Immunol.* **143**, 79–83.

Dua, H. S., Gregerson, D. S., and Donoso, L. A. (1992). Inhibition of experimental autoimmune uveitis by retinal photoreceptor antigens coupled to spleen cells. *Cell. Immunol.* **139**, 292–305.

Egwuagu, C. E., Bahmanyar, S., Mahdi, R. M., Brezin, A. P., Nussenblatt, R. B., Gery, I., and Caspi, R. R. (1992). Vβ8.3 gene usage in experimental autoimmune uveoretinitis. *Clin. Immunol. Immunopathol.* **65**, 152–160.

Faure, J. P. (1980). Autoimmunity and the retina. *Curr. Topics Eye Res.* **2**, 215–301.

Fujino, Y., Okumura, A., Nussenblatt, R. B., Gery, I., and Mochizuki, M. (1988). Cyclosporine-induced specific unresponsiveness to retinal soluble antigen in experimental autoimmune uveoretinitis. *Clin. Immunol. Immunopathol.* **46**, 234–248.

Gery, I., Robinson, W. G., Jr., Shichi, H., El-Saied, M., Mochizuki, M., Nussenblatt, R. B., and Williams, R. M. (1985). Differences in susceptibility to experimental autoimmune uveitis among rats of various strains. *In* "Advances in Immunology and Immunopathology of the Eye (Proceedings of the Third International Symposium on Immunology and Immunopathology of the Eye)" (J. W. Chandler and G. R. O'Conner, Eds.), Chap. 59, pp. 242–245. Masson Publishing, New York.

Gery, I., Mochizuki, M., and Nussenblatt, R. B. (1986a). Retinal specific antigens and immunopathogenic processes they provoke. *Prog. Retinal Res.* **5**, 75–109.

Gery, I., Wiggert, B., Redmond, T. M., Kuwabara, T., Crawford, M. A., Vistica, B. P., and Chader, G. J. (1986b). Uveoretinitis and pinealitis induced by immunization with interphotoreceptor retinoid-binding protein. *Invest. Ophthalmol. Vis. Sci.* **27**, 1296–1300.

Gregerson, D. S., Fling, S. P., Obritsch, W. F., Merryman, C. F., and Donoso, L. A. (1989). Identification of T cell recognition sites in S-antigen: Dissociation of proliferative and pathogenic sites. *Cell. Immunol.* **123**, 427–440.

Gregerson, D. S., Merryman, C. F., Obritsch, W. F., and Donoso, L. A. (1990). Identification of a potent new pathogenic site in human retinal S-antigen which induces experimental autoimmune uveoretinitis in LEW rats. *Cell. Immunol.* **128**, 209–219.

Gregerson, D. S., Fling, S. P., Merryman, C. F., Zhang, X. M., Li, X. B., and Heber-Katz, E. (1991). Conserved T cell receptor V gene usage by uveitogenic T cells. *Clin. Immunol. Immunopathol.* **58**, 154–161.

Hirose, S., Ogasawara, K., Natori, T., Sasamoto, Y., Ohno, S., Matsuda, H., and Onoe, K. (1991). Regulation of experimental autoimmune uveitis in rats—Separation of MHC and non-MHC gene effects. *Clin. Exp. Immunol.* **86**, 419–425.

Iwase, K., Fujii, Y., Nakashima, I., Kato, N., Fujino, Y., Kawashima, H., and Mochizuki, M. (1990). A new method for induction of experimental autoimmune uveoretinitis (EAU) in mice. *Curr. Eye Res.* **9**, 207–216.

Kawashima, H., Fujino, Y., and Mochizuki, M. (1990). Antigen-specific suppressor cells induced by FK506 in experimental autoimmune uveoretinitis in the rat. *Invest. Ophthalmol. Vis. Sci.* **31**, 2500–2507.

Kotake, S., Wiggert, B., Zhang, X. Y., Redmond, T. M., Chader, G. J., and Gery, I. (1990a). Stimulation in vitro of lymphocytes for induction of uveoretinitis without any significant proliferation. *J. Immunol.* **145**, 534–539.

Kotake, S., Wiggert, B., Redmond, T. M., Borst, D. E., Nickerson, J. M., Margalit, H., Berzofsky, J. A., Chader, G. J., and Gery, I. (1990b). Repeated determinants within the retinal interphotoreceptor retinoid-binding protein (IRBP): Immunological properties of the repeats of an immunodominant determinant. *Cell. Immunol.* **126**, 331–342.

Kotake, S., Redmond, T. M., Wiggert, B., Vistica, B., Sanui, H., Chader, G. J., and Gery, I. (1991a). Unusual immunologic properties of the uveitogenic interphotoreceptor retinoid-binding protein-derived peptide R23. *Invest. Ophthalmol. Vis. Sci.* **32**, 2058–2064.

Kotake, S., de Smet, M. D., Wiggert, B., Redmond, T. M., Chader, G. J., and Gery, I. (1991b). Analysis of the pivotal residues of the immunodominant and highly uveitogenic determinant of interphotoreceptor retinoid-binding protein. *J. Immunol.* **146**, 2995–3001.

Li, Q., Fujino, Y., Caspi, R. R., Najafian, F., Nussenblatt, R. B., and Chan, C. C. (1992). Association between mast cells and the development of experimental autoimmune uveitis in different rat strains. *Clin. Immunol. Immunopathol.* **65**, 294–299.

Merryman, C. F., Donoso, L. A., Zhang, X. M., Heber-Katz, E., and Gregerson, D. S. (1991). Characterization of a new, potent, immunopathogenic epitope in S-antigen that elicits T cells expressing V beta 8 and V alpha 2-like genes. *J. Immunol.* **146**, 75–80.

Mirshahi, M., Boucheix, C., Collenot, G., Thillaye, B., and Faure, J. P. (1985). Retinal S-antigen epitopes in vertebrate and invertebrate photoreceptors. *Invest. Ophthalmol. Vis. Sci.* **26**, 1016–1021.

Mizuno, K., Clark, A. F., and Streilein, J. W. (1989). Ocular injection of retinal S antigen: Suppression of autoimmune uveitis. *Invest. Ophthalmol. Vis. Sci.* **30**, 772–774.

Mochizuki, M., Kuwabara, T., Chan, C. C., Nussenblatt, R. B., Metcalfe, D. D., and Gery, I. (1984). An association between susceptibility to experimental autoimmune uveitis and choroidal mast cell numbers. *J. Immunol.* **133**, 1699–1701.

Mochizuki, M., Kuwabara, T., McAllister, C., Nussenblatt, R. B., and Gery, I. (1985). Adoptive transfer of experimental autoimmune uveoretinitis in rats. Immunopathogenic mechanisms and histologic features. *Invest. Ophthalmol. Vis. Sci.* **26**, 1–9.

Nussenblatt, R. B., and Palestine, A. G. (1989). "Uveitis: Fundamentals and Clinical Practice." Year Book Medical Publishers, Inc.

Nussenblatt, R. B., Caspi, R. R., Mahdi, R., Chan, C. C., Roberge, F., Lider, O., and Weiner, H. L. (1990). Inhibition of S-antigen induced experimental autoimmune uveoretinitis by oral induction of tolerance with S-antigen. *J. Immunol.* **144**, 1689–1695.

Pfister, C., Chabre, M., Plouet, J., Van Tuyen, V., DeKozak, Y., Faure, J. P., and Kühn, H. (1985). Retinal S antigen identified as the 48K protein regulating light-dependent phosphodiesterase in rods. *Science* **228**, 891–893.

Rizzo, L. V., Silver, P. B., Hakim, F., Chan, C. C., Wiggert, B., and Caspi, R. R. (1993). Establishment and characterization of an IRBP-specific T cell line that induces EAU in B10.A mice. *Invest. Ophthalmol. Vis. Sci.* **34**(suppl.), p. 1143.

Roberge, F. G., Xu, D., and Chan, C. C. (1992). A new effective and non-harmful chemical adjuvant for the induction of experimental autoimmune uveoretinitis. *Curr. Eye Res.* **11**, 371–376.

Robison, W. G. J., Kuwabara, T., and Zwaan, J. (1983). Eye research. *In* "The Mouse in Biomedical Research" (H. Foster, et al., Eds.), Vol. IV, pp. 69–95. Academic Press, New York.

Sanui, H., Redmond, T. M., Hu, L. H., Kuwabara, T., Margalit, H., Cornette, J. L., Wiggert, B., Chader, G. J., and Gery, I. (1988). Synthetic peptides derived from IRBP induce EAU and EAP in Lewis rats. *Curr. Eye Res.* **7**, 727–735.

Sanui, H., Redmond, T. M., Kotake, S., Wiggert, B., Hu, L. H., Margalit, H., Berzofsky, J. A., Chader, G. J., and Gery, I. (1989). Identification of an immunodominant and highly immunopathogenic determinant in the retinal interphotoreceptor retinoid-binding protein (IRBP). *J. Exp. Med.* **169**, 1947–1960.

Sasamoto, Y., Kawano, Y. I., Bouligny, R., Wiggert, B., Chader, G. J., and Gery, I. (1992). Immunomodulation of experimental autoimmune uveoretinitis by intravenous injection of uveitogenic peptides. *Invest. Ophthalmol. Vis. Sci.* **33**, 2641–2649.

Schalken, J. J., Winkens, H. J., van Vugt, A. H., Bovée-Geurts, P. H., de Grip, W. J., and Broekhuyse, R. M. (1988). Rhodopsin-induced experimental autoimmune uveoretinitis: Dose-dependent clinicopathological features. *Exp. Eye Res.* **47**, 135–145.

Silver, P. B., Rizzo, L. V., Chan, C. C., Donoso, L. A., Wiggert, B., and Caspi, R. R. (1993). Identification of a putative epitope in the IRBP molecule that is uveitogenic for mice of the H-2b haplotype. *Invest. Ophthalmol. Vis. Sci.* **34**(suppl.), p. 1482.

Silver, P. B., Rizzo, L. V., Chan, C. C., Donoso, L. A., Wiggert, B., and Caspi, R. R. (1994). Identification of a major pathogenic epitope in the irbp molecule recognized by mice of the H-2^r haplotype. *Invest. Ophthalmol. Vis. Sci.* **35** (suppl.), 2061.

Singh, V. K., Nussenblatt, R. B., Donoso, L. A., Yamaki, K., Chan, C. C., and Shinohara, T. (1988). Identification of a uveitopathogenic and lymphocyte proliferation site in bovine S-antigen. *Cell. Immunol.* **115**, 413–419.

Stanford, M. R., Brown, E. C., Kasp, E., Graham, E. M., Sanders, M. D., and Dumonde, D. C. (1987). Experimental posterior uveitis. I: A clinical, angiographic, and pathological study. *Br. J. Ophthalmol.* **71**, 585–592.

Thurau, S. R., Chan, C. C., Suh, E., and Nussenblatt, R. B. (1991). Induction of oral tolerance to S-antigen induced experimental autoimmune uveitis by a uveitogenic 20mer peptide. *J. Autoimmun.* **4**, 507–516.

Whitcup, S. M., DeBarge, L. R., Caspi, R. R., Harning, R., Nussenblatt, R. B., and Chan, C. C. (1993). Monoclonal antibodies against ICAM-1 (CD54) and LFA-1 (CD11a/CD18) inhibit experimental autoimmune uveitis. *Clin. Immunol. Immunopathol.*, **67**, 143–150.

Chapter 6

Experimental Autoimmune Myasthenia Gravis

Angela Vincent

Neurosciences Group, Department of Clinical Neurology, Institute of Molecular Medicine, University of Oxford, Oxford OX3 9DU, United Kingdom

I. Introduction

It is now 20 years since the first report of a disorder of neuromuscular transmission in rabbits induced by injection of xenogeneic acetylcholine receptor in Freund's complete adjuvant (Patrick and Lindstrom, 1973). Experimental autoimmune myasthenia gravis (EAMG) as it became known, followed

Autoimmune Disease Models:
A Guidebook

immunization with affinity-purified acetylcholine receptor (AChR) extracted from the electric organ of *Electrophorus electricus*. The anti-AChR antibodies formed cross-reacted with the rabbits' own AChRs at the neuromuscular junction and caused a defect in neuromuscular transmission which was evident as severe weakness. This responded dramatically to treatment with an intravenous antiacetylcholinesterase drug.

The main interest in EAMG is its similarity to the human disorder myasthenia gravis (MG; for general reviews see Vincent, 1980; Drachman, 1987; Lindstrom *et al.*, 1988). This acquired condition has a peak incidence during the second and third decade but can occur at any age. Antihuman AChR antibodies, which are detectable by a radioimmunoassay using human muscle AChR as antigen in over 85% of patients, are immunoglobulin G (IgG) and high-affinity and heterogeneous in their subclass, light chain, and in their reactivity with different regions on the surface of the AChR (see Vincent, 1991, for a review). They are thought to be responsible for the loss of AChR that underlies weakness in this disease, and are not found in healthy individuals or in other neurological diseases.

The diagnosis of MG rests on a history of fatigable weakness, improvement following the administration of a short-acting anti-AChE drug, a positive anti-AChR antibody assay (>0.5 nM), and the presence of a decremental response to repetitive stimulation (usually at 3 Hz) during electromyography, or increased "jitter" on single-fiber studies. There are genetic factors in the etiology. MG is more common in females, particularly in cases presenting before the age of 40 years, and these cases are often associated with the major histocompatibility complex (MHC) antigens HLA-B8 and DR3, and with thymic changes which include the presence of germinal centers and T-cell areas. These "hyperplastic" thymuses frequently synthesize anti-AChR antibody in a spontaneous fashion. Patients presenting later (>40 years) are more often HLA-B7 and DR2, with atrophic or normal thymus tissue. A third group of patients have a thymic tumor (for a review, see Wilcox and Vincent, 1988).

MG is not a very common disease, the prevalence being about 1:10,000, and it can be treated fairly satisfactorily with anticholinesterase drugs, and by thymectomy and immunosuppression. Research into MG and EAMG, however, has been considerable, partly because of the interest in ion channels and receptors of the nervous system, and the accessibility of the neuromuscular junction to physiological studies. The AChR was the first known autoantigen to be purified, cloned, and sequenced (Claudio, 1989) and this has enabled detailed studies at the molecular level not only of its function as a ligand-gated ion channel, but also of the T- and B-cell epitopes involved in autoimmune responses (Tzartos *et al.*, 1991; Willcox *et al.*, 1993). These factors have made EAMG one of the best model autoimmune diseases in which to study immunogenetic factors, and to test the applicability of nonspecific and antigen-specific immunotherapy.

II. Immunization against Purified Electric Organ AChR

A. Antigen Preparation

The electric organs of certain electric rays are very good sources of AChR ($10-100$ μg/g), which can be extracted in detergent, usually 1% Triton X100, from membrane preparations and purified by affinity chromatography using Sepharose columns to which one of the cobra (*Naja naja*) α-neurotoxins has been attached (Vincent, 1980; Lindstrom, 1979). These toxins bind specifically and with high affinity (about 0.1 nM k_d) to electric organ AChR, and to muscle AChR (except in the mongoose and some other snake-eating species!). The toxin is usually coupled at about 0.2 mg/ml of resin. A higher density is inadvisable since the AChR has two binding sites for α-toxins and if both are occupied, it will be difficult to elute the AChR. Elution is generally performed using the cholinergic ligand, carbamylcholine, at 1 M. Detergent can be changed, before eluting, to 1% cholate, which is easier to remove by dialysis. Dialysis is needed in any case to remove the ligand. Extensive dialysis against nondetergent solutions will result in aggregation of the protein; this may be helpful for immunization, but is not good for subsequent studies. It is very important to add protease inhibitors, such as phenyl methyl sulfonyl fluoride or pepstatin, throughout the procedure. If using poor sources of AChR, such as mammalian muscle, it is helpful to pass the extract through a "dummy" Sepharose column to absorb lipids and proteins that bind nonspecifically and will otherwise contaminate the final preparation. Further purification, if required, can be achieved by using lectin (concanavalin A, ConA or wheat germ agglutinin) or positively charged ion-exchange (DEAE) columns. The final product can be assayed by binding of [125I]α-bungarotoxin or other α-neurotoxins (Vincent, 1980; Patrick *et al.*, 1973; Lindstrom *et al.*, 1976a). The activity should be about 8 nmoles/mg of protein (i.e. one binding site/125,000 K_D molecular mass). The purified preparation can be stored satisfactorily at $-70°C$, but deteriorates at $-20°C$.

The AChR is a membrane protein (Figure 1) consisting of $\alpha_2, \beta, \gamma, \delta$ subunits, with an ϵ taking the place of the γ in normal innervated muscle. There is homology between the subunits, but the α-subunits contain the α-BuTx binding sites and the main immunogenic region (see later discussion).

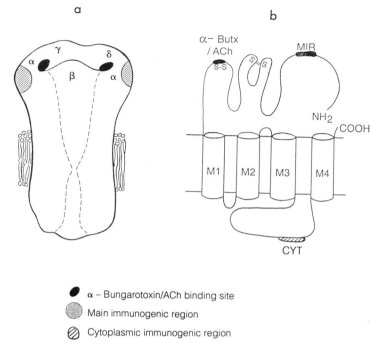

Figure 1   Diagram representing the acetylcholine receptor with its five subunits.
(a) As it appears in the membrane. (b) The transmembrane topography of the α-
subunit. The main immunogenic region, MIR, involves α67–76, and α-BuTx/ACh
binding sites (involving α185–196) are situated extracellularly. Another immunogenic
region is found within the cytoplasmic loop (CYT), but antibodies directed toward
this region will not be able to cause disease *in vivo*.

B. Species, Adjuvants, Clinical Course, and Symptoms

Many species, including rabbits, rats, mice, and monkeys, have been immunized with purified AChR using 25 to 600 μg in Freund's complete adjuvant
(FCA; see Table I). The protein solution (for instance, in 0.1% Triton or 0.2%
cholate–phosphate buffer) should be emulsified (water in oil) in an equal
volume of FCA using standard procedures. Droplets of the final emulsion
should be able to float undispersed on water. The number of injections required to produce a clinical effect varies according to the species, some becoming clearly weak after one or two injections (e.g., rabbits) whereas others
show few symptoms even after four or more. High antibody levels can be
obtained against the fish AChR, although the proportion that cross-react
with the recipient's AChR is only about 1–2% (see later discussion).

Table I

Immunization against Purified Electric Fish Acetylcholine Receptors

Species/strain	AChR source	Dose[a] (μg)	No. injections/ frequency (day)	Clinical signs at day (day)	Anti-AChR[b]	Other investigations performed	References
Rabbits							
NZW (f)[c]	E. electricus	300	2–3/14	+++ 35	1 μM	Edrophonium responsive, EMG decrement	Patrick and Lindstrom (1973)
Dutch	T. marmorata	200	2–3/21	+++ 25	1.5 μM	Mepp amplitudes and [125I] α-BuTx binding reduced	Green et al. (1975)
Chinchilla	T. marmorata	300	3–4/7	+++ 20	Immunoelectrophoresis	EMG decrement	Heilbronn et al. (1975)
NZW	T. californica	25	>2	+++ 22	Immunodiffusion	Mepp amplitudes reduced	Sanders et al. (1977)
White (f)	N. japonica	300	>5	+ –> +++	2 μM		Ueno et al. (1980)
Rats							
Lewis(f)	E. electricus	25–50[a]	1	Acute 8–11 Chronic >30	Low 5–11 μM	Cellular infiltration Antibody-mediated changes	Lennon et al. (1975)
Wistar	T. marmorata	200	2–3	Negligible	1 μM	Mepp amplitudes and [125I] α-BuTx binding reduced	Green et al. (1975)
Lewis	T. californica	40	1–4	Negligible	Immunodiffusion		Sanders et al. (1977)
Guinea pigs							
Albino (f)	E. electricus	150	1	– to +++ 42	Immunodiffusion	EMG decrement	Lennon et al. (1975)
Monkey							
Macaca mulatta (f)	T. californica	100–200	4	+++ 50	Hemagglutination	EMG decrement	Tarrab-Hazdai et al. (1975a)
Mice see Table IV							

[a] Additional adjuvant used (Lennon et al., 1985).
[b] Titer against the immunizing AChR.
[c] (f) = female.

Lennon and her colleagues have used a single dose of antigen in FCA (sometimes with additional *Mycobacterium butyricum* and *M. tuberculosis*), given by multiple intradermal (i.d.) injection, with a separate injection of 10^{10} *Bordetella pertussis* organisms as additional adjuvant (Lennon *et al.*, 1975, 1976). With this protocol, female Lewis rats were highly susceptible to EAMG and developed two phases of illness. The first, acute stage, began around 8–10 days and was followed by a recovery stage during which serum anti-AChR rose to high levels. A chronic phase was found after about 30 days. The pathophysiology of this EAMG model has been described in great detail (Lennon *et al.*, 1975; Engel *et al.*, 1976; Lindstrom *et al.*, 1976b). No other groups have routinely used this procedure.

In contrast, most species of animals injected without additional adjuvants do not develop any clinical signs until at least 20 days after the first injection (Table I). Rabbits are more vulnerable to clinical EAMG than other species; within 10–12 days of a second injection or within 40 days of a single one, they develop a flaccid paralysis, lying with unsupported head and extended limbs. They have difficulty in breathing and swallowing. Anti-AChE treatment produces temporary improvement at first but many die within 10–12 days. Monkeys show the most human-like symptoms, with ptosis, dysphagia, and opthalmoplegia progressing to death within a few weeks. Guinea pigs, and some strains of rats and mice (see later discussion), are more resistant to clinical weakness, but they may show hypoactivity and weight loss progressing to respiratory failure. Weakness of the facial muscles has been demonstrated in α-bungarotoxin-treated rats (see later discussion) and may be a useful sign in EAMG animals as well.

No standard grading system is in use, but some groups have used the following guide in rats and other small species: +, weak cry or grip; ++, abnormal posture; +++, obvious weakness, no cry or grip, tremulous, weight loss, moribund or dead.

C. Anti-AChR Assays

Initially several different assays were used to detect the presence of anti-AChR against the immunogen (Table I); with the most quantitative—immunoprecipitation of $[^{125}I]$α-BuTx-AChR—micromolar levels of antibody were found. However, these weren't very helpful since they didn't indicate the level of antibody reacting with muscle AChR, and in only a few studies do anti-fish AChR levels correlate with severity of the disease (Green *et al.*, 1975; Ueno *et al.*, 1980). Subsequent studies have used crude detergent extracts of normal or denervated mammalian muscle from the immunized species as a source of the antigen (Lindstrom, 1976b). The presence of the $[^{125}I]$α-BuTx attached to the AChR α-subunits does not prevent anti-AChR antibodies from binding since most are directed at other sites on the surface of the molecule (Patrick *et al.*, 1973). The assay is sensitive and quantitative values can be obtained by titrating the sera. Values >0.5 nmoles of $[^{125}I]\alpha$-BuTx binding sites precipitated per liter of serum are usually considered significant but, as in the human disease, there is not necessarily a good correlation between anti-AChR levels and clinical or pathological findings in individual animals.

III. Assessment of EAMG and the Safety Factor

As indicated above, the clinical expression of EAMG can be quite variable. This is because of the nature of neuromuscular transmission, which has an inbuilt safety margin that differs among species. The transmission of impulses from nerve to muscle depends on the release of acetylcholine, in packets, from the nerve terminal which binds to the AChRs on the postsynaptic muscle membrane. This leads to opening of the AChR-associated ion channel and depolarization of the membrane. If this depolarization is above a certain threshold, voltage-gated sodium channels open and the impulse is conducted along the muscle fiber and results in contraction. If the depolarization is subthreshold, no contraction will result in that fiber; in most voluntary muscles there is an "all or none" phenomenon (in certain fibers of the extraocular muscles this does not apply). Thus the safety factor depends on the number of ACh packets released, the number and density of AChRs, and the threshold for activation (see Engel, 1992, for further discussion). These differ between, for instance, mice which release large numbers of ACh quanta and have a low threshold, and rabbits, in which the number of packets is quite large but the threshold is much higher. The amplitude of the miniature end plate potential (mepp), which is the depolarization caused by release of an individual ACh packet, is an easily measured parameter of neuromuscular function which reflects the density of the AChRs on the muscle membrane; it does not give information about the safety margin.

In those animals in which clinical weakness is evident, improvement following intravenous administration of tensilon is very characteristic. In those without clinical weakness, decremental responses to repetitive nerve stimulation, under general anesthesia, are also diagnostic of a defect in neuromuscular transmission (see Table I). However, clearly both these tests will depend partly on the safety factor of the species. *In vitro* stimulation of muscle, particularly in the presence of *d*-tubocurarine, which reduces AChR function and thereby decreases the safety factor, may be helpful (Thompson *et al.*, 1992). An alternative, but less easy, method of assessing the effect of immunization is to measure the number of muscle AChRs by $[^{125}I]\alpha$-BuTx binding to muscle extracts (Lindstrom *et al.*, 1976b). In this case one can also assess by immunoprecipitation the proportion of AChRs that have antibody bound to them (Lindstrom *et al.*, 1976b; Verschuuren *et al.*, 1992). Alternatively, incubation of diaphragm muscle in [^{125}I]α-BuTx allows estimation of specific binding to the neuromuscular junction (end plate) AChRs after subtraction of binding to extrajunctional regions (Green *et al.*, 1975). Better still, miniature end plate potential amplitude provides a standardized measure of AChR function. In most normal muscles, the mepp amplitude is around 0.5–1.0 mV. In EAMG, or MG, mepp amplitudes can be as low as 0.2, with many mepps lost in the background "noise" (Green *et al.*, 1975; Sanders *et al.*, 1977; Lambert *et al.*, 1976; Albuquerque *et al.*, 1979).

One has to decide, depending on the reasons for inducing EAMG, whether clinical weakness is the most important outcome or whether measurement of AChR numbers or of mepp amplitudes will be a more useful and quantitive indicator of loss of AChR.

IV. Immunization against Purified Mammalian AChR

The amount of AChR in normal adult mammalian muscle is very small; about 0.025–0.1 μg/gram of tissue. It can be increased 5- to 40-fold by prior denervation. The TE671 (rhabdomyosarcoma) cell line could also be used as a source of human AChR, but large quantities of cells would be required since the yield of AChR is usually around 0.1 μg per large flask. Muscle AChR is relatively difficult to purify and there have been fairly few studies (Table II). Surprisingly, very small amounts (0.1–10 μg) of closely related or even syngeneic AChR are successful immunogens coupled with FCA (Lindstrom *et al.*, 1976b; Granato *et al.*, 1976) or without adjuvant (see below). Although the levels of antibody against the immunogen are not always as high using mammalian AChR, the cross-reactivity with the animals' own AChR is usually very good (Table II) and impressive clinical and electromyographic evidence of EAMG has been obtained.

V. Immunization without Adjuvant

A few studies have attempted with surprising success to induce anti-AChR in mice with injections of AChR without Freund's adjuvant. The first studies used intrasplenic (i.s.) injections of membranes prepared from the BC3H1 cell line (Scadding *et al.*, 1986). This comes from a mouse tumor and expresses a muscle-type AChR. The BALB/c mice did not become weak but showed antimouse AChR and reduced mepp amplitudes. Similar effects were achieved in several strains of mice intrasplenically injected with 1 μg of

Table II

Immunization against Purified Mammalian Acetylcholine Receptor

Species	AChR source	Dose[a] (μg)	Clinical effect	Anti-AChR[b] (immunogen) (nM)	Anti-AChR[c] (autoantigen) (nM)	Other findings
Lewis rat (f)[d]	Normal rat muscle	2–3[a]	+++	100	100	AChR loss and antibody complexed with AChR Lindstrom et al. (1976b)
Lewis rat (f)	Human ischemic muscle	2–10[a]	+++	90	18	AChR loss, small mepp amplitudes, antibody complexed with AChR Lennon et al. (1991)
BALB/c mouse	Denervated rat	5–10	+, ++	300	200	EMG decrement Granato et al. (1976)
BALB/c mouse	BC3H1 cell line	0.1	+, +++	0–1000	0–700	End plate AChR loss Jermy et al. (1993)

[a] Additional adjuvant used.

[b] Titer against immunizing AChR.

[c] Titer against immunized species muscle AChR (nonimmunized mice give values <0.5 nM).

[d] (f) = female.

Torpedo AChR followed by intraperitoneal injections (Jermy *et al.*, 1989), and even in BALB/c mice with affinity-purified BC3H1 AChR (Jermy *et al.*, 1993). In the latter case, antimouse AChR levels were high (from 0 to 700 nM) and there was obvious weakness, some deaths, and substantially reduced AChR numbers in the surviving mice. The advantage of these models is the ease with which auto-antibodies are induced and the hope that they may provide a particularly suitable model for trying therapeutic strategies aimed at making the immune system tolerant to self ACLR.

VI. Genetics of EAMG in Rats and Mice

In both rats and mice there are clear strain differences in susceptibility to induction of EAMG. What is not so clear is the extent to which these depend on nonimmune factors or on the autoimmune response to AChR. In rats, for instance, a thorough study by Biesecker and Koffler (1988) using 100 μg of *Torpedo* AChR in fortnightly injections (without additional adjuvants) showed marked differences in clinical evidence (Table III), with little difference in either anti-AChR levels or the amount of AChR remaining at the end plate. However, the proportion of AChRs that had antibody bound did seem to correlate with disease susceptibility, particularly as indicated by the amount of curare required to produce an electromyogram (EMG) decrement in the immunized animals. These observations suggest that the specificity of the anti-AChR may partly account for the different susceptibility of, for instance, Wistar Furth and Wistar Munich rats. Clonotypic analysis of anti-AChR from Lewis and Wistar Furth rats confirmed some difference in antibody characteristics (Zoda *et al.*, 1991), and two subsets of differing pathogenicity have been identified (Thompson and Krolick, 1992).

In mice the picture is more complicated (Table IV). Several groups have found C57B1/6 and AKR strains to be susceptible; use of allogenic and congenic strains suggested that the presence of both *H-2^b* and *Ig-1^b* produced the highest susceptibility whereas *H-2^d* and *Ig-1^a* mice were relatively resistant (Berman and Patrick, 1980a,b; Christadoss *et al.*, 1979). Nevertheless, when immunizing with *Torpedo* AChR without adjuvant, a different pattern of susceptibility was found (Jermy *et al.*, 1989). There was little correlation between anti-AChR levels and clinical evidence of EAMG within any of these studies (Fuchs *et al.*, 1976; Berman and Heinemann, 1984; Christadoss *et al.*, 1979) although antibody specificity may underlie part of the difference between C57B1/6 and C3H/Hej mice (Marzo *et al.*, 1986). In addition, C5-deficient mice are much less susceptible than coisogenic, C5 sufficient, mice (for review see Christadoss and Shenoy, 1992). However, it is possible that other genetic factors are involved. Dawkins and his colleagues (Degli-Eposti *et al.*,

Table III

Immunization of Different Rat Strains with *Torpedo* AChR[a]

Immunogen	Strain	Incidence of severe weakness or death	Curare sensitivity, μg required to produce decrement	Anti-AChR (nM)	AChR (% control)	% of AChR with antibody bound
T. californica AChR, affinity-purified, 100 μg m.s., plus 3×50 μg s.c. at 2, 4, and 6 weeks	Wistar Furth	0/8	8.0	51.7	39%	36%
	Copenhagen	0/5				
	Wistar Kyoto	1/6				
	ACI	1/4				
	Brown Norway	2/4				
	Buffalo	3/4				
	Lewis	6/8				
	Fisher	6/6	4.5	35.6	54%	63%
	Wistar Munich	6/6	2.7	52.8	33%	82%
Nonimmunized or other controls		0/0	26–30	Not given	100	Not given

[a]From Biesecker and Koffler (1988).
m.s., multiple sites.
s.c., subcutaneous.

Table IV
Immunogenetics and Responses of Different Mouse Strains Immunized with *Torpedo* AChR

Strain	*H-2*	IgCh	γ-Subunit polymorphism[a]	Hanging time (s)[a]	Clinical effect, frequency of clinical disease		AChR loss induced without adjuvant[a]	Anti-(mouse)AChR positive[a]
C57B1/6	*b*	*b*	s	10	0.7[b]	0.7[c]	+++	5/5
AKR/J	*k*	*d*	s		0.5[b]	1.0[c]	−	0/2
SJL/j	*s*	*b*	r		0.64[b]	0.0[c]	++	4/4
A/J	*a*	*e*			0.13[b]	0.2[c]	++	3/4
C3H/Hej	*k*	*a*	r	3.2	0.11[b]	0.4[c]	−	0/2
BALB/c	*d*	*a*	s		0.07[b]	0.4[c]	++	0/3
DBA/1	*q*		r	4.6		0.0[c]	+++	1/3

[a] s or r designates the particular polymorphic phenotype found. In fact, neuromuscular function, as determined by hanging times, was better in C57B1/6 mice than in C3H/Hej mice. Therefore, these findings are unlikely to underlie susceptibility to induction of EAMG (Degli-Eposti *et al.*, 1992).

[b] Berman and Patrick (1980b).

[c] Fuchs *et al.* (1976).

[d] Jermy *et al.* (1989).

1992) have found a polymorphism in the AChR γ-subunit gene between some strains of mice, which seems to correlate with their neuromuscular function as shown by "hanging times" (Table IV).

The partial resistance of AKR/J mice to EAMG is associated with $I\text{-}A_\alpha{}^k$ and may result from Mlsla-mediated deletion of the $V_\beta 6^+$ T-cell receptor subset (Krco *et al.*, 1991). The $I\text{-}A_\beta{}^b$ gene causes susceptibility to EAMG but when paired with $I\text{-}A_\alpha{}^k$ (introduced transgenically) the result is protective (Christadoss *et al.*, 1992). The $I\text{-}A^{bm12}$ mutation confers resistance to EAMG, apparently by changing the T-cell repertoire and preventing recognition of the T-cell epitope α*146-162* (Infante *et al.*, 1991; Bellone *et al.*, 1991b). Monoclonal antibody analysis does not indicate restricted use of particular V_H gene families in mice, but showed some restriction in rats (Graus *et al.*, 1993a,b).

VII. T- and B-Cell Epitopes in EAMG

There have been a number of studies of T- and B-cell epitopes, which are summarized in Table V. Thus in Lewis rats, α108–116 is a dominant T-cell epitope (Fujii and Lindstrom, 1988a), and T cells responding to this peptide can provide help for specific (AChR-induced) B cells (Fujii and Lindstrom, 1988b). In one study, cells from α100–116 immunized rats could provide help for anti-AChR production in naive rats (Yeh and Krolick, 1990). Moreover, some improvement in AChR-immunized rats can be achieved by making cells sensitive to this peptide tolerant to it (see later discussion). In inbred strains of mice, however, the T-cell epitopes seem more diverse and no clearly dominant ones have emerged (Table V).

B-cell epitopes have been difficult to define. A high proportion of monoclonal and polyclonal antibodies bind to a region on the extracellular surface of the native AChR called the main immunogenic region (MIR; Tzartos and Lindstrom, 1980) (see Fig. 1). Some of these antibodies bind to α67–76, but they do so with low affinity and probably other sequences contribute to the MIR in the native molecule (see Tzartos *et al.*, 1991). Very few binding sites for other anti-AChR monoclonal antibodies have been determined. In contrast, antibodies to denatured AChR or isolated α-subunits bind strongly to a region of the AChR α-subunit which is cytoplasmic in the native state (Figure 1) (Tzartos and Remoundos, 1992; Palace *et al.*, 1994).

Anti-AChR antibodies from MG patients have also been very difficult to map using synthetic peptides. Competition experiments, however, indicate that a variable but quite high proportion of MG antibodies compete with anti-MIR MAbs. Other epitopes or regions on the surface of human AChR, including the α-BuTx binding sites, are also involved in the human anti-AChR response (Tzartos *et al.*, 1991; Vincent, 1991).

Table V

T- and B-Cell Epitopes on AChR

Species, strain	Immunogen	Main T cell	B cell
Rat			
Lewis	*Torpedo* AChR	α100–116[a]	Not investigated in different strains; mainly conformation dependent and directed at extracellular epitopes (i.e. α1–210). However, α67–76 contributes to the main immunogenic region as defined by rat monoclonal antibodies.[b]
Wistar Furth		α152–167[a]	
Brown Norway		α172–205[a]	
Buffalo		α52–70[a]	
Mouse			
C57B1/6	*Torpedo* AChR	α146–162[c], α150–169[d], α182–198[c], α181–200[d], α360–378[d]	
C3H		α67–82, α146–162[c]	
SWR		α1–16, α67–82[c]	
SJL		α67–82, α111–126[c]	
BALB/c		α1–20, α304–322[d]	
Outbred			Many sequences within α1–210[e]
Mouse			
SJL	Recombinant human α37–429[f]	α40–65, α84–98, distal to α347[f]	α309–368[f]
C57B1/6		Distal to α347	α309–368, α137–168
BALB/c		Distal to α347	α309–368
SWR		Distal to α347	α309–368

[a] Fujii and Lindstrom (1988).
[b] Tzartos *et al.* (1991).
[c] Bellone *et al.* (1991a).
[d] Yokoi *et al.* (1987).
[e] Mulac-Jericivec *et al.* (1987).
[f] Palace *et al.* (1994).

VIII. Immunization against Denatured AChR Subunits, Recombinant or Synthetic Peptides

Table VI summarizes a number of attempts to induce electrophysiological or clinical evidence of EAMG by immunization with denatured, recombinant, or synthetic preparations of AChR sequences. In general, these preparations have been unsuccessful in inducing convincing signs of weakness, and the reduction in mepp amplitudes or $[^{125}I]\alpha$-BuTx binding sites has been at best moderate. For instance, even immunization against a composite peptide consisting of the MIR sequence, $\alpha67-76$, and the T-cell epitope $\alpha107-116$, did not produce consistent evidence of EAMG in Lewis rats (Takamori et al., 1992). These results are perhaps not surprising since, from the mapping results described above, one would not expect antipeptide antibodies to bind well to the animals' own AChRs, with the exception of those to the cytoplasmic region, which would not have access to their target in vivo.

One pool of peptides, representing $\alpha138-199$ ($\alpha138-167$, $\alpha157-188$, 185–199), induced clear clinical signs of EAMG in NZW rabbits after two injections in FCA (Jacobson et al., 1993). The rabbits had significant anti-rabbit AChR titers and mepp amplitudes were reduced in the diaphragm muscle. Interestingly, titers against rabbit AChR were higher than those against human AChR and anti-α-138-199 antibodies could be separated from anti-rabbit AChR antibodies suggesting that true "autoimmunity" had been induced, perhaps by determinant spreading (Vincent et al., 1994). None of the rabbits immunized against other extracellular sequences became weak.

IX. Resistance to EAMG

Immunogenetic factors clearly affect disease susceptibility (see earlier discussion) although in most instances the basis for intraspecies differences is not fully understood. A comparison of EAMG in brown Norway rats showed an interesting resistance of aged animals (>100 weeks) compared with younger ones (10 weeks), which appeared to be due mainly to an increased resistance of the neuromuscular junction to the effects of antibodies, rather than a difference in anti-AChR titers, and lack of macrophage infiltration in the older animals (Graus et al., 1993c). MG is more common in females, and many EAMG studies have been performed using female animals (see Table I), but there have been no definitive studies indicating sex-linked susceptibility.

Table VI

Immunization against Denatured AChR Subunits, Recombinant α-Subunit, or Synthetic Peptides

Source	Species	No. of injections	Clinical effect	Anti-AChR against immunized species (nM)	Other investigations
AChR					
Torpedo α, β, γ, δ PAGE purified[a]	Rat Lewis (f)[a]	4–5	+		Required repeated immunization to achieve AChR loss and EAMG[b]
Human α1–210 recombinant	Lewis (f)	1+	Variable	17.1	Mepps reduced; blocking and modulating antibodies found[c]
Human α37–429 recombinant	Mouse C57B1/6 SJL SWR BALB/c	2–3	Nil	0–25 0–13 0–11 0–64	Antibodies directed mainly to intracellular epitopes[d]
	BKTO (outbred)	5	Nil	18	No significant loss of AChR[e]
Synthetic peptides (human sequence)	Rat				
α107–116–NPGG–α190–205	Lewis (f)	3	Nil	Blocking antibody only	Curare sensitivity increased; mepps reduced[f]
α125–143	Lewis (f)	1+	1/12	0.3	Mepp amplitude reduced by 42%[g]
α127–147	Lewis (f)	1+	Nil	0–10	Only 2/10 rats had anti-AChR, but IgG detected at end plates[h]
α107–116–α67–76–α107–116	Lewis (f)	3	Nil	0.6	Mepps slightly reduced[i]
α183–200	Lewis (f)	3	Nil	Blocking antibody only	Mepps reduced 40% in 4/7[j]
Synthetic peptide pools (human sequences)	Rabbit				
α1–50, α51–65, α61–114	NZW	2–4	Nil	<1	Nil
α125–143			Nil	<1	Nil
α138–199			++,+++	10	Mepps reduced by 50%[k]
α309–368			Nil	807	Nil

[a] (f) = female.
[b] Lindstrom et al. (1978).
[c] Lennon et al. (1991).
[d] Palace et al. (1994).
[e] Jermy et al. (1993).
[f] Takamori et al. (1990).
[g] McCormick et al. (1987).
[h] Matsuo et al. (1992).
[i] Takamori et al. (1992).
[j] Takamori et al. (1988).
[k] Vincent et al., (1994).

X. Alternative Models

A. Spontaneous MG in Dogs and Cats

A large number of cases of canine (Shelton *et al.*, 1988) and feline (Indrieri *et al.*, 1983) MG have now been reported. The anti-AChR against the appropriate muscle AChR is raised in a proportion of cases, and the characteristics of the antibody have been shown to be similar to those in MG and EAMG (Shelton *et al.*, 1988). However, these cases are sporadic, and no strong hereditary factors have yet been identified. Idiopathic magaesophagus in dogs may also be associated with anti-AChR antibodies (Shelton *et al.*, 1990). It should be noted that in the Jack Russel terrier, a congenital, hereditary form of myasthenia has been described. This form is not autoimmune, and is probably similar to the congenital myasthenic syndromes identified in humans (Palmer *et al.*, 1980; Engel *et al.*, 1992; Shillito *et al.*, 1993).

B. Passive Transfer of EAMG or MG Antibodies

An interesting parallel with the human disease is the transient neonatal EAMG in offspring of EAMG rats. Whereas in human MG, placental transfer of antibodies between the mother and fetus is probably most important for development of neonatal MG, in the rats, antibodies are transferred through the milk (Sanders *et al.*, 1978).

The pathogenic potential of anti-AChR was shown by transfer of EAMG serum from Lewis rat to nonimmunized littermates (Lindstrom *et al.*, 1976c). However, they achieved a relatively short-lived effect, similar to the acute phase of EAMG (Engel *et al.*, 1979), and did not initiate a secondary autoanti-AChR production in the recipient. Transfer of monoclonal anti-AChR antibodies, directed at various extracellular epitopes, has also been effective in many instances (e.g., Lennon and Lambert, 1980; Richman *et al.*, 1980; Gomez and Richman, 1985; Tzartos *et al.*, 1987). $F(ab')_2$ fragments induced less AChR loss than whole anti-MIR monoclonal antibody, and complement depletion also reduced clinical EAMG (Loutrari *et al.*, 1992). Transfer of EAMG by adoptive cell transfer, rather than by antibody, has been demonstrated in a few cases (Tarrab-Hazdai *et al.*, 1975b; Jermy *et al.*, 1989).

Passive transfer of IgG prepared from MG patients has been used to demonstrate the relevance of their antibodies. Daily injections of 10 mg/mouse for 10–15 days, or 3 days of 60 mg/mouse, can achieve substantial levels of human IgG in the recipient animal and reproduce some of the pathology of the disease (Toyka *et al.*, 1977; Mossman *et al.*, 1988).

C. Use of Idiotype Networks

Of particular interest was the induction of anti-AChR antibodies in rabbits (Wasserman *et al.*, 1982) and mice (Cleveland *et al.*, 1983) by immunization with Bis-Q, a cholinergic analog which binds to the ACh binding site on the AChR. Antibodies against Bis-Q were able to induce anti-idiotype antibodies, some of which bound to the AChR and caused EAMG symptoms.

D. Use of SCID Mice

There have only been two reports of successful induction of EAMG in mice given tissue from MG patients. Schöenbeck *et al.* (1992) showed that injection of dissociated MG thymic cells into severe combined immunodeficiency (SCID) mice led to anti-AChR production, but it was not sustained beyond 3–10 weeks; in contrast, implantation of intact MG thymus tissue beneath the kidney capsule produced a slower rise in anti-AChR which appeared to be sustained for much longer. They were able to identify human IgG at the end plates of the mice. This procedure looks very promising and may be the ideal model for testing therapeutic strategies. A similar model has been described by Martino *et al.* (1993).

E. Nonimmunological Models of MG Induced by α-Neurotoxins

Several groups have shown that injections of α-neurotoxins into experimental animals produce many of the symptoms and signs of EAMG by reducing the number of functional end plate AChRs. A system which depends on alternate-day injections of α-BuTx into Wistar rats has been used to examine the pharmacology of myasthenic weakness. This regime does not cause severe weakness or respiratory failure and can be continued for several months without undue hardship to the animals concerned. The authors have established sensitive and noninvasive tests of muscle function, such as measuring the drooping of the lower lip, which may be applicable to autoimmune models (see Molenaar *et al.*, 1991, for details).

F. Penicillamine-Induced EAMG

Although it is clear that penicillamine treatment for rheumatoid arthritis often induces myasthenia gravis, as well as other autoimmune disorders in immunogenetically susceptible individuals (see Vincent, 1980), attempts to induce anti-AChR spontaneously in laboratory animals have been largely unsuccessful.

XI. Use of EAMG for Therapeutic Studies

The effect of various immunosuppressive regimes on EAMG has been studied with predictable results (Pachner, 1987; De Silva *et al.*, 1990). More interesting is the use of this model to test the feasibility of strategies designed to reverse or counteract the defect in neuromuscular transmission, or to specifically target the cells involved in the autoimmune response. Some of the more interesting applications are summarized in Table VII. These include approaches aimed at the activated immune system, block of specific class II molecules, or antigen- or epitope-specific procedures. Ultimately it will be important to test these approaches in a model that is dependent on the human immune responses (SCID or transgenic mice).

XII. Relation to Human Disease

The clinical, immunohistological, and electrophysiological findings in EAMG closely mirror those in the human disease and have been reviewed thoroughly elsewhere (Vincent, 1980; Lindstrom, 1979; Lindstrom *et al.*, 1988). There are probably minor differences between the specificity of the antibodies and the mechanisms by which they act on the end plate AChRs at the neuromuscular junction (see Engel and Fumagalli, 1982; Sahashi *et al.*, 1978), but considering the heterogeneity of the antibodies in the human disease, the similarities far outweigh the differences. In both conditions a combination of complement-mediated postsynaptic damage, increased degradation of AChR, and some pharmacological block of AChR, combine to cause the loss of AChR function which underlies the electrophysiological findings (Engel and Fumagalli, 1982). Many additional findings in EAMG, such as altered presynaptic function (Takamori *et al.*, 1984), are probably also relevant in MG. Moreover, the general lack of correlation between anti-AChR levels in animals and their clinical state reflects the similar findings in MG.

Other aspects of EAMG may be of relevance to the human disease. For instance, a compensatory increase in AChR gene expression has been found (Asher *et al.*, 1990). On the other hand, thymic changes have not usually been found (e.g., Meinl *et al.*, 1991), emphasizing the fact that an artificially induced experimental disease cannot reproduce etiological factors that may be responsible for the human condition.

XIII. Conclusions

EAMG is very similar to MG in its anti-AChR characteristics (Tzartos *et al.*, 1991) and pathophysiology (Engel and Fumagalli, 1982; Drachman, 1987).

Table VII

Effect of Some Experimental Treatment Strategies on EAMG

Model	Treatment	Results	References
Prevention of AChR degradation/antigen processing			
NZW rabbits	Leupeptin–protease inhibitor	Reduced clinical signs	Valderrama et al. (1987)
Depletion of complement			
Passive transfer	Antibody to complement C6	Reduced weakness and AChR loss	Biesecker and Gomez (1989)
Depletion of activated T cells			
C57B1/6 mice	I1-2-diphtheria toxin conjugate	Anti-AChR levels reduced 50%	Balcer et al. (1991)
Block of class II presentation			
SJL mice	*In vivo* anti-I-A antibody	Clinical EAMG reduced	Waldor et al. (1983)
Antigen specific			
C57B1/6	AChR-induced suppressor T cells	Reduced clinical and electrophysiological changes	Pachner and Kantor (1984)
Lewis rats	Ricin-AChR conjugate treatment	Reduced AChR responses *in vitro*	Killen and Lindstrom (1984); Olsberg et al. (1985)
Sprague-Dawley rats	[125I] AChR preimmunization	Reduced EAMG	Sterz et al. (1985)
Lewis rats	Fixed AChR-loaded spleen cells	Reduced T cell responses *in vitro*, and reduced EAMG	McKintosh and Drachman (1992); Reim et al. (1992)
Epitope specific			
B6 mice	Neonatal tolerance to α146–162	Less EMG decrement and anti-α146–162, but no effect on anti-AChR	Shenoy et al. (1993)
C57B1/6 mice	Glycol-conjugated peptide	Specific suppression	Atassi et al. (1992)
Lewis rats	MHC Class II-α100–116 complex	Reduced deaths from EAMG	Spack et al. (1994)

The studies in rats and inbred mice show how difficult it is to establish the true basis for genetic susceptibility to clinical disease even when immunizing against a purified antigen in immunogenetically defined animals. However, EAMG provides a useful model for testing therapy; in particular the nonadjuvant model and use of SCID mice should be indispensable as systems in which to test the effects of antigen-specific treatment with potential clinical application to humans.

XIV. Lambert-Eaton Myasthenic Syndrome

In Lambert-Eaton myasthenic syndrome (LEMS), another autoimmune disorder of neuromuscular transmission, autoantibodies against voltage-gated Ca^{2+} channels (VGCCs) on the motor nerve terminal result in a reduction in release of the neurotransmitter, ACh. About 50% of patients have LEMS in association with small cell cancer of the lung. VGCCs have been purified from both muscle and neuronal tissues from a number of species, and can be extracted from neuronal cell lines and small cell cancer lines, but no animal model for immunization has yet been established. Some features of LEMS can, however, be induced by immunization with *Torpedo* cholinergic nerve terminal proteins (Chapman *et al.*, 1990) and with N-terminal peptides of the vesicle-associated protein synaptotagmin (Takamori *et al.*, 1994). It is also possible to passively transfer LEMS to experimental mice or rats by daily injection of patients' IgG (Vincent and Newsom-Davis, 1993).

References

Albuquerque, E. X., Eldefrawi, A. T., Oliveira, A. C., Copio, D. S., Eldefrawi, M. E. (1979). *Exp. Neurol.* **66**, 109–122.

Asher, O., Neumann, D., Witzemann, V., and Fuchs, S. (1990). *FEBS Lett.* **267**, 231–235.

Atassi, M. Z., Ruan, K.-H., Jinnai, K., Oshima, M., and Ashizawa, T. (1992). *Proc. Natl. Acad. Sci. USA* **89**, 5852–5856.

Balcer, L. J., McIntosh, K. R., Nichols, J. C., and Drachman, D. B. (1991). *J. Neuroimmunol.* **31**, 115–122.

Bellone, M., Ostlie, N., Lei, S., and Conti-Tronconi, B. M. (1991a). *Eur. J. Immunol.* **21**, 2303–2310.

Bellone, M., Ostlie, N., Lei, S., Wu, X.-D., and Conti-Tronconi, B. M. (1991b). *J. Immunol.* **147**, 1484–1491.

Berman, P. W., and Heinemann, S. F. (1984). *J. Immunol.* **132**, 711–717.

Berman, P. W., and Patrick, J. (1980a). *J. Exp. Med.* **151**, 204–223.

Berman, P. W., and Patrick, J. (1980b). *J. Exp. Med.* **152**, 507–520.

Biesecker, G., and Gomez, C. M. (1989). *J. Immunol.* **142**, 2654–2659.

Biesecker, G., and Koffler, D. (1988). *J. Immunol.* **140**, 3406–3410.

Bogen, S., Mozes, E., and Fuchs, S. (1984). *J. Exp. Med.* **159**, 292–304.

Chapman, J., Rabinowitz, R., Korcsyn, A., and Michaelson, D. (1990). *Muscle Nerve* **13**, 726–733.

Christadoss, P., and Shenoy, M. (1992). *Reg. Immunol.*, **4**, 314–320.

Christadoss, P., David, C. S., and Keve, S. (1992). *Clin. Immunol. Immunopathol.* **62**, 235–239.

Christadoss, P., Lennon, V. A., and David, C. (1979). *J. Immunol.* **123**, No. 6, 2540–2543.

Claudio, T. (1989). *In* "Molecular Neurobiology" (D. M. Glover and B. D. Hames, Eds.), pp. 63–142. IRL Press, Oxford University Press, Oxford.

Cleveland, W. L., Wassermann, N. H., Sarangarajan, R., Penn, A. S., and Erlanger, B. F. (1983). *Nature* **305**, 56–57.

De Silva, S., McIntosh, K., Blum, J. E., Order, S., Mellits, D., and Drachman, D. B. (1990). *J. Neuroimmunol.* **29**, 93–103.

Degli-Eposti, M. A., Dallas, P. B., and Dawkins, R. L. (1992). *Muscle Nerve* **15**, 543–549.

Drachman, D. B. (Ed.) (1987). *Ann. N.Y. Acad. Sci.* **505**, 1–914.

Engel, A. G. (1992). *In* "Neuromuscular Transmission: Basic and Clinical Aspects" (A. Vincent and D. Wray, Eds.). Pergamon Press, Oxford, UK.

Engel, A. G., and Fumagalli, G. (1982). *In* "Receptors, Antibodies and Disease" (Ciba Foundation symposium 90), pp. 197–224. Pitman, London.

Engel, A. G., Tsujihata, M., Lambert, E. H., Lindstrom, J. M., and Lennon, V. A. (1976). *J. Neuropathol. Exp. Neurol.* **25**, 569–587.

Engel, A. G., Sakakibara, H., Sahashi, K., Lindstrom, J. M., Lambert, E. H., and Lennon, V. A. (1979). *Neurology* **29**, 179–188.

Fuchs, S., Nevo, D., and Tarrab-Hazdai, R. (1976). *Nature* **263**, 329–330.

Fujii, Y., and Lindstrom, J. (1988a). *J. Immunol.* **140**, No. 6, 1830–1837.

Fujii, Y., and Lindstrom, J. (1988b). *J. Immunol.* **141**, No. 10, 3361–3369.

Gomez, C. M., and Richman, D. P. (1985). *J. Immunol.* **135**, 234–235.

Gomez, C. M., and Richman, D. P. (1987). *J. Immunol.* **139**, No. 1, 73–76.

Granato, D. A., Fulpius, B. W., and Moody, J. F. (1976). *Proc. Natl. Acad. Sci. USA* **73**, No. 8, 2872–2876.

Graus, Y. M. F., Van Breda Vriesman, P. J. C., and De Baets, M. H. (1993a). *Clin. Exp. Immunol.*, **92**, 506–513.

Graus, Y. M. F., Verschuuren, J. J. G. M., Bos, N. A., Van Breda Vriesman, P. J. C., and De Baets, M. H. (1993b). *J. Neuroimmunol.*, **43**, 113–124.

Graus, Y. M. F., Verschuuren, J. J. G. M., Spaans, F., Jennekens, F., Van Breda Vriesman, P. J. C., and De Baets, M. H. (1993c). *J. Immunol.*, **150**, 4093–4103.

Green, D. P. L., Miledi, R., and Vincent, A. (1975). *Proc. R. Soc. Lond. B* **189**, 57–68.

Heilbronn, E., Mattsson, C. H., Stalberg, E., and Hilton-Brown, P. (1975). *J. Neurol. Sci.* **24**, 59–64.

Indrieri, R. J., Creighton, S. R., Lambert, E. H., and Lennon, V. A. (1983). *J. Am. Vet. Med. Assoc.* **182**, 57–60.

Infante, A. J., Thompson, P. A., Krolick, K. A., and Wall, K. A. (1991). *J. Immunol.* **146**, 2977–2982.

Jacobson, L., Vincent, A., Shillito, P., and Newsom-Davis, J. (1993). *Ann. N.Y. Acad. Sci. USA* **681**, 295–297.

Jermy, A. C., Fisher, C. A., Vincent, A. C., Willcox, N. A., and Newsom-Davis, J. (1989). *J. Autoimmun.* **2**, 675–688.

Jermy, A., Beeson, D., and Vincent, A. (1993). *Eur. J. Immunol.* **23**, 973–976.

Killen, J. A., and Lindstrom, J. M. (1984). *J. Immunol.* **133**, 2549–2553.

Krco, C. J., David, C. S., and Lennon, V. A. (1991). *J. Immunol.* **147**, 3303–3305.

Lambert, E. H., Lindstrom, J. M., and Lennon, V. A. (1976). *Ann. N.Y. Acad. Sci.* **274**, 300–318.

Lennon, V. A., and Lambert, E. H. (1980). *Nature* **285**, No. 5762, 238–240.

Lennon, V. A., Lindstrom, J. M., and Seybold, M. E. (1975). *J. Exp. Med.* **141**, 1365–1375.

Lennon, V. A., Lindstrom, J. M., and Seybold, M. E. (1976). *Ann. N.Y. Acad. Sci.* **274**, 283–299.

Lennon, V. A., Lambert, E. H., Leiby, K. R., Okarma, T. B., and Talib, S. (1991). *J. Immunol.* **146**, 2245–2248.

Lindstrom. J. (1979). *Adv. Immunol.* **27**, 1–50.

Lindstrom. J. M., Lennon, V. A., Seybold, M. E., and Whittingham, S. (1976a). *Ann. N.Y. Acad. Sci.* **274**, 254–274.

Lindstrom, J., Einarson, B. L., Lennon, V. A., and Seybold, M. E. (1976b). *J. Exp. Med.* **144**, 726–738.

Lindstrom, J. M., Engel, A. G., Seybold, M. E., Lennon, V. A., and Lambert, E. H. (1976c). *J. Exp. Med.* **144**, 739–753.

Lindstrom, J., Einarson, B. L., and Merlie, J. (1978). *Proc. Natl. Acad. Sci. USA* **75**, 769–773.

Lindstrom, J., Shelton, D., and Fujii, Y. (1988). *Adv. Immunol.* **42**, 233–284.

Loutrari, H., Kokla, A., and Tzartos, S. J. (1992). *Eur. J. Immunol.* **22**, 2449–2452.

McCormick, E. J., Griesmann, G. E., Huang, Z.-X., Lambert, E. H., and Lennon, V. A. (1987). *J. Immunol.* **139**, 2615–2619.

Martino, G., DuPont, B. L., Wollmann, R. L., Bongioanni, P., Anastasi, J., Quintans, J., Arnason, B. G. W., Grimaldi, L. M. E. (1993). *Ann. Neurol.* **34**, 48–56.

Marzo, A. L., Garlepp, M. J., Schon-Hegard, M., and Dawkins, R. L. (1986). *Clin. Exp. Immunol.* **64**, 101–106.

Matsuo, H., Tsujihata, M., Satoh, A., Takeo, G., Yoshimura, T., and Nagataki, S. (1992). *Muscle Nerve* **15**, 282–287.

McIntosh, K. R., and Drachman, D. B. (1992). *J. Neuroimmunol.* **38**, 75–84.

Meinl, E., Klinkert, W. E. F., and Wekerle, H. (1991). *Am. J. Pathol.* **139**, 995–1008.

Molenaar, P. C., Oen, B. S.-S., Plomp, J. J., Van Kempen, G. Th. H., Jennekens, F. G. I., and Hesselmans, L. F. G. M. (1991). *Eur. J. Pharmacol.* **196**, 93–101.

Mossman, S., Vincent, A., and Newsom-Davis, J. (1988). *J. Neurol. Sci.* **84**, 15–27.

Mozes, E., Dayan, M., Zisman, E., Brocke, S., Arieh, L., and Pecht, I. (1989). *EMBO J.* **8**, 4049–4052.

Mulac-Jericivac, B., Kurisaki, J., and Atassi, M. Z. (1987). *Proc. Natl. Acad. Sci. USA* **84**, 3633–3637.

Olsberg, C. A., Mikiten, T. M., and Krolick, K. A. (1985). *J. Immunol.* **135**, 3062–3067.

Pachner, A. R. (1987). *Yale J. Biol. Med.* **60**, 169–177.

Pachner, A. R., and Kantor, F. S. (1984). *Clin. Exp. Immunol.* **56**, 659–668.

Palace, J., Vincent, A., Beeson, D., and Newsom-Davis, J. (1994). *J. Autoimmun.*, in press.

Palmer, A. C., Lennon, V. A., Beadle, C., and Goodyear, J. V. (1980). *J. Small Anim. Pract.* **21**, 359–364.

Patrick, J., and Lindstrom, J. (1973). *Science* **180**, 871–872.

Patrick, J., Lindstrom, J., Culp, B., and McMillan, J. (1973). *Proc. Natl. Acad. Sci. USA* **70**, No. 12, 3334–3338.

Reim, J., McIntosh, K., Martin, S., and Drachman, D. B. (1992). *J. Neuroimmunol.* **41**, 61–70.

Richman, D. P., Gomez, C. M., Berman, P. W., Burres, S. A., Fitch, F. W., and Arnason, B. G. W. (1980). *Nature* **286**, 738–?.

Sahashi, K., Engel, A. G., Lindstrom, J. M., Lambert, E. H., and Lennon, V. A. (1978). *J. Neuropathol. Exp. Neurol.* **27**, 212–223.

Sanders, D. B., Johns, T. R., Eldefrawi, M. E., and Cobb, E. E. (1977). *Arch. Neurol.* **34**, 75–79.

Sanders, D. B., Cobb, E. E., and Winfield, J. B. (1978). *Muscle Nerve* **1**, 146–150.

Scadding, G., Calder, L., Vincent, A., Prior, C., Wray, D., and Newsom-Davis, J. (1986). *Immunology* **58**, 151–155.

Schönbeck, S., Padberg, F., Hohlfeld, R., and Wekerle, H. (1992). *J. Clin. Invest.* **90**, 245–250.

Shelton, G. D., Cardinet, G. H., and Lindstrom, J. M. (1988). *Neurology* **38**, 1417–1423.

Shelton, G. D., Willard, M. D., Cardinet, G. H., and Lindstrom, J. (1990). *J. Vet. Int. Med.* **4**, 281–284.

Shenoy, M., Oshima, M., Atassi, M. Z., and Christadoss, P. (1993). *Clin. Immunol. Immunopathol.*, **66**, 230–238.

Shillito, P., Vincent, A., Newsom-Davis, J. (1993). *Neuromusc. Disord.* **3**, 183–190.

Spack, E. G., Passmore, D., Nag, B., Kopa, D., and Sharma, S. D. (1994). Manuscript submitted for publication.

Sterz, R. K. M., Biro, G., Rajki, K., Filipp, G., and Peper, K. (1985). *J. Immunol.* **134**, 841–846.

Takamori, M., Okumura, S., Komai, K., and Satake, R. (1990). *J. Neurol. Sci.* **99**, 219–227.

Takamori, M., Hamada, T., Komai, K., Takahashi, M., Yoshida, A. (1994). *Ann. Neurol.* **35**, 74–80.

Takamori, M., Hamada, T., and Okumura, S. (1992). *J. Neurol. Sci.* **109**, 82–187.

Takamori, M., Sakato, S., and Okumura, S. (1984). *J. Neurol. Sci.* **66**, 245–253.

Takamori, M., Okumura, S., Nagata, M., and Yoshikawa, H. (1988). *J. Neurol. Sci.* **85**, 121–129.

Tarrab-Hazdai, R., Aharanov, A., Silman, I., and Fuchs, S. (1975a). *Nature* **256**, 128–130.

Tarrab-Hazdai, R., Aharanov, A., Abramsky, O., Yaar, I., and Fuchs, S. (1975b). *J. Exp. Med.* **142**, 785–789.

Thompson, P. A., and Krolick, K. (1992). *Clin. Immunol. Immunopathol.* **62**, 199–209.

Thompson, P. A., Barohn, R. A., and Krolick, K. A. (1992). *Muscle Nerve* **15**, 94–100.

Toyka, K. V., Drachman, D. B., Griffin, D. E., Pestronk, A., Winkelstein, J. A., Fischbeck, K. H., and Kao, I. (1977). *N. Engl. J. Med.* **296**, 125–131.

Tzartos, S., and Lindstrom, J. L. (1980). *Proc. Natl. Acad. Sci. USA* **77**, 755–759.

Tzartos, S. J., and Remoundos, M. S. (1992). *Eur. J. Biochem.* **207**, 915–922.

Tzartos, S., Hochschwender, S., Vasquez, P., and Lindstrom, J. (1987). *J. Neuroimmunol.* **15**, 185–194.

Tzartos, S. J., Barkas, T., Cung, M. T., Kordossi, A., Loutrari, H., Marraud, M., Papadouli, I., Sakarellos, C., Sophianos, D., and Tsikaris, V. (1991). *Autoimmunity* **8**, 259–270.

Ueno, S., Kang, J., Takeuchi, H., Takahashi, M., and Tarui, S. (1980). *Exp. Neurol.* **68**, 512–520.

Valderrama, R., Chang, V. K., Stracher, A., Maccabee, P. J., and Kaldany, R.-R. J. (1987). *J. Neurol. Sci.* **82**, 133–143.

Verschuuren, J. J. G. M., Graus, Y. M. F., Theunissen, R. O. M., Yamamoto, T., Vincent, A., Van Breda Vriesman, P. J. C., and De Baets, M. H. (1992). *J. Neuroimmunol.* **36**, 117–125.

Vincent, A. (1980). *Physiol. Rev.* **60**, 756–824.

Vincent, A. (1991). *Biochem. Soc. Trans.* **19**, 180–183.

Vincent, A., Jacobson, L., Shillito, P. (1994). *Immunol. Lett.* **39**, 269–275.

Vincent, A., and Newsom-Davis, J. (1994). *In* "Immunology of Neuromuscular Diseases" (R. Hohlfeld, Ed.). Academic Press, London.

Vincent, A., and Wood, H. (1988). *Monogr. Allergy* **25**, 33–40.

Waldor, M. K., Sriram, S., McDevitt, H. O., and Steinman, L. (1983). *Proc. Natl. Acad. Sci. USA* **80**, 2713–2717.

Wassermann, N. H., Penn, A. S., Freimuth, P. I., Treptow, N., Wentzel, S., Cleveland, W. L., and Erlanger, B. F. (1982). *Proc. Natl. Acad. Sci. USA* **79**, 4810–4814.

Willcox, H. N. A., and Vincent, A. (1988). *In* "B Lymphocytes in Human Disease" (G. Bird and J. E. Calvert, Eds.), pp. 469–506. Oxford University Press, Oxford, UK.

Willcox, N., Baggi, F., Batocchi, A.-P., Beeson, D., Harcourt, G., Hawke, S., Jacobson, L., Matsuo, H., Moody, A.-M., Nagvekar, N., Nicolle, M., Ong, B., Pantic, N., Newsom-Davis, J., and Vincent, A. (1993). *Ann. N.Y. Acad. Sci.* **681**, 219–237.

Wood, H., Beeson, D., Vincent, A., and Newsom-Davis, J. (1989). *Biochem. Soc. Trans.* **17**, 220–221.

Yeh, T.-M., and Krolick, K. A. (1990). *J. Immunol.* **144**, 1654–1660.

Yokoi, T., Mulac-Jericevic, B., Kurisaki, J.-I., and Atassi, M. Z. (1987). *Eur. J. Immunol.* **17**, 1697–1702.

Zoda, T., Yeh, T.-M., and Krolick, K. A. (1991). *J. Immunol.* **146**, 663–670.

Chapter 7

The Obese Strain of Chickens with Spontaneous Autoimmune Thyroiditis as a Model for Hashimoto Disease

G. Wick,[1] R. Cole,[2] H. Dietrich,[1] Ch. Maczek,[1] P.-U. Müller,[1] and K. Hála[1]

[1] Institute for General and Experimental Pathology, University of Innsbruck Medical School, Innsbruck, Austria
[2] New York State College of Agriculture and Life Sciences, Department of Poultry and Avian Sciences, Cornell University, Ithaca, New York 14853

I. Introduction

Autoimmune diseases (AID) that are experimentally induced in normal animals by immunization with various antigens and appropriate adjuvants have greatly contributed to our understanding of the immunological mechanisms underlying this large group of diseases (Rose and Witebsky, 1956). Nevertheless, animal models that develop AID spontaneously generally parallel the human situation more closely. This is especially true for the obese strain (OS) of chickens, which are afflicted with a spontaneously occurring hereditary autoimmune thyroiditis that resembles Hashimoto thyroiditis in most clinical, immunological, and endocrinological aspects. Several elaborate reviews have been written on the OS, covering various aspects of this interesting model (Cole et al., 1970; Wick et al., 1974; Rose et al., 1976; Wick et al., 1981; Wick et al., 1982a; Wick et al., 1985; Wick et al., 1986; Wick et al., 1989).

As will be detailed below, chickens have certain advantages over mammals for immunological studies, such as the extramaternal development and thus easy accessibility of the embryo, the clear-cut anatomical division of the immune system into a T- and B-dependent portion, the large number of offspring that can be produced from a single pair of parents, the expression of major histocompatibility complex (MHC–B-complex in chickens) antigens on erythrocytes and thus testability by simple hemagglutination methods, the nucleated erythrocytes that serve as a convenient source of DNA for molecular biological investigations and, last, but not least, the enormous economic importance of this species. On the other hand, chickens also have certain disadvantages, above all the considerable costs of their breeding and maintenance and the relative scarcity of immunological reagents, such as monoclonal antibodies against cell-surface antigens. The latter shortcoming is, however, rapidly improving (Cooper et al., 1991).

II. History and Development of the OS

The origin and development of the OS as a model for the study of an AID was a good case of serendipity. In 1955, three females among about 800 examined at 150 days of age showed an abnormal condition of obesity, silky feathers, and small body size. They belonged to one of two strains of white Leghorns (Cole and Hutt, 1973) being selected for resistance to disease and economically important traits. The fact that two of them were full sisters suggested that the trait might be hereditary. Because these birds were not normal and the basic project involved genetic resistance to disease, a follow-up seemed appropriate. In 1956, two dams that had survived and came into egg production were mated to one of the sires that had produced an affected pullet the previous year. Both matings yielded phenotypically obese females, 1 of 3 and 2 of 10. The progeny from these matings and other obese females recovered from the Cornell C strain (CS) in 1956 and 1957 were used in an attempt to increase the number of affected birds so that the nature and cause of the "defect" might be determined. The incidence of the trait increased but involved only females.

In 1958, matings of normal sons from obese dams to obese hens recovered from the CS in 1957 yielded two sons that showed the obese syndrome. When mated to obese dams and daughters of such dams, they yielded progeny showing a tremendous increase in frequency of the trait, 64–72% in females and 17–18% in males. A hereditary basis for the trait was clearly established (Cole, 1966).

The major defect found at necropsy involved the thyroid glands. Although essentially normal at hatching, by the age when the symptoms became evident, the glands were small and histologically abnormal. Lack of thyroid-stimulating hormone (TSH) was proven not to be a factor. The use of dietary low level of iodinated casein (Protamone) was shown to provide adequate thyroid hormone and thus supplemented adult hens would commence to lay or lay at a better rate. This made it possible to produce a sufficient number of obese birds. From then on birds selected as breeders had to show the trait and come from families showing the highest frequency among siblings. Since the expression of the syndrome varied in degree, preference was given to those birds that were more severely affected. Subsequently, families selected to provide breeders, especially males, were those in which a high percentage showed the syndrome very well developed.

The presence of specific circulating autoantibodies against chicken thyroglobulin was then demonstrated in each of the 10 obese females tested but was not found in normal birds from other strains (Cole *et al.*, 1968). Thus, the autoimmune basis for the condition was clearly established. Since this autoimmune thyroiditis was of genetic origin, the further development and improvement of the OS chicken for use as a model to study autoimmunity, especially that of Hashimoto disease in humans, was started and continues.

Ensuring the availability of a breeding stock that can produce a sufficient number of experimental animals that will show well-developed autoimmune thyroiditis requires that the selection be for both the trait and also for several other genetic traits related to efficient reproduction and survival. These selection criteria include the number and size of eggs produced, fertility, and hatchability. The more severely affected birds tend to be quite small in size and to lay eggs of small size, which leads to the need for compromise in breeder selection. When an abnormal condition is observed in any species, attempts should be made to determine if it has a genetic background. If so, a follow-up by appropriate studies might yield a model of value for research on a human abnormality of similar type. The OS chicken model is a good example.

III. Clinical Symptoms and Pathohistology

Soon after hatching, OS chickens develop severe clinical and functional symptoms of hypothyroidism (Figure 1), such as small body size but relatively high body weight, due to subcutaneous and abdominal fat deposits (hence

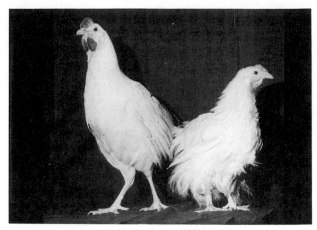

Figure 1   Six-month-old NWL (left) and OS chickens (right). Note phenotypic symptoms of hypothyroidism in the latter, such as smaller body size; small comb and wattles; long, silky, and ruffled (cold sensitivity!) feathers.

the name), lipid serum, small combs and wattles, long silky feathers, cold sensitivity, low fertility of both roosters and dams, and poor hatchability of the fertilized eggs. The underlying reason is a severe mononuclear cell infiltration of the thyroid glands (chickens have two separate thyroid lobes attached to the *arteria carotis communis* in close proximity to the last thymus lobe). At present in the history of the strain, this infiltration starts during the first to second week after hatching and leads to almost complete destruction of the thyroid architecture at the age of 3 to 5 weeks. Infiltration begins multifocally and perivascularly, and a high number of well-developed germinal centers are a hallmark of spontaneous autoimmune thyroiditis (SAT), which is similar to the findings in Hashimoto thyroiditis in man, but in contrast to the appearance of experimentally (with adjuvant)-induced autoimmune thyroiditis (EAT) (Wick and Burger, 1971).

The severity of SAT is classified according to a standard schedule in which 0 = no infiltration, $1+$ = up to 25% of the total histological thyroid cross section occupied by mononuclear cell infiltrate, $2+$ = 25–50% of the cross section infiltrated, $3+$ = 50–75% infiltration, and $4+$ = 75% to total infiltration (Figures 2a–2d).

IV. Immunological Parameters

A detailed account of immunological parameters can be found in the most recent elaborate review by the authors and the references cited therein (Wick *et al.*, 1989).

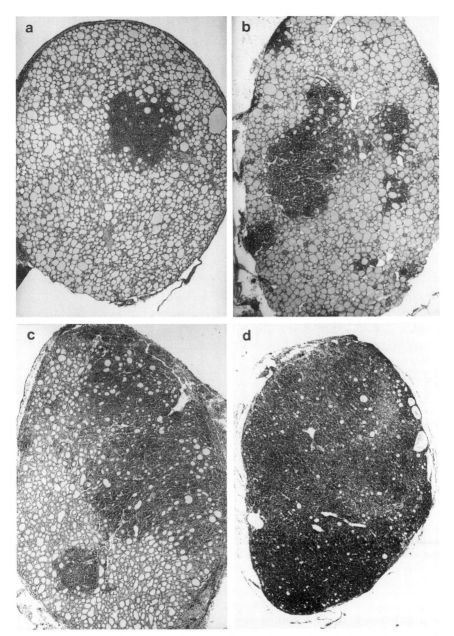

Figure 2 Hematoxilin-eosin stained paraffin sections of thyroid glands from 2-week-old OS chickens exemplifying different degrees of SAT: (a) 1+, (b) 2+, (c) 3+, (d) 4+. For details see text. ×100.

A. Autoantibodies

Over 75% of the sera of 10- to 12-week-old OS chickens contain autoantibodies to thyroglobulin (TgAAbs) that can be assessed by passive hemagglutination or enzyme linked immunosorbent assay (ELISA) techniques. About 50% of the sera is also positive in precipitation tests by double diffusion in gel. A lower percentage also contains autoantibodies to thyroid microsomal antigens (26%) as well as to the thyroid hormones T3 and T4. No thyroid-stimulating immunoglobulins (TSIs) have been found. In addition to thyroid antigen-specific AAbs, some OS sera also contain AAbs against nonthyroid antigens, such as proventricular parietal cells, exocrine and endocrine (islets of Langerhans) constituents of the pancreas, the adrenal cortex, and the parathyroid gland. However, there are no concomitant pathological lesions.

B. Cellular Immune Reactions

The first cells to infiltrate thyroid glands are activated CD4[+], interleukin-2 receptor (IL-2R)[+], T-cell receptor α/β (TCR α/β)[+] cells. Later, B cells and fully developed plasma cells as well as macrophages also contribute to the infiltrate. Adoptive transfer experiments have shown that thyroid-infiltrating lymphocytes (TIL) are most effective in transferring disease into histocompatible recipients of the CS, the nearly normal mother strain from which the OS was originally developed by selective breeding.

In vitro mitogen stimulation tests revealed a significant hyperreactivity of OS T cells toward concanavalin A (ConA) and phytohemagglutinin (PHA). Most important, OS TIL, spleen cells, and peripheral blood lymphocytes (PBL) display a significant hyperproduction of IL-2 and also an increased expression of IL-2R compared with various normal strains. In spleen cells, this alteration can be observed before the development of SAT. As a matter of fact, these latter observations provided the basis for the establishment of a new concept of the role of IL-2 in the development of AID (Kroemer and Wick, 1989). The OS immune system shows a general humoral and cellular hyperreactivity not only against thyroid antigens but also against exogenous antigens such as sheep red blood cells and Rous sarcoma virus (RSV). This hyperreactivity may in part be due to an imbalance between effector cells and suppressor cells (see later discussion) but also to the intrinsic hyperproduction of IL-2.

C. Potential Effector Mechanisms

Originally, SAT was considered to be mainly an antibody-mediated disease because neonatal or *in ovo* bursectomy resulted in a decrease in the frequency and severity of thyroiditis. Furthermore, hormonal bursectomy by treatment of 3-day-old embryos with testosterone or androgen analogs prevented the development of SAT, and chemical bursectomy by neonatal cyclophospha-mide treatment delayed the beginning of infiltration for several weeks. In addition, TgAAbs are vertically transferred from the mother hen to the em-bryo and Tg containing immune complexes can be found in thyroid glands of newly hatched chickens.

In contrast, neonatal thymectomy of OS chicks not only failed to amelio-rate SAT but actually resulted in the development of more severe disease and increased frequency and titers of TgAAbs. On the other hand, this treat-ment was known to abolish the susceptibility of chickens for EAT and enceph-alomyelitis (EAE) (Jankovic *et al.*, 1965). This disease-precipitating effect of neonatal thymectomy was shown to be due to an altered kinetic behavior of T cells, where—for still-unknown reasons—suppressor cells fail to leave the thymus on time, and are thus removed by thymus ablation, while effector T and helper cells are already present in sufficient numbers in the periphery. However, later experiments of DeCarvalho *et al.* (1981), which involved neo-natal thymectomy plus depletion of peripheral T cells with specific antibod-ies, led to a complete prevention of SAT. This could, of course, have been due to either the elimination of T effector cells, or of T-helper (Th) cells involved in AAb production. Final proof that SAT is T-cell mediated came from exper-iments in which OS chickens that were depleted of B cells, and thus the capacity for AAb production, by neonatal cyclophosphamide treatment, still had the capacity for splenic and even more effectively, TIL, to transfer auto-immune thyroiditis into histocompatible CS recipients. It was thus concluded that SAT is primarily mediated by T cells and that TgAAbs play an aggravat-ing role.

D. Disturbed Immunoregulation

Immunoregulation in the OS is altered at two levels: on one hand there is an intrinsic hyperreactivity of the immune system and on the other, a disturbed interaction between the immune and the neuroendocrine system. The abnor-malities intrinsic to the immune system are, for example, reflected in the increased mitogen responsiveness of T cells, the intrinsic hyperproduction of IL-2 and increased expression of IL-2R, the general humoral and cellular hyperreactivity against exogenous antigens, and the occurrence of auto-antibodies against nonthyroid antigens, albeit in rather low frequency, as mentioned earlier. T-cell hyperfunction *in vitro* is complemented by similar observations *in vivo*, such as increased antiviral responses, accelerated allo-transplant rejection, and graft-versus-host reaction.

As mentioned, the disease-accelerating effect of neonatal thymectomy was interpreted as being due to the removal of suppressor cells. This hypothesis was later substantiated in cocultivation experiments of OS thymocytes with autologous PBL, which showed an increased suppressive potential of the latter on mitogen and cytotoxic responses of PBL compared with similar combinations in normal white Leghorn (NWL) controls. The different mechanisms of T-cell hyperreactivity observed so far in various suspensions of mononuclear cell preparations of OS chickens are summarized in Table I.

In addition to these disturbances intrinsic to the immune system, the OS also displays alterations of immune regulation by glucocorticoids. First, OS chickens have a decreased glucocorticoid tonus: the baseline of peripheral glucocorticoid (corticosterone) serum levels in OS chicken is normal but the biologically active concentration is significantly decreased owing to an age- and sex-independent increase of corticosteroid binding globulin (CBG).

Second, the OS chicken was the first animal model of an autoimmune disease in which an altered immunoendocrine feedback regulation via the hypothalamo–pituitary–adrenal axis was observed. Immunization of OS chickens with exogenous antigens or injection of immune system-derived glucocorticoid-increasing factors (GIF), for example IL-1, leads to a significantly lower surge of peripheral glucocorticoid levels compared to normal controls. This decreased glucocorticoid response correlates well with the increased mitogen responsiveness of PBL. Interestingly, this defect is significantly associated with the presence of a new endogenous virus locus, *ev22*, that is only found in the OS but not in any other chicken strain.

Table I
Different Mechanisms of T-Cell Hyperreactivity Operative in OS Thymus, PBL, Spleen, and TIL[a]

	Thymus	Spleen	PBL	TIL
ConA- or PHA-driven proliferation	↑	↑	↑	—
Spontaneous proliferation	↑	↑	(↑)[b]	—
ConA-induced IL-2 production	ND	↑	↑	—
Spontaneous IL-2 secretion	ND	ND	ND	↑
ConA-activatable cells	ND	—	↑	ND
IL-2 receptor+ cells	—	—	—	↑
Overall cellularity	↓	↓	—	ND
ConA binding capacity	—	↑	↑	ND

[a] Data from Wick *et al.* (1989).
Arrows indicate significant increase or decrease of the parameters compared with the respective control group (NWL or CS cells for OS thymocytes, splenocytes, and PBL; OS PBL for thyroid-infiltrating lymphocytes). —, no difference; ND, not determined. All comparisons were done with 1–4-week-old chickens.
[b] () = weak.

Third, there is preliminary evidence that OS thymocytes are relatively resistant against glucocorticoid-induced apoptosis. Together with the fact that OS chickens show a significant deficiency of so-called thymic nurse cells (large complexes of thymic epithelial cells containing intact T cells enclosed within membrane-lined vacuoles), which have been shown to be sites for positive and perhaps also negative T-cell selection, the latter finding may perhaps be an explanation for an insufficient negative T-cell selection process, and thus hyperautoreactivity, in the OS (Wick *et al.*, 1992a).

E. Endocrinology

The clinical symptoms of hypothyroidism due to autoimmune thyroid gland destruction are based on low T3 and T4 serum levels. The symptoms can be reversed by appropriate hormonal substitution. Sundick (1989) has shown an iodine organification defect in OS chickens as well as a TSH-independent autonomous hyperfunction of the thyroid preceding the development of SAT. Furthermore, depleting OS chickens of dietary iodine significantly decreases the development of SAT, while resupplementation of iodine leads to a fast reemergence of the disease. The reasons for these disturbances of iodine metabolism, which seem to be closely related to the emergence of SAT, are still unknown. A thyrotropic virus infection would, for example, be a good candidate for a genetically determined factor underlying alterations in iodine metabolism and thus predisposing to the pathogenesis of autoimmune thyroiditis. The disturbed immunoendocrine dialogue via the hypothalamo-pituitary-adrenal axis in the OS has been discussed in the last section. Other endocrine functions have not yet been studied in depth in the OS, with the exception of androgen metabolism and tonus, which are both normal.

F. Evidence for Primary Target Organ Susceptibility

Based on studies in the OS, we have developed a new concept for the pathogenesis of autoimmune diseases in general and autoimmune thyroiditis in particular that can be summarized as follows: A given autoimmune disease can only develop in an individual that possesses two sets of essential genes that, on one hand, code for an abnormal autoreactivity in the immune system and on the other, for a primary susceptibility of the target organ to an attack by humoral and/or cellular immunological effector mechanisms; the final outcome of the disease is then fine tuned by additional modulatory factors that can act either on the immune system or on the target organ itself (Wick *et al.*, 1987). Examples for modulatory factors acting on the immune system are glucocorticoid hormones. An example for a modulatory factor involving the target organ is, of course, dietary iodine. Only if both sets of essential genes are present and an individual carries a sufficient load of modulatory aggravating factors does severe autoimmune thyroiditis develop. Classic genetic cross-breeding experiments as well as passive transfer studies have revealed that a single autosomal gene seems to be coding for this target organ susceptibility. There is evidence that a thyrotropic virus infection constitutes a primary target organ alteration that renders the thyroid gland susceptible to an autoimmune process (Wick *et al.*, 1992b; Kühr *et al.*, 1994).

V. Breeding and Management of OS Chickens

Successful propagation of the OS, especially in a small population, can be done only if rigid precautions are taken with respect to animal care and housing, the selection of adequate parental animals, and proper management of breeding matters (Dietrich, 1989).

A. Food and Cages

After hatching, chickens are housed in commercial cages and adequate space in relation to their age. The chicks are given free access to drinking water in plastic dishes and to commercial chick food in troughs. In our Animal Unit the food is G-1 (Pillermühle, Austria, registration number A 3403) containing 18% protein, energy 11.5 MJ/kg and amprolium as a coccidiostatic drug. From the age of 8–20 weeks, G-3 food for growing chickens (Pillermühle, Austria, registration number A 3402, protein 14%, energy 11 MJ/kg) is used and the birds are offered drinking water via an automatic nipple system. (Warning: Chickens will only drink from nipples if they are trained to do so at a young age!)

To alleviate the symptoms of hypothyroidism, adult OS chickens receive a G-5 diet for laying hens (Pillermühle, Austria, registration number A 4209) containing 17% protein, energy 11.2 MJ/kg, supplemented with 100 g/1000 kg (100 ppm) Protamone (iodinated casein, Agri Tech. Inc., Kansas City, Missouri; lot Sp-790917) which is metabolized in the chickens to T3 and T4. Protamone contains 7% total iodine, of which 1% is inorganic and 0.65% is incorporated into a thyroxine-like component. As an alternative to Protamone supplementation, thyroxine (T4) can be used, mixing a premix (1 g T4/1000 kg food) to a final concentration of 250 μg T4/kg food (Sundick *et al.*, 1979).

For our breeding management, the commercially available chicken cage systems are not suitable with respect to cage size, floor wire design, and ease of cleaning procedures. Parental OS chickens are therefore housed individually in cages which were designed and manufactured in our laboratory. The floor in each unit measures 30 × 50 cm (larger than those for commercial purposes) and the cage heights are 62 cm for sires and 42 cm for dams. Sliding galvanized wire doors on each cage permit easy and gentle handling of chickens, especially for semen collection from roosters and the artificial insemination procedure for hens. Aluminum troughs for food are placed in the front of the cages and in the back a commercially available automatic nipple system offers fresh drinking water. Tar-coated paper rolls are placed below the chickens to remove feces.

B. Selection Procedure for Breeders

The selection criteria in our OS population are based on blood typing for *B*-complex antigens, TgAAbs and the phenotypic trait of the OS syndrome, as well as avoiding brother-sister matings to maintain a high degree of heterozygosity. To determine the *B*-haplotype, specific antisera are raised against surface determinants of chicken red blood cells (Plachy *et al.*, 1992) and all OS chickens are monitored for the three haplotypes, *B13B13*, *B5B5*, and *B15B15*, known to be present in this strain (Bacon *et al.*, 1974). TgAAbs in the sera of 10- to 12-week-old birds are evaluated using a specific ELISA technique (Kofler *et al.*, 1984) and precipitating Tg-AAbs are determined by double diffusion in gel (Witebsky *et al.*, 1969).

The phenotypical selection procedure for the parental generation is based on a two-step classification scheme at 10 and 20 weeks of age, respectively. The birds are classified according to their clinical appearance as being phenotypically normal (0), slightly affected (1+ = somewhat smaller than normal controls), strongly affected (2+ = showing all characteristic traits as described above and depicted in Fig. 1), severely hypothyroid dwarfs (3+ = known to rarely reach a reproductive stage, even with hormonal supplementation). The expression of the characteristic "obese trait" (Fig. 1) is classified as 2+ for sires and dams, which are then housed, two at a time in one cage, until the second selection step at 20 weeks. From this time on, reselected roosters and hens with a 2+ OS phenotype are housed in individual cages. The egg productivity of dams and semen quality of sires are individually recorded. Artificial insemination programs are started to produce chickens for experimental purposes and as progeny for the next mating generation. Semen samples are carefully obtained from the selected roosters and placed in the magnum of hens according to the mating schedule.

The fertilized eggs are gently collected several times each day and the wing tag number and *B*-haplotype of the hen as well as the collecting date are marked with a pencil on the egg shell. Eggs are stored under optimal conditions at 14–16°C and 60–70% relative humidity in a special thermostat with the blunt egg pole upward. Storage time should be limited to 14 days under these conditions because embryonal mortality increases thereafter.

After a 30-min formaldehyde vapor disinfection period, breeding eggs are incubated under standardized and optimal conditions for temperature and relative humidity, and the eggs are turned on their longitudinal axis every 2 hrs. On embryonic day 8, all eggs are candled and the number of fertilized eggs, the embryonal mortality rate, and the percentage of nonfertilized eggs are recorded for each parental pair. The hatching conditions for temperature and relative humidity are optimized as described by Dietrich (1989), and hatchability rates are calculated for the progeny of each parental pair. On the day of hatching, the combs of all chickens are trimmed with scissors to retard growth, in particular in adult roosters. For security reasons, all hatched chickens receive two wing tags, one on each side. The date of hatching and the wing tag numbers and B-haplotype are noted accurately in a master logbook and these records are used for pedigree protocols and the selection of suitable OS birds for future breeding stock.

VI. Immunogenetics

SAT is a multigenic disease. As discussed above, at least four groups of functional abnormalities are involved in its development (Kroemer et al., 1989): (1) a target organ susceptibility to autoaggressive effector cells encoded by a single, autosomal, recessive gene; (2) a general hyperreactivity of T cells (elevated proliferation, IL-2 secretion, and IL-2R expression upon stimulation with Con A), regulated by a dominant, autosomal gene; (3) a decreased glucocorticoid tonus due to an elevated plasma concentration of CBG, inherited as an autosomal recessive trait; (4) an autosomal dominant trait, $ev22$, that cosegregates with a deficient increase in plasma corticosterone in response to antigen or injection of GIF, for example, IL-1.

Initially, the B-locus haplotype was discussed as a possible essential factor governing the outcome of SAT (Bacon et al., 1974, 1977, 1981). Later, however, it became clear that the MHC type plays only a modulatory role (Bacon and Rose, 1979) since, for example, high responder (high TgAAb titers and severe SAT) and low responder (absent TgAAb and low degree of SAT) sublines, both homozygous for $B15$ could be developed (Hála, 1988).

To calculate the number of genes responsible for a certain trait (SAT), we assumed a simple Mendelian type of inheritance (Neu et al., 1985, 1986; Kroemer et al., 1989), based on the calculation of percentages of F_2 hybrids (crosses of OS female × CB inbred male F_1) chickens exhibiting the OS trait, for example, in this case the infiltration of thyroid glands by lymphoid cells.

Histological analyses for SAT in 4-month-old F_2 animals revealed lymphoid infiltration (1+ and more) in 24%; among these, 8% had severe disease (over 2+). If two recessive genes were involved, 6.25% of the F_2 birds should exhibit SAT. If one dominant and one recessive gene were involved, about 18.75% of the animals could be expected to be afflicted. Since we have only recently begun to develop a completely leucosis virus-free chicken colony, we have not taken into account animals with minor lymphoid foci in their thyroid gland but rather included only those with $\geq$2+ SAT for genetic analyses, that is, 8% in an F_2 generation. This percentage is compatible with the existence of two recessive genes (expected frequency of birds with SAT, 6.25%) or four dominant and one recessive gene (expected frequency, 8%) regulating the development of SAT. As mentioned earlier, we have placed these genes into two groups, one regulating the abnormality of the target organ, the second coding for a pathological increased autoreactivity of the immune system (Hála, 1988). The relative importance of different genetic factors for the development of SAT has shifted considerably with time since the original establishment of the OS, as summarized in Table II.

VII. Comparison of SAT and EAT

As mentioned in the introductory section, spontaneously occurring autoimmune diseases of susceptible animals as well as experimentally induced diseases in primarily normal animal strains both constitute important models for human autoimmune thyroiditis. To examine the pathogenetic mechanisms in these two forms of thyroiditis, comparative studies were made be-

Table II
Factors Considered to Influence the Development of SAT in the OS

Type of OS population	Years of selection	Approx. age with max. infiltration	Apparent dominating gene(s)	Modulating factors
"Stone Age"	1956–1970	7–12 weeks	Sex	Age
"Middle Age"	1971–1983	5–10 weeks	MHC	Non-MHC immune response genes
"Present-Day Age"	1984–	2–4 weeks	T-cell hyperreactivity, target organ susceptibility (dietary iodine), environmental influence (virus, bacteria)	Glucocorticoid, tonus, IL-2 hyperproduction, environmental influence (virus, bacteria), MHC

tween EAT in NWL chickens induced by immunization with thyroid antigens and adjuvant, and SAT in OS chickens. Immunization of NWL chickens with saline thyroid extract and complete Freund's adjuvant (CFA) leads to production of high titers of TgAAb and infiltration of the thyroid glands by mononuclear cells. The degree of this EAT shows a wide interindividual variation and, in contrast to SAT, both infiltration and TgAAb production are selflimiting. Thus EAT in NWL does not lead to complete destruction of the thyroid architecture and clinical manifestation of hypothyroidism. This fact is possibly due to a normalization of the T-helper/T-suppressor ratio after a few weeks. Progression of the disease can only be obtained by repeated immunization. Comparative histopathological investigations demonstrate further differences concerning the thyroid infiltrate; specifically, the appearance of germinal centers is typical for SAT (and Hashimoto disease), but cannot be observed in EAT.

F$_1$ hybrids between *B15B15* OS birds and normal inbred *B12B12* CB chickens are not susceptible to SAT, although a high proportion produces TgAAb (Neu *et al.*, 1986). Injection of Tg in CFA causes development of severe EAT and TgAAb production in these F$_1$ birds. Interestingly, in these crosses thyroid infiltration is accompanied by formation of a few germinal centers and so partly resembles the SAT infiltrate (Maczek *et al.*, 1992).

Taken together, SAT and EAT in chickens are both characterized by TgAAb production and thyroid infiltration, but exact analysis of these parameters also reveals principal differences. These are: (1) the self-limiting nature of EAT and (2) the different histopathology. Distinct pathogenetic mechanisms seem to be responsible for these discrepancies as was demonstrated for EAE in comparison to SAT (Wick and Steiner, 1972). Different epitopes on Tg may, for example, play a role in the two forms of thyroiditis. Comparison of these two models in chickens with human Hashimoto thyroiditis supports our previous notion that the spontaneously occurring type is the more appropriate animal model for the human disease.

VIII. Use of the OS for the Development of New Therapeutic Strategies

Owing to the rapid development of SAT within the first 2 weeks after hatching, the possibility of starting treatment in the embryo or after full emergence of the disease, and the relatively easy and unequivocal readout parameters (i.e., histopathological assessment of SAT and determination of autoantibodies against thyroid antigens), the OS lends itself as a perfect model for testing new therapeutic approaches for the treatment of autoimmune thyroiditis. The data obtained so far have been summarized in a recent review (Wick *et al.*, 1990). Thus, SAT has been successfully prevented by induction of tolerance to thyroglobulin, by dietary iodine depravation, and by treatment with glucocorticoids and androgens. With respect to the latter, newly designed androgen analogs, which retain their immunosuppressive potential but are devoid of unwanted endocrinological side effects, are of special interest. Finally, the OS was the first example of an animal model with a spontaneously occurring autoimmune disease in which treatment with cyclosporin A has been shown not only to be not beneficial, but rather even aggravate the disease (Wick *et al.*, 1982b), an observation that was also later corroborated, for example, for collagen type II arthritis (Kaibara *et al.*, 1983) and streptocotocin-induced diabetes in mice (Iwakiri *et al.*, 1987).

IX. Conclusions

The OS is an animal model for Hashimoto thyroiditis that parallels the human counterpart in all aspects that have been studied so far. It is perfectly suited for studying the essential mechanisms leading to the development of SAT as well as the various modulatory factors that determine the final outcome of the disease. Owing to the extremely fast development of severe thyroiditis—2 weeks after hatching, and the easy histopathological and serological readout parameters, the OS is also a useful tool for studying new therapeutic avenues for thyroiditis in particular and organ-specific autoimmune diseases in general.

Acknowledgments

The work by the authors was supported by several consecutive grants of the Austrian Research Council, the Jubiläumsfonds of the Austrian National Bank, and the Kamillo Eisner-Foundation, Hergiswil, Switzerland. We would like to take this opportunity to thank the technical staff of our Central Laboratory Animal Facilities for many years of good professional care of our chicken colonies and Mr. E. Rainer for excellent technical assistance.

References

Bacon, L. D., and Rose, N. R. (1979). *Proc. Natl. Acad. Sci. USA* **76**, 1435–1437.
Bacon, L. D., Kite, J. H., and Rose, N. R. (1974). *Science* **186**, 274–275.
Bacon, L. D., Kite, J. H., and Rose, N. R. (1977). *In* "Avian Immunology" (A. A. Benedict, Ed.), pp. 309–315. Plenum Press, New York.
Bacon, L. D., Polley, C. R., Cole, R. K., and Rose, N. R. (1981). *Immunogenetics* **12**, 339–349.
Cole, R. K. (1966). *Genetics* **53**, 1021–1023.
Cole, R. K., and Hutt, F. B. (1973). *Anim. Breeding Abstr.* **41**, 103–118.

Cole, R. K., Kite, J. H., Jr., and Witebsky, E. (1968). *Science* **160**, 1357–1358.

Cole, R. K., Kite, J. H., Jr., Wick, G., and Witebsky, E. (1970). *Poultry Sci.* **49**, 480–488.

Cooper, M. D., Chen, C.-L. H., Bucy, R. P., and Thompson, C. B. (1991). *Adv. Immunol.* **50**, 87–117.

DeCarvalho, P. L. C., Wick, G., and Roitt, I. M. (1981). *J. Immunol.* **126**, 750–753.

Dietrich, H. M. (1989). *Lab. Anim.* **23**, 345–352.

Hála, K. (1988). *Immunobiology* **177**, 354–373.

Iwakiri, R., Nagafuchi, S., Kounone, E., Nakano, S., Koya, T., Nakayama, M., Nakamura, M., and Niko, Y. (1987). *Experientia* **43**, 324–326.

Jankovic, B. D., Isvaneski, M., Popeskovic, L., and Mitrovic, K. (1965). *Int. Arch. Allergy* **26**, 18–33.

Kaibara, N., Hotokebuchi, T., Takagishi, K., and Katsuki, I. (1983). *J. Exp. Med.* **158**, 2007–2015.

Kofler, H., Kofler, R., Wolf, H., Müller, P. U., and Wick, G. (1984). *J. Immunol. Meth.* **69**, 243–252.

Kroemer, G., and Wick, G. (1989). *Immunol. Today* **10**, 246–251.

Kroemer, G., Neu, N., Kühr, Th., Dietrich, H., Fässler, R., Hála, K., and Wick, G. (1989). *Clin. Immunol. Immunopathol.* **52**, 202–213.

Kühr, Th., Hála, K., Dietrich, H., Herold, M., and Wick, G. (1994). *J. Autoimmun.* **7**, 13–25.

Maczek, Ch., Neu, N., Wick, G., and Hála, K. (1992). *Autoimmunity* **12**, 277–284.

Neu, N., Hála, K., Dietrich, H., and Wick, G. (1985). *Clin. Immunol. Immunopathol.* **37**, 397–405.

Neu, N., Hála, K., Dietrich, H., and Wick, G. (1986). *Int. Arch. Allergy Appl. Immunol.* **80**, 168–173.

Plachy, J., Pink, J. R. L., and Hála, K. (1992). *Crit. Rev. Immunol.* **12**, 47–79.

Rose, N. R., and Witebsky, E. (1956). *J. Immunol.* **76**, 417–427.

Rose, N. R., Bacon, L. D., and Sundick, R. S. (1976). *Transplant. Rev.* **31**, 264–285.

Sundick, R. S. (1989). *Immunol. Res.* **8**, 39–60.

Sundick, R. S., Bagchi, N., Livezey, M. D., Brown, T. R., and Mack, R. E. (1979). *Endocrinol.* **105**, 493–.

Wick, G., and Burger, H. (1971). *Z. Immun.-Forsch.* **142**, 54–70.

Wick, G., and Steiner, R. (1972). *J. Immunol.* **109**, 1031–1035.

Wick, G., Sundick, R. S., and Albini, B. (1974). *Clin. Immunol. Immunopathol.* **3**, 272–300.

Wick, G., Boyd, R. L., Hála, K., de Carvalho, L., Kofler, R., Müller, P.-U., and Cole, R. K. (1981). *Curr. Top. Microbiol. Immunol.* **91**, 109–128.

Wick, G., Boyd, R. L., Hála, K., Thunhold, S., and Kofler, H. (1982a). *Clin. Exp. Immunol.* **47**, 1–18.

Wick, G., Müller, P.-U., and Schwarz, S. (1982b). *Eur. J. Immunol.* **12**, 877–881.

Wick, G., Möst, J., Schauenstein, K., Krömer, G., Dietrich, H., Ziemiecki, A., Fässler, R., Schwarz, S., Neu, N., and Hála, K. (1985). *Immunol. Today* **6**, 359–364.

Wick, G., Hála, K., Wolf, H., Ziemiecki, A., Sundick, R. S., Stöffler-Meilicke, M., and DeBaets, M. (1986). *Immunol. Rev.* **94**, 113–136.

Wick, G., Kroemer, G., Neu, N., Fässler, R., Ziemiecki, A., Müller, R. G., Ginzel, M., Béladi, I., Kühr, Th., and Hála, K. (1987). *Immunol. Lett.* **16**, 249–258.

Wick, G., Brezinschek, H.-P., Hála, K., Dietrich, H., Wolf, H., and Kroemer, G. (1989). *Adv. Immunol.* 433–500.

Wick, G., Hu, Y., and Gruber, J. (1992a). *Trends Endocrinol. Metabol.* **3**, 141–146.

Wick, G., Hu, Y., Gruber, J., Kühr, Th., Wozak, E., and Hála, K. (1992b). *Intern. Rev. Immunol.* **9**, 77–89.

Wick, G., Dietrich, H., Kroemer, G., Fässler, R., Brezinschek, H.-P., and Schuurs, A. H. W. (1990). *In* "Organ-Specific Autoimmunity" (P. E. Bigazzi, G. Wick, and K. Wicher, Eds.), pp. 191–211. Marcel Dekker, New York.

Witebsky, E., Kite, J. H., Wick, G., and Cole, R. K. (1969). *J. Immunol.* **103**, 708–715.

Chapter 8

Experimental Autoimmune Thyroiditis in the Mouse and Rat

Yi-chi M. Kong[1] and Alvaro A. Giraldo[2]

[1]Department of Immunology and Microbiology, Wayne State University School of Medicine, Detroit, Michigan 48201

[2]Division of Immunopathology, St. John Hospital, Detroit, Michigan 48236

I. Experimental Autoimmune Thyroiditis in the Mouse

A. History of the Model

Murine experimental autoimmune thyroiditis (EAT) became a firmly established model for Hashimoto's thyroiditis (HT) in 1971, when susceptible and resistant strains were segregated according to the major histocompatibility complex (MHC), the mouse *H-2* (Vladutiu and Rose, 1971), and particular attention was paid to preparing ingredients in complete Freund's adjuvant (CFA) for emulsion with the thyroid antigen (Rose *et al.*, 1971; Vladutiu and Rose, 1972). Although it is the last animal model to be described (Rose, 1976), it has proven the most useful in obtaining an understanding of the genetic and T-cell regulation of autoimmune diseases because of parallel advances in our knowledge of mouse immunogenetics and the immune network (Kong, 1986).

B. The Animals

For optimal induction of EAT with mouse thyroglobulin (MTg), female mice of the k (e.g., CBA, C3H) or s (e.g., SJL, A.SW) haplotype are used at 2–3 months of age. Males tend to yield less severe or uniform autoimmune responses and are more influenced by hormonal effects than females (Okayasu *et al.*, 1981b), and mice immunized after 4 months have a lower incidence of disease (Okayasu *et al.*, 1989). The normal diet of Purina mouse (5015) or rodent lab (5001) chow is used. If breeding is desired, half the pellet mixture is Purina breeder chow, given only to breeders; this would eliminate any potential effect of diet on susceptibility to EAT (Bhatia *et al.*, 1993). All animals are maintained on acidified water (0.008 N HCl), and housed in cages with tops equipped with paper filters; both protocols allow the manipulation of the immune system with little increased risk of infection, and protect against possible transmission of infection into the cage. It is worth noting that EAT studies *in vivo* have not been affected by infection with mouse hepatitis virus in the past, but animals free of common mouse pathogens are used if they are available.

C. Genetic Considerations

1. MHC Genes

   a. Class II genes.   Susceptibility to EAT induction with MTg is mapped to the *I-A* subregion of the *H-2* complex whether the independent haplotypes are on different (Vladutiu and Rose, 1971) or B10 (Beisel *et al.*, 1982a) background genes. Whereas $H-2^{b, d}$ strains are resistant, $H-2^{k, s}$ strains are susceptible regardless of the adjuvant used (Esquivel *et al.*, 1977; Kong *et al.*, 1985) or even if no adjuvant is used (ElRehewy *et al.*, 1981). The MHC-based susceptibility also holds true when heterologous Tgs, such as human (H) (Tomazic and Rose, 1976; Simon *et al.*, 1985, 1986; Krco *et al.*, 1990) or rabbit Tg (Tomazic and Rose, 1976), are compared. The recent demonstration that the transfer of A_α and A_β genes from susceptible k mice into resistant B10.M ($H-2^f$) mice results in thyroiditis after immunization further supports the major role of *H-2A* in susceptibility, most likely involving antigen presentation (Kong *et al.*, 1992). Susceptibility to EAT is dominant; ($k \times d$)F$_1$ mice develop EAT after immunization (Vladutiu and Rose, 1975). It should be noted that F_1 mice and mice of the q haplotype generally develop less severe thyroiditis than the k and s strains, when lipopolysaccharide (LPS) (Beisel *et al.*, 1982a), a finer discriminator than CFA (Vladutiu and Rose, 1971), is used as adjuvant.

The influence of *H-2E* is less clear and may vary from strain to strain; k strains express H-2E while s strains do not. *I-E* restriction in k strains has been observed in the responses of T cells to HTg (Krco *et al.*, 1990) and a Tg epitope (Chronopoulou and Carayanniotis, 1993). In E^- B10.S mice, the introduction of the E_α^k transgene to form a stable $E_\alpha^k E_\beta^s$ molecule results in clonal deletion of T-cell receptor (TCR) $V_\beta 5^+$ and $V_\beta 11^+$ T cells, as well as resistance to EAT. The reduction in EAT severity of immunized B10.S(E$^+$) mice could implicate these T cells in the autoimmune repertoire (Kong *et al.*, 1992).

b. Class I genes. Evidence accumulated thus far indicates the participation of class I genes primarily at the effector/target cell level. The use of *K*- and *D*-end recombinant strains has shown the *D* allele to play a prominent role in reducing autoantibody titers and/or thyroiditis, depending on the *I-A* (*k* or *s* allele) combination (Kong *et al.*, 1979). The *K* region can also exert an influence on autoantibody level, and incidence or severity of thyroiditis (Beisel *et al.*, 1982a). Such influences are more readily discernible when recombinant strains on the same B10 background genes are tested and when LPS is used as adjuvant. Since cytotoxic T cells (Tc) kill thyroid epithelial cells in a class I antigen-restricted manner (Creemers *et al.*, 1983; Salamero and Charreire, 1985), the *H-2* compatibility between the thyroid target and effector cells is demonstrably important (Ben-Nun *et al.*, 1980; Okayasu and Hatakeyama, 1983).

2. Non-MHC Genes

Compared with the MHC genes, non-*H-2* background genes play a relatively minor role in influencing antibody levels and disease incidence and severity, which are discernible when LPS rather than CFA is used as adjuvant (Beisel *et al.*, 1982b). Regardless of the adjuvant, however, mice on B10 background are generally poorer responders, and their T cells do not proliferate consistently upon MTg stimulation (Christadoss *et al.*, 1978; Krco *et al.*, 1990). They are less suitable for studies requiring *in vitro* activation (Section I,D,5).

As to the specific role of TCR genes, thyroiditogenic T cells infiltrating the thyroid are mostly TCR α/β^+ (Fuller *et al.*, unpublished data). The involvement of TCR genes has not been determined. However, susceptibility to EAT induction with MTg is undiminished in k or s strains with *mls* deletion (CBA) or 50% genomic deletion (SJL, C57BR) of V_β^+ T cells (Vladutiu and

Rose, 1971; Tomazic and Rose, 1976). The extent of participation of various TCR genes will be determined when the thyroiditogenic epitopes on MTg have been identified (Section I,D,2).

D. The Disease

1. Spontaneous Development in the Nonobese Diabetic Mouse

There is no spontaneous model in murine AT (SAT) except for the coexistence of mononuclear cell infiltration in endocrine organs, such as the salivary and thyroid glands, in the nonobese diabetic (NOD) mouse, a recent model for insulin-dependent, Type I diabetes (Asamoto *et al.*, 1986). The incidence of thyroiditis varies from colony to colony, from about 18% (Asamoto *et al.*, 1986) to >77% (Bernard *et al.*, 1992) with no predilection for females or aged mice, as observed for diabetes. Where tested in the colony with high incidence, no MTg autoantibodies were found. The class II genes of the NOD mouse are different from susceptible haplotypes, but EAT can be induced in these mice (Y. M. Kong and C. S. David, unpublished data).

2. Autoantigens for Active Induction

a. MTg preparation. Because homologous MTg contains MTg-unique epitope(s) in addition to those shared with other heterologous Tgs (Kong *et al.*, 1986; Simon *et al.*, 1986; Nabozny *et al.*, 1990), this self-autoantigen has long been known to be a superior inducer of EAT (Tomazic and Rose, 1976). It is a dimer of 660 kDa and is prepared from pooled thyroids which have been stored at −70°C while still attached to the tracheae (Kong *et al.*, 1979).

On the day of column fractionation, both lobes of 300–500 thyroids are detached from the tracheae with curved forceps, and kept moist with borate-buffered saline (BBS), pH 8.2, in a petri dish on ice. They are then gently homogenized in 4–5 ml of BBS with a glass homogenizer placed in ice. After centrifugation at 100,000g for 60 min to remove membranous materials and MTg aggregates, the thyroid extract is recovered from the first peak off a Sephadex G-200 column (2.3 × 90 cm). The concentration of MTg is determined spectrophotometrically at 280 nm and usually ranges from 1.5 to 2.5 mg/ml, with a total yield of 30–60 mg. The MTg is stored at −20°C in 2-ml aliquots of ≤2.0 mg/ml.

Repeated freezing and thawing as well as lyophilization cause loss of antigen in the form of aggregates. About 0.5 ml is concentrated to 10–15 mg/ml for immunoelectrophoresis against rabbit hyperimmune antiserum to crude thyroid extract and rabbit antiserum to mouse serum. Purity is assured when an arc is seen only with antiserum to thyroid extract. Because we use MTg for induction of resistance (Section I,F) and *in vitro* stimulation, LPS-free disposable ware and glassware (which has been heated at 200°C for 30 min) are used throughout. All MTg preparations are checked for LPS contamination with *Limulus* amebocyte lysate as described (ElRehewy *et al.*, 1981); 200 μg MTg, the highest dose injected, contains <10 ng LPS. MTg for injection is diluted in nonpyrogenic saline.

A number of laboratories use thyroid extract without purification (Ben-Nun *et al.*, 1980; Braley-Mullen *et al.*, 1985). An estimate of 50% thyroid extract being Tg or 50 μg Tg/lobe appears adequate.

b. Pathogenic peptides.   Unlike other heterologous Tgs, MTg has not been cloned and its sequence is not known. However, two synthetic peptides, a large 40-mer of 1672–1711 derived from HTg (Texier *et al.*, 1992b) and a 17-mer of 2495–2511 (TgP1) from rat (R) Tg (Chronopoulou and Carayanniotis, 1992), have been shown to induce EAT in susceptible mice. The 17-mer peptide does not appear to be a dominant thyroiditogenic epitope on MTg, since it and MTg do not cross-stimulate lymph node cells (LNC) primed *in vivo* with the other, and curiously, nor does it do so with RTg. Another thyroxine (T_4)-containing synthetic 12-mer of 2549–2560 derived from HTg cannot induce EAT but does prime and cross-stimulate with MTg for adoptive transfer (Hutchings *et al.*, 1992). These studies support the concept that MTg contains unique and conserved epitopes, all of which contribute to its pathogenicity (Simon *et al.*, 1986; Nabozny *et al.*, 1990).

3. Active Induction Protocols

a. MTg and LPS.   The most uniform induction of EAT in terms of incidence has resulted when LPS is used as adjuvant (Esquivel *et al.*, 1977) and has been adopted in other laboratories (Braley-Mullen *et al.*, 1985; Parish *et al.*, 1988). The standard protocol is 20 or 40 μg MTg, followed 3 hr later by 20 μg LPS (*Salmonella enteritidis* or *Escherichia coli*, trichloroacetic acid-precipitated); both are given i.v. in 0.1 ml on days 0 and 7. Severity of thyroiditis is dose-dependent; 20 μg MTg is adequate but >40 μg gives greater thyroid involvement. (Note: 10 μg LPS is sufficient for SJL and A.SW strains and less toxic.)

b. MTg and CFA.   The standard protocol is a refinement of the original (Rose *et al.*, 1971). The MTg dose is 30 or 60 μg/0.1 ml of emulsion, given s.c. to alternate inner thighs on days 0 and 7 (Nabozny *et al.*, 1990). To achieve this final concentration, 0.6 or 1.2 mg MTg/ml is emulsified in Difco CFA containing *Mycobacterium tuberculosis* H37Ra (3 mg/ml) at a 1:1 ratio. (Note: Difco CFA #3113 contains 1 mg/ml, to which is added 2 mg desiccated H37Ra, #3114; all must be finely dispersed.) To achieve a good emulsion which does not disperse when a drop is tested in water, we load the MTg and CFA separately into two glass syringes and mix rapidly in a three-way plastic stopcock. The valve openings are then partially closed to increase resistance for the final 30-min mixing. The third opening may be used for testing the emulsion. Injection is made by loading the emulsion into a 1-ml syringe. This mixture is also suitable for 0.05 ml injection into the hind footpad or 0.1 ml into the base of the tail (Section I,D,5).

   c. **Thyroid lobe and LPS.** Under pentobarbital anesthesia, one fresh thyroid lobe is implanted under alternate kidney capsules on days 0 and 7 (Okayasu and Hatakeyama, 1983). The incision is closed with Autoclips and 20 μg LPS is injected i.v. 6 hr after each implant.

4. Course of Disease

   Thyroid infiltration is the hallmark of EAT and distinguishes susceptible from resistant strains (Vladutiu and Rose, 1971). After immunization with MTg and LPS or CFA on days 0 and 7, lesions are easily discerned in histologic sections by day 21 (Esquivel et al., 1977), although mononuclear cells can be recovered from pooled thyroid suspensions on day 13 (Creemers et al., 1984). Depending somewhat on the dose and strain, maximal infiltration is usually reached by day 28 and maintained for at least 2 months thereafter (Kong et al., 1989b). Long-term observations after EAT induction reveal a chronic state for up to 12 (C3H) or 18 (CBA) months (Okayasu et al., 1989). This is in contrast to induction with heterologous Tgs, such as porcine (P) Tg, which results in milder lesions that resolve after day 28 (Tang et al., 1990).

   Earlier monitoring by *in vitro* proliferative response to MTg, which correlates with subsequent detection of thyroid pathology (Okayasu et al., 1981a), can begin with popliteal or inguinal lymph nodes by days 7–8 (Christadoss et al., 1978; Okayasu et al., 1981a) or the spleen by day 14 (Simon et al., 1986) after MTg/CFA or MTg/LPS immunization respectively. The level of IgG antibodies to MTg usually plateaus between days 14 and 21 and lasts for many months (Okayasu et al., 1989), but it is not a predictor of infiltration (Vladutiu and Rose, 1971; Esquivel et al., 1977).

5. Transfer of Disease

   Both spleen cells (SC) and LNC effectively transfer disease to normal syngeneic recipients after the appropriate immunization and *in vitro* activation (Simon et al., 1986; Flynn et al., 1989); the recipients do not need to be irradiated first, as reported by others (Williams et al., 1987; Parish et al., 1988). MTg in BBS, pH 8.2, is first dialyzed with PBS, pH 7.2, and filter-sterilized after dilution. The culture medium is RPMI 1640 containing 25 mM HEPES buffer, supplemented with 2 mM glutamine, 50 μM 2-mercaptoethanol, 1% normal mouse serum (stored frozen in 25 μM 2-mercapto-ethanol), penicillin (100 U/ml), streptomycin (100 μg/ml), and Fungizone (optional, 2.5 μg/ml). Day 14 SC or days 10–12 LNC from MTg/LPS- or MTg/CFA-primed CBA mice (Section I,D,3) are cultured in flasks with MTg (20–40 μg/ml). After 3 days at 37°C in 5% CO_2, the cells are washed and transferred i.v. into recipient mice at 2×10^7 SC or 1×10^7 LNC/mouse (Flynn *et al.*, 1989). An aliquot of cultured cells is plated in a 96-well plate to measure the proliferative response by [³H]thymidine uptake.

Concanavalin A (ConA) at 3 μg/ml (Okayasu, 1985; Simon *et al.*, 1986) and HTg, PTg, and bovine (B) Tg at 40 μg/ml (Kong *et al.*, 1986) can also be used to activate MTg-primed cells for transfer of thyroiditis. Con A activation is the least efficient for cell transfer, requiring about three times the cell number per mouse (Simon *et al.*, 1986).

T-cell lines (Maron *et al.*, 1983) and clones (Romball and Weigle, 1987) obtained after *in vivo* priming and *in vitro* activation have transferred thyroid-itis to irradiated recipients but unfortunately these lines have not remained stable. Recently, CD4⁺ cell lines and clones have been generated from thy-roid lesions to transfer disease to irradiated recipients (Sugihara *et al.*, 1993). The thyroidal T cells are derived from "B" mice (thymectomized and T-cell-depleted, then irradiated and bone marrow-reconstituted) which have been given a CD5^bright T-cell-depleted population. Curiously, only the thyroid is affected in these mice, although the CD5^dull population has not been enriched for thyroid antigens (Sugihara *et al.*, 1988).

The course of disease in recipients of cell transfer is generally rapid, with some infiltrating cells detectable at 4 (Braley-Mullen *et al.*, 1985) and 7 (Con-away *et al.*, 1990) days, and reaching maximum at 14–18 days. With little antigenic stimulation in the recipient, the anti-MTg titers are generally low.

6. Granulomatous Thyroid Lesion

After MTg/CFA immunization, mice of certain strains show both mono-nuclear and polymorphonuclear cell infiltration and, by the 4th week, also display granulomatous lesions resembling human subacute (de Quervain's) thyroiditis (Imahori and Vladutiu, 1983, 1984). Recently, MTg/LPS-primed SC cultured *in vitro* with both MTg and monoclonal antibodies (MAbs) to interleukin-2 (IL-2) receptor or interferon-γ (IFNγ) have been shown to transfer granulomatous thyroiditis to irradiated recipient mice (Braley-Mullen *et al.*, 1991; Stull *et al.*, 1992). Anti-MTg titers are also increased in such recipients.

E. Quantitation

In this section, the three basic parameters of EAT evaluation are described. Detailed methods for additional parameters are referenced.

1. Thyroid Infiltration

a. Basic histology. The extent of mononuclear cell infiltration in both thyroid lobes of each animal is determined by examining 60–70 sections from 10–12 step levels (about 30 hematoxylin and eosin sections/slide), and expressed as a pathology index (Rose *et al.*, 1971) or as percentage of thyroid involvement (Nabozny *et al.*, 1991) as follows: 0, no infiltration; 0.5, >0–10% with definite perivascular foci of infiltration; 1.0, >10–20% infiltration with follicular destruction; 2.0, >20–40% infiltration; 3.0, >40–80% infiltration; and 4.0, >80% infiltration. Statistical differences in pathology indices among groups are determined by the nonparametric Mann–Whitney U test (Kong *et al.*, 1979, 1989b).

   b. In situ analysis.   Typically, the infiltrate has <6% B cells and few polymorphonuclear cells at any given time. Macrophages vary from about 30 to 40%, partly because there are usually fewer T cells in the infiltrate after active immunization (31–46%) (Conaway *et al.*, 1989) than after adoptive transfer (35–56%) (Conaway *et al.*, 1990). The infiltrating T cells are largely TCR α/β^+ (Fuller *et al.*, unpublished data). Of particular interest are time-dependent changes in the composition of the T-cell subset. Thus, the CD4 : CD8 ratio fluctuates primarily because the $CD8^+$ T cells undergo cyclic variation. The kinetics can be analyzed by immunohistochemical labeling with appropriate MAbs. The technique of using various rat anti-mouse CD45 and other T- and B-cell markers, followed by treatment with biotinylated anti-rat IgG and avidin–biotin–peroxidase conjugate, has been detailed (Conaway *et al.*, 1989). Instead of frozen sections, freeze-dried, paraffin-embedded sections (Kong *et al.*, 1989b) can also be prepared from thyroid lobes in tissue embedding medium, quick-frozen in liquid nitrogen, and stored at −70°C.

2. *In Vitro* T-Cell Functional Assays

   a. Basic proliferative response.   As described earlier for adoptive transfer (Section I,D,5), SC or LNC from MTg-primed mice are assayed *in vitro* in 96-well plates at 4–6×10^5 cells/well in 0.2 ml of medium containing 40 μg/ml of various Tgs for 4–5 days. For the last 18 hr of culture, 1.2 μCi [^{3}H]thymidine is added. The cells are then harvested onto glass fiber filters, and counts per minute (cpm) determined (Flynn *et al.*, 1989). Stimulation indices are calculated by dividing the experimental mean cpm by the control mean cpm. The majority of the proliferating cells is $CD4^+$ (Stull *et al.*, 1988; Flynn *et al.*, 1989).

   b. Recognition of Tg epitopes.   T-cell clones and hybridomas have been derived from LNC of HTg-immunized (Krco *et al.*, 1990) or MTg-immunized (Champion *et al.*, 1987, 1991) mice to examine cross-reactivity with homologous and heterologous Tgs. In general, the clones do not transfer disease and are therefore not thyroiditogenic, and they recognize shared or conserved rather than MTg-unique epitopes. Two hybridomas derived from MTg-immune T-cell lines recognize a $T_4(2553)$-containing synthetic peptide on HTg (Champion *et al.*, 1991), which can activate primed cells *in vitro* for adoptive transfer (Hutchings *et al.*, 1992; Section I,D,2).

c. Cytotoxicity assay. CD8[+] Tc develop by day 5 *in vitro* after *in vivo*-primed LNC have been cultured with MTg (Creemers *et al.*, 1983; Simon *et al.*, 1986) or HTg (Simon *et al.*, 1986), and kill thyroid epithelial cells in a class I antigen-restricted manner. A cytotoxic T-cell hybridoma derived from PTg-immunized mice has also been described (Remy *et al.*, 1989). The specialized methods are detailed in the references.

3. Autoantibody Assay

a. Basic MTg antibody measurement. Anti-MTg antibody level is an indicator of priming and not thyroiditis. It is most useful as a measure of suppression after tolerance induction and challenge (Section I,F). In our hands, the passive hemagglutination assay is more sensitive than the ELISA for detecting low levels of IgM and IgG antibodies. Anti-MTg titers (with or without treatment with 0.1 M 2-mercaptoethanol) are determined with human group O erythrocytes coupled to MTg by $CrCl_3$ (.$6H_2O$) (Poston, 1974). In brief, the entire test is carried out in saline without phosphate. In quick mixing order, 0.2 ml MTg (1 mg/ml) is added to 0.2 ml packed erythrocytes, followed by 0.2 ml of 0.125% freshly prepared $CrCl_3$. After 4 min, the reaction is stopped with cold saline. After washing with diluent (1:150 normal rabbit serum in saline), an equal volume of the resuspended erythrocytes (1:80) is added to twofold dilutions of mouse antisera. Antibody levels are expressed in log_2 titers. ELISA for antibody titers is used in several laboratories (Williams *et al.*, 1987; Parish *et al.*, 1988).

b. Cross-reactive antibody measurement. The sensitive hemagglutination procedure is used to measure cross-reactive antibodies, for example, between MTg and HTg after cross-induction of tolerance (Nabozny *et al.*, 1990), and among MTg, HTg, and rabbit Tg after EAT induction with each Tg (Tomazic and Rose, 1976). With a panel of MAbs raised in mice against MTg (standard allogeneic mixture), it can detect alloantigenic differences on MTg (Kong *et al.*, 1980). The ELISA has also been used to test for cross-reactivity (Chronopoulou and Carayanniotis, 1992).

F. Natural and Acquired Resistance

1. Induction of Resistance (Suppression) with MTg

a. Pretreatment with exogenous MTg. Deaggregated (d) MTg is injected i.v. at 100 μg/0.1 ml of nonpyrogenic saline into susceptible (CBA) mice. It is either used directly off the column without centrifugation or is derived by ultracentrifuging stock MTg (1.5–2.0 mg/ml) at 100,000g for 60 min (an approximate loss of 30%) and adjusting the concentration at

280 nm (Lewis *et al.*, 1987). After two doses of dMTg 7 days apart (days −10, −3), challenge with the standard doses of 20 or 40 μg MTg + 20 μg LPS i.v. is carried out 3 days later (days 0, 7) and thyroiditis assayed on day 28 according to the above parameters (Section I,E). Both T and B cells are usually tolerant, with little MTg antibody production, no *in vitro* proliferation, and minimal thyroid infiltration (Kong *et al.*, 1982; Lewis *et al.*, 1987). The strong suppression is correlated with increased circulatory Tg level for ≥2–3 days (Lewis *et al.*, 1987), operates at the afferent phase to prevent EAT induction, and is demonstrable for at least 73 days (Fuller *et al.*, 1993). The abrogation of suppression of thyroiditis development by depleting CD4$^+$, but not CD8$^+$, cells prior to challenge shows that MTg-induced resistance is mediated by CD4$^+$ suppressor T cells (Ts) (Kong *et al.*, 1989a). Administration of 10,000 U of human recombinant IL-1β or polyadenylic·polyuridylic acid complex 3 hr after dMTg interferes with induction of resistance (Kong *et al.*, 1982; Nabozny and Kong, 1992).

   b. Pretreatment with endogenous MTg. Administration of thyroid-stimulating hormone (TSH) to release endogenous MTg in susceptible CBA mice also results in reduced thyroiditis after EAT induction with MTg/LPS (Lewis *et al.*, 1987; Fuller *et al.*, 1993). An Alzet mini-osmotic pump containing bovine TSH (about 0.21 ml at 10.4 U/ml) is placed in the peritoneal cavity under brief ether anesthesia, and the incision closed with Autoclips. Each pump delivers TSH at the rate of 0.25 U/day for 7–8 days. Because a 3½-day delivery is sufficient, the pump is usually removed on day 4 and placed in another mouse which becomes similarly resistant to EAT induction. At 6 hr after pump implantation, each mouse is given i.v. 20 μg *E. coli* LPS (if the challenge adjuvant is *S. enteritidis* LPS), which serves to delay MTg clearance (Lewis *et al.*, 1992). Compared with exogenous MTg doses, the raised MTg level is insufficient to induce complete B-cell tolerance and MTg antibody titers are observed in many animals after challenge, but thyroiditis is markedly reduced. TSH-induced resistance lasts for at least 66 days (Fuller *et al.*, 1993) and is also mediated by CD4$^+$ Ts (Kong *et al.*, 1989a).

2. Induction of Resistance with Idiotype-Bearing T Cells

   Vaccination with irradiated, MTg-primed, MTg-activated T cells, given i.v. 14 days apart at 2–3 × 10^7/dose, also reduces thyroiditis in challenged mice without necessarily lowering antibody production (Flynn and Kong, 1991), as first reported with T-cell lines (Maron *et al.*, 1983). Both CD4$^+$ and CD8$^+$ Ts are implicated in the suppression (Flynn and Kong, 1991). Another group uses a PTg-derived hybridoma, which induces resistance to PTg immunization by stimulating an anti-idiotype network against the shared epitope(s) (Texier *et al.*, 1992a).

3. Natural Resistance

In addition to demonstrating naturally existing Ts in susceptible mice by stimulating or expanding them with MTg as described above, natural resistance can be overcome by neonatal thymectomy, which results in the spontaneous development several months later of MTg autoantibodies and thyroiditis in 25% females and 6% males (Kojima *et al.*, 1976). However, treatment with cyclophosphamide, ostensibly depleting Ts, neither enhances EAT induction in naive mice nor abrogates established MTg-induced resistance (Kong *et al.*, 1989a).

In certain EAT-resistant strains, on the other hand, cyclophosphamide administration has resulted in the development of thyroid lesions following immunization, presumably by inhibiting suppressor activity in these animals (Vladutiu, 1982). Moreover, by cell transfer into *nu/nu* or "B" mice, the removal of the Lyt-1$^+$,2,3$^-$ or CD5^{bright} T-cell subset respectively from EAT-resistant (Sakaguchi *et al.*, 1985; Sakaguchi and Sakaguchi, 1990) or F$_1$ responder (Sugihara *et al.*, 1988, 1993) donors enables the remaining T cells to induce thyroiditis. These studies indicate that, in certain susceptible and resistant strains, Ts are normally present to inhibit SAT (Section III,B).

Recently, a synthetic peptide, 774–788, derived from porcine thyroid peroxidase (TPO) has been shown to induce thyroiditis in an EAT-resistant (C57BL/6) strain (Kotani *et al.*, 1992), thus distinguishing it from Tg peptides. The antibodies produced do not stain mouse, but do stain porcine thyroid sections. About 10–25% of this strain also display some infiltration after CFA immunization. Further confirmatory studies will determine if a model to another thyroid antigen is being established.

II. Experimental Autoimmune Thyroiditis in the Rat

A. History of the Model

Both an induced and a spontaneous model have been used to study rat EAT. EAT induced with RTg and CFA was first described in 1961 and the inflammatory lesions were noted to regress with time (Jones and Roitt, 1961). Subsequent use of pertussis vaccine as co-adjuvant shows that disease can progress with little evidence of regression (Paterson and Drobish, 1968; Twarog and Rose, 1969), and this method of induction is now used by most groups. However, because of the lack of recombinant strains and general immunologic reagents, more studies have continued in the mouse than in the rat.

The Buffalo (BUF) rat strain has been used as the spontaneous model with an incidence of 54% first noted in males at about 8 months (Hajdu and Rona, 1969). From the many studies performed by Rose and co-workers (see Rose *et al.*, 1977), we have learned that: autoantibodies to RTg appear with thyroid infiltration; females are affected three times more frequently than males; 30–60 weeks are optimal for thyroiditis with an incidence of 48%; and methylcholanthrene or neonatal thymectomy accelerates disease. However, in recent years, the incidence has decreased such that neonatal thymectomy needs to be used to promote SAT (Cohen *et al.*, 1988). The increased susceptibility to infection has made this a much less used model.

As seen in the NOD mouse (Section I,D,1), the BioBreeding/Worcester (BB/W) rat, a model for spontaneous Type I diabetes, also develops thyroiditis. The first colony had 59% incidence reported in 8- to 10-month-old diabetic rats, and 11% in the nondiabetic (Sternthal *et al.*, 1981). However, this strain was not inbred and was highly lymphopenic. Recent sublines derived from it show 5–100% incidence of SAT at 3 months of age, compared to 30–75% for diabetes, an obvious dissociation (Rajatanavin *et al.*, 1991).

B. The Animals

General guidelines described for mouse EAT are applicable here; standard rat or rodent lab chow and tapwater are used for the induced model. Special care for thymectomized BUF strain or other thymectomy and irradiation-induced models (Section II,F), as well as for the diabetic BB rat, should be followed. Some genetic considerations are summarized in Section II,C, but female rats, 8–12 weeks of age, of strains AUG(RT.1^c), LEW(RT.1^l), WKY(RT.1^k), and WF(RT.1^u), are generally susceptible.

C. Genetic Considerations

With induced EAT, strain differences in susceptibility (Rose, 1975) as well as strain variations within the same genotype (Penhale *et al.*, 1975b) have been reported, but the extent of MHC influence on susceptibility as observed in the mouse (Vladutiu and Rose, 1971) continues to be controversial. The lack of congenic strains made the contribution of MHC genes at first seemed less important (Lillehoj *et al.*, 1981; Lillehoj and Rose, 1982), but the recent use of congenic strains has segregated the susceptible (RT.1^c) from the resistant (RT.1^u) haplotype (De Assis-Paiva *et al.*, 1989). However, the observations that RT.1^u on different background genes is susceptible indicate the involvement of non-MHC genes.

Cross-breeding studies between the BUF(RT.1^b) strain and BB(RT.1^u) strain has linked SAT to the RT.1^b haplotype, dissociating it from pancreatic

Warning!

The due date of your books may change due to a RECALL!

- All materials checked out are subject to recall if needed by another borrower or by Reserves.
- Once recalled, a notice will be sent via email or mail. The material is now due on the *new due date* printed on the notice.
- Return the book promptly to avoid being fined. The minimum recall fine is $11.00 for the first late day plus $1.00 for each day thereafter.
- Being out of town does not excuse recall fines. If you are to be away from UCR for more than one week, return the material before you leave or arrange to have a friend or colleague return the material in your absence.
- If material is recalled and you still need it, ask at the Circulation Desk for further information.

This recall policy applies to all borrowers.

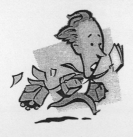
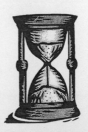

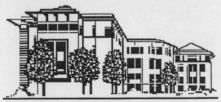
Science Library

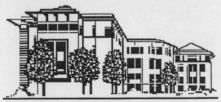
UCR Science Library

*For Further
Information About
Recalls*

Please Contact Us:
Science Library
Circulation:
(951) 827-3701
scicirc@library.ucr.edu

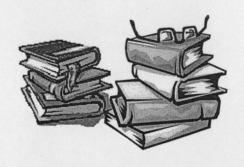

insulitis governed by RT.1^u (Colle *et al.*, 1985). Thyroiditis occurs equally in both sexes, in contrast to the predilection for BUF females (Rose *et al.*, 1977).

D. The Disease

1. Spontaneous Development in the BUF and BB Rat

As mentioned above, the BUF strain has undergone changes due to unknown genetic and/or environmental factors, and the incidence of SAT has decreased drastically from 17 to 50% (depending on age) to near 0% unless the animals are thymectomized or immunized with RTg/CFA (Cohen and Weetman, 1987), resembling more an induced model. Thymectomy is usually performed within 24 hr of birth and raises the incidence to >30% (Cohen and Weetman, 1987; Allen and Braverman, 1990). Although TSH levels show some increases as seen in HT, germinal centers, also found in HT, and originally observed in 33% of BUF rats with SAT (Silverman and Rose, 1978), are no longer discernible (Cohen and Weetman, 1987).

Increase in dietary iodine enhances SAT in both BUF (Cohen and Weetman, 1988; Allen and Braverman, 1990) and BB/W (Rajatanavin *et al.*, 1991) rats. In the BB/W rat (Banovac *et al.*, 1988), the effect of T_4 in the drinking water is immunosuppressive, lowering RTg and TPO antibody titers and incidence of thyroiditis, whereas T_4 has little effect on induced EAT (Weetman *et al.*, 1982b).

2. Autoantigens for Active Induction

a. RTg preparation. Essentially the same procedure for MTg (Section I,D,2) is used to prepare RTg (Lillehoj *et al.*, 1981) and the same precautions apply.

b. Pathogenic peptide. The same synthetic peptide, a 17-mer peptide of 2495–2511 (TgP1) from RTg, which induces EAT in susceptible mice (Chronopoulou and Carayanniotis, 1992), also induces EAT in susceptible rats (Balasa and Carayanniotis, 1993). However, it does not cross-stimulate RTg-primed LNC.

3. Active Induction Protocol

Preparation of the RTg/CFA emulsion is similar to MTg/CFA (Section I,D,3), but Difco CFA containing 1 mg/ml *M. butyricum* (or *M. tuberculosis* H37Ra) is adequate, since killed *Bordetella pertussis* is used as co-adjuvant (Lillehoj *et al.*, 1981). RTg at 10 mg/ml is mixed with CFA at a 1:1 ratio. Each rat receives 1 mg in 0.2 ml emulsion divided into the four footpads on each of days 0 and 7. On day 0 only, 2×10^8 pertussis bacilli in 0.4 ml are injected in divided doses onto the dorsal side of the footpads. The animals are killed for thyroid pathology on days 28–30.

4. Course of Disease

Thyroid infiltration reaches maximum by day 21 and shows no regression until after day 30 (Twarog and Rose, 1969; Lillehoj and Rose, 1982). Depending on the strain, anti-RTg is detectable by days 7–14, and, as in mouse EAT, there is no correlation between RTg antibody titers and pathology (Rose, 1975). *In vitro* proliferative response of LNC to RTg increases by day 21 and reaches maximum by day 30 (Lillehoj and Rose, 1982).

5. Transfer of Disease

LNC are obtained from Lewis donors 10 days after immunization with RTg/CFA, and 4.8×10^8 cells are transferred into normal recipients. High incidence is observed without irradiation of recipients (350–550 rads reduce severity), and incubation for 60 min with 0.3 mg RTg enhances severity in the recipients (Rose *et al.*, 1973). As in mouse EAT, antibody levels are very low and thyroiditis develops more rapidly compared with active induction. Infiltration is observed at 1 day after transfer, becoming severe in 3–7 days.

In the diabetic model, thyroiditis can be transferred from BB/W rats to MHC-compatible *nu/nu* recipients with 4×10^7 SC which have been activated *in vitro* with ConA (5 µg/ml) for 3 days. An incidence of 59% is observed (McKeever *et al.*, 1990).

E. Quantitation

The same three basic parameters for EAT evaluation in the mouse are applicable to the rat and are briefly described. Additional parameters are referenced.

1. Thyroid Infiltration

a. Basic histology. The grading of pathology on a scale from 0 to 4 (Twarog and Rose, 1969) is similar to mouse EAT (Section I,E,1).

b. In situ analysis. Immunohistochemical analysis of the leukocyte composition in the thyroid is carried out by several laboratories with the appropriate MAbs for rat antigens to measure class II antigen expression, T-cell subsets, and macrophages. The avidin-biotin-peroxidase technique has been used for SAT in neonatally thymectomized BUF rats (Cohen *et al.*, 1988), and dual-specificity staining with biotinylated and indirect immunofluorescence described for induced EAT (De Assis-Paiva *et al.*, 1989). Similar to mouse EAT (Conaway *et al.*, 1989), there are few B cells, but a high proportion of T cells belong to the CD8+ subset (De Assis-Paiva *et al.*, 1989).

2. *In Vitro* T-Cell Functional Assays

a. Basic proliferative response. As with mouse EAT, T-cell proliferative response to RTg correlates well with thyroiditis and the footpad immunization used for induction prepares the popliteal and inguinal LNC for this response (Lillehoj and Rose, 1982; Balasa and Carayanniotis, 1993). The medium used is similar to mouse EAT (Section I,D,5) except 10% fetal calf serum is used. LNC are obtained 14–30 days after immunization and cultured at $2–4 \times 10^5$ cells/well with RTg (50 μg/ml) for 3–4 days. At 18 hr prior to harvest, 1 μCi [^{3}H]thymidine is added and cpm are determined.

b. Recognition of Tg epitopes. T-cell clones recognizing shared epitopes between rat and mouse Tg have been generated from LNC obtained from Tg-primed (BUF × Fisher) F_1 rats (Hirose and Davies, 1988). The clones are CD4$^+$ and exhibit either helper or suppressor activity for B cells, and, as seen in mouse EAT (Section I,E,2), are unlikely to be thyroiditogenic *in vivo*.

3. Autoantibody Assay

a. Basic RTg antibody measurement. Antibody levels do not correlate with thyroiditis and are measured primarily as an indicator of sensitization. Both passive hemagglutination with RTg coupled to erythrocytes with CrCl$_3$ (Lillehoj and Rose, 1982; Section I,E,3) and a standard ELISA detailed in Weetman *et al.* (1982a) are used.

b. Cross-reactive antibody measurement. The sensitive hemagglutination procedure has been used to measure alloantigenic differences among RTgs from several strains (Rose, 1975). Lacking the MAb technology applied later to MTg (Kong *et al.*, 1980; Section I,E,3), these workers could not use the polyclonal antibodies to determine whether the antigenic differences were qualitative and/or quantitative.

4. Thyroid Functional Assay

The availability of a rat standard TSH has prompted the measurement of circulatory T_4 or TSH level as an indicator of thyroid dysfunction. Despite the sensitivity of radioimmunoassay, neither has proven reliable as a gauge for thyroid inflammation in induced EAT since both the rat and mouse appear to compensate well for the follicular destruction.

In SAT, neonatal thymectomy of the BUF strain induces higher TSH levels than immunization (Cohen and Weetman, 1987). With both neonatal thymectomy and supplemental dietary iodine, TSH levels and the incidence of thyroiditis are increased (Allen and Braverman, 1990).

In the BB/W sublines with the incidence of thyroiditis varying from 5 to 100%, there are no consistent differences in serum T_4 or TSH level (Rajatanavin *et al.*, 1991). Only when iodine intake is increased for 8 weeks are

TSH levels elevated, and only in the 100% incidence subline are both levels affected.

F. Natural and Acquired Resistance

Acquired resistance induced by specific antigens in rat EAT has not received the attention extended to mouse EAT (Section I,F,1). Instead, natural resistance has been reduced by neonatal thymectomy in the BUF rat to promote SAT (Cohen et al., 1988). Also, in female rats of susceptible strains, adult thymectomy at 3 weeks followed by repeated low-dose irradiation (200 rads four times at 2-week intervals) leads to 80–100% incidence of spontaneous thyroiditis and production of Tg autoantibodies after 60 days (Penhale et al., 1975a, 1975b). As described for mouse EAT (Section I,F,3), reconstitution studies show a regulatory T cell suppressing SAT in these strains (Penhale et al., 1976).

In studies with the diabetic BB/W model, the removal of a RT6$^+$ regulatory T-cell subset from SC donors enables the remaining population to transfer diabetes and thyroiditis to *nu/nu* recipients (McKeever et al., 1990). However, the incidence of one does not correlate with the other, and the sublines of BB/W vary greatly (5–100%) in their incidence of thyroiditis (Rajatanavin et al., 1991). Thus, it is unknown to what extent the RT6$^+$ cell may contribute to suppressing SAT in these strains.

III. Lessons

A. Expert Experience

The features important in establishing the EAT model for study have been incorporated into the appropriate sections. Additional points salient to understanding the uses of this model are given here.

1. EAT as A Prototype Autoimmune Disease

Not only is EAT the first autoimmune disease to be shown to correlate with human thyroid disease, it remains the primary autoimmune disease with known autoantigens for induction similar to HT, its human counterpart. The antigens, HTg and TPO, have now been cloned, and a study with porcine TPO to construct a potential animal model is beginning (Kotani et al., 1992). Although the need for hundreds of mouse thyroids has prevented some groups from using homologous MTg, it is well known that MTg induces more severe and chronic disease than heterologous Tgs, lasting for 12–18 months (Okayasu et al., 1989). And, MTg contains unique epitope(s) (Nabozny et al.,

1990), besides those shared and/or conserved on HTg, PTg, and BTg (Kong et al., 1986; Section I,D,2); the recently defined epitopes are all shared (Hutchings et al., 1992; Texier et al., 1992b; Balasa and Carayanniotis, 1993). One contains a T_4 hormonogenic site (Hutchings et al., 1992) and one lacks any iodine (Chronopoulou and Carayanniotis, 1992), indicating that iodination (Champion et al., 1991) is not a requirement for immunogenicity. None of them is immunodominant, suggesting that EAT induction may result from several thyroiditogenic epitopes.

As to choosing between an induced or a spontaneous model, it is necessary to realize that neonatal thymectomy is now necessary to have a baseline incidence of >30% for the BUF rat. The appeal of the diabetic BB/W or NOD model for autoimmune endocrine disease featuring both diabetes and thyroiditis should be tempered by variations among colonies and sublines unless the factors, for example, genetic or environmental, relating to each disease entity become better understood (Sections I,D,1; II,D,1).

2. Study of Pathogenic Mechanisms

For both induced mouse and rat EAT, the in vitro proliferative response to Tg correlates well with thyroiditis development but not severity. The measurements of serum T_4 and TSH levels, on the other hand, are not reliable indicators of thyroid dysfunction (Section II,E,4). Thus, as in other autoimmune disease models, target organ pathology remains the most reliable index of disease.

In in situ analysis of the cellular infiltrate, the cyclic increase and decline of $CD8^+$ T cells (Conaway et al., 1989; 1990) indicate that a single time point cannot be used to determine the efficacy of various treatment modalities in influencing subset composition. For detection of $CD4^+$ and $CD8^+$ subsets in the infiltrate or depletion in vivo of a particular subset, we use synergistic pairs of rat MAbs, which recognize different epitopes on the same CD4 or CD8 molecule, thereby increasing their efficiency (Kong et al., 1989a, 1989b). These studies show that regulatory T cells are $CD4^+$, the subsets in the infiltrate are independent of each other, and the most efficacious immunotherapy requires the administration of MAbs to both subsets.

3. Study of Regulatory Mechanisms

An induced model provides the opportunity to study underlying mechanisms of self-tolerance prior to disease induction. Since thyroid hormone and circulatory MTg levels are controlled by TSH stimulation, its administration is used to study the mechanisms of normal regulation in a natural, physiological manner (Lewis et al., 1987, 1992). That $CD4^+$ Ts are involved in suppression of mouse EAT in susceptible mice (Kong et al., 1989a) has been confirmed for other autoimmune diseases. Other methods of depleting regulatory T cells and using *nu/nu* (Sakaguchi *et al.*, 1985) or "B" (Sugihara *et al.*, 1988) recipients, and of using thymectomized and sublethally irradiated mice (Ansar Ahmed and Penhale, 1981) lead to low incidence in relatively resistant hosts, and represent more extreme manipulations and probably fairly extreme human conditions. Such studies serve to illustrate that the weight of MHC-based regulation can be diminished and that there could exist different levels of tolerance in polygenic humans under a variety of environmental conditions.

B. Relationships to Hashimoto's Thyroiditis

A discussion of the early years during which work on mouse EAT and its counterpart HT drew from each other has been presented (Kong, 1986). As mentioned earlier (Section III,A,1), since the animal models and HT have Tgs as self-antigens with a high degree of homology, the potential relevance of animal studies to HT is increased. A few more recent features will be highlighted here.

1. Importance of MHC and Non-MHC Genes

In mouse EAT we see the classic demonstration of the first autoimmune disease in which the MHC is highly influential (Vladutiu and Rose, 1971), as verified recently in the rat (De Assis-Paiva *et al.*, 1989). Many HLA associations with autoimmune thyroid disease, including Graves' disease (Farid, 1991), and other autoimmune diseases, have followed, with relative risks varying with the particular disease. The relatively weak association of the HLA complex with HT in no way diminishes the importance of the MHC for a number of reasons. Autoimmune thyroid disease is a composite of several entities which exist in familial clusters and display ethnic differences in HLA association.

Recent transgenic studies reaffirm the extent of class II gene involvement by showing the *H-2A* genes transferring susceptibility to a resistant strain, presumably promoting antigen presentation (Kong *et al.*, 1992), and the E_α gene rendering an E^--susceptible strain resistant (Section I,C,1). As our knowledge of the HLA class II genes is incomplete, more studies that include families are needed in HT. In addition, studies with synthetic epitopes shared with MTg have not revealed any immunodominant sites (Section III,A,1). The involvement of several thyroiditogenic epitopes would make the demonstration of HLA association more difficult, but the conserved epitopes illustrate their potential usefulness for human studies.

Less important but nevertheless demonstrable are the class I and non-*H-2* gene effects in mouse EAT (Section I,C,2). These studies support the polygenic influences seen in HT.

2. Correlation in T Cell Functions

The demonstration of T-cell mediation of EAT (Vladutiu and Rose, 1975) has been followed by *in vitro* proliferative response to Tg (Okayasu *et al.*, 1981a; Lillehoj and Rose, 1982), the transfer of EAT with T-cell lines and clones, and killing of thyroid target cells by $CD8^+$ Tc, differentiated *in vitro* and restricted by class I antigen (Section I,D; II,D). These studies have led to reports of peripheral T cells from HT responding to HTg (Canonica *et al.*, 1984; Weetman *et al.*, 1985) and thyroidal T-cell clones responding to and cytotoxic for thyroid cells (Mackenzie *et al.*, 1987).

The *in situ* analysis of thyroidal T-cell composition shows further correlation in the high proportion of the $CD8^+$ subset in HT (Canonica *et al.*, 1985), mouse EAT (Conaway *et al.*, 1989, 1990), and rat EAT (De Assis-Paiva *et al.*, 1989). The importance of both $CD4^+$ and $CD8^+$ T cells in mouse EAT is seen by the efficacy of combined immunotherapy of advanced disease with CD4 and CD8 MAbs (two doses in 4 days), clearing many thyroids of all T cells and macrophages (Kong *et al.*, 1989b).

3. Regulatory T-Cell Analogy

For obvious reasons, *in vivo* regulatory T-cell studies can only be conducted in animal models. Since the triggering mechanisms for HT are unknown, it is generally considered a spontaneous disease. However, since many individuals with the proper genetic predisposition, circulating antigen, and periodic polyclonal stimuli do not develop disease, or only harbor Tg autoantibodies without overt thyroid dysfunction, HT could be closer to an "induced" disease than previously realized. Manipulations, such as increased dietary iodine and/or neonatal thymectomy, enhance thyroiditis only in highly prone strains (BB/W and BUF strains; Section II,D,1), and thymectomy + irradiation doses result in a <10% incidence of SAT in certain mouse strains (Ansar Ahmed and Penhale, 1981). Other transfers of SAT also require the depletion of certain T-cell subsets and the use of T-cell-deficient hosts (Sakaguchi *et al.*, 1985; Sugihara *et al.*, 1988; Section I,D,5).

These studies illustrate the strong, normally existing regulatory influence and support our hypothesis of clonal balance between Ts and autoreactive inducer T cells (Ti), with Ts normally in dominance (Kong *et al.*, 1982; Kong, 1986). The effect of Ts can be overridden when sufficient immunogenic signals stimulate the Ti toward autoimmunity, as seen when IL-1 is given with dMTg (Nabozny and Kong, 1992). To simulate human conditions, TSH is infused for several days to raise circulatory MTg levels for 2–3 days (Lewis *et al.*, 1987, 1992; Section I,F,1). The resultant $CD4^+$ Ts suppress thyroid infiltration, but not necessarily Tg autoantibody production, in immunized mice. Thus, we postulate that a possible function of circulatory MTg is to maintain the dominance of Ts and raise the defense when appropriately stimulated to a level higher than normal, and higher than the level provided by "vaccination" *in vivo* by idiotype-bearing cells, which may also exist in low numbers after triggering (Roubaty *et al.*, 1990; Flynn and Kong, 1991; Section I,F,2).

In summary, EAT and HT have many characteristics in common: the same antigen in Tg, shared epitopes, T-cell proliferation to and cytotoxicity for thyroid epithelial target cells, and, by inference, regulatory T cells operating at several levels to prevent autoreactive T cells from being triggered and/or expanded.

Acknowledgments

This work is supported by the National Institute of Diabetes, and Digestive and Kidney Diseases, DK 45960, and St. John Hospital, Detroit. The expert assistance of Brian Fuller both in performing experiments and preparing the manuscript is gratefully acknowledged.

References

Allen, E. M., and Braverman, L. E. (1990). *Endocrinology* **127**, 1613–1616.

Ansar Ahmed, S., and Penhale, W. J. (1981). *Experientia* **37**, 1341–1343.

Asamoto, H., Oishi, M., Akazawa, Y., and Tochino, Y. (1986). *In* "Insulitis and Type I Diabetes: Lessons from the NOD Mouse" (S. Tarui, Y. Tochino, and K. Nonaka, Eds.), pp. 61–71. Academic Press, Tokyo.

Balasa, B., and Carayanniotis, G. (1993). *Cell. Immunol.* **148**, 259–268.

Banovac, K., Ghandur-Mnaymneh, L., Zakarija, M., Rabinovitch, A., and McKenzie, J. M. (1988). *Int. Arch. Allergy Appl. Immunol.* **87**, 301–305.

Beisel, K. W., David, C. S., Giraldo, A. A., Kong, Y. M., and Rose, N. R. (1982a). *Immunogenetics* **15**, 427–430.

Beisel, K. W., Kong, Y. M., Babu, K. S. J., David, C. S., and Rose, N. R. (1982b). *J. Immunogenet.* **9**, 257–265.

Ben-Nun, A., Maron, R., Ron, Y., and Cohen, I. R. (1980). *Eur. J. Immunol.* **10**, 156–159.

Bernard, N. F., Ertug, F., and Margolese, H. (1992). *Diabetes* **41**, 40–46.

Bhatia, S. K., Rose, N. R., Schofield, B., Lafond-Walker, A., and Kuppers, R. C. (1993). *J. Immunol.* **150**, 162A.

Braley-Mullen, H., Johnson, M., Sharp, G. C., and Kyriakos, M. (1985). *Cell. Immunol.* **93**, 132–143.

Braley-Mullen, H., Sharp, G. C., Bickel, J. T., and Kyriakos, M. (1991). *J. Exp. Med.* **173**, 899–912.

Canonica, G. W., Cosulich, M. E., Croci, R., Ferrini, S., Bagnasco, M., Dirienzo, W., Ferrini, O., Bargellesi, A., and Giordano, G. (1984). *Clin. Immunol. Immunopathol.* **32**, 132–141.

Canonica, G. W., Caria, M., Bagnasco, M., Cosulich, M. E., Giordano, G., and Moretta, L. (1985). *Clin. Immunol. Immunopathol.* **36**, 40–48.

Champion, B. R., Page, K., Rayner, D. C., Quartey-Papafio, R., Byfield, P. G., and Henderson, G. (1987). *Immunology* **62**, 255–263.

Champion, B. R., Page, K. R., Parish, N., Rayner, D. C., Dawe, K., Biswas-Hughes, G., Cooke, A., Geysen, M., and Roitt, I. M. (1991). *J. Exp. Med.* **174**, 363–370.

Christadoss, P., Kong, Y. M., ElRehewy, M., Rose, N. R., and David, C. S. (1978). *In* "Genetic Control of Autoimmune Disease" (N. R. Rose, P. E. Bigazzi, and N. L. Warner, Eds.), pp. 445–454. Elsevier–North Holland, New York.

Chronopoulou, E., and Carayanniotis, G. (1992). *J. Immunol.* **149**, 1039–1044.

Chronopoulou, E., and Carayanniotis, G. (1993). *Immunogenetics* **38**, 150–153.

Cohen, S. B., and Weetman, A. P. (1987). *Clin. Exp. Immunol.* **69**, 25–32.

Cohen, S. B., and Weetman, A. P. (1988). *J. Endocrinol. Invest.* **11**, 625–627.

Cohen, S. B., Dijkstra, C. D., and Weetman, A. P. (1988). *Cell. Immunol.* **114**, 126–136.

Colle, E., Guttmann, R. D., and Seemayer, T. A. (1985). *Endocrinology* **116**, 1243–1247.

Conaway, D. H., Giraldo, A. A., David, C. S., and Kong, Y. M. (1989). *Clin. Immunol. Immunopathol.* **53**, 346–353.

Conaway, D. H., Giraldo, A. A., David, C. S., and Kong, Y. M. (1990). *Cell. Immunol.* **125**, 247–253.

Creemers, P., Rose, N. R., and Kong, Y. M. (1983). *J. Exp. Med.* **157**, 559–571.

Creemers, P., Giraldo, A. A., Rose, N. R., and Kong, Y. M. (1984). *Cell. Immunol.* **87**, 692–697.

De Assis-Paiva, H. J., Rayner, D. C., Roitt, I. M., and Cooke, A. (1989). *Clin. Exp. Immunol.* **75**, 106–112.

ElRehewy, M., Kong, Y. M., Giraldo, A. A., and Rose, N. R. (1981). *Eur. J. Immunol.* **11**, 146–151.

Esquivel, P. S., Rose, N. R., and Kong, Y. M. (1977). *J. Exp. Med.* **145**, 1250–1263.

Farid, N. R. (1991). *In* "The Immunogenetics of Autoimmune Diseases" (N. R. Farid, Ed.), Vol. II, pp. 163–177. CRC Press, Boca Raton, FL.

Flynn, J. C., and Kong, Y. M. (1991). *Clin. Immunol. Immunopathol.* **60**, 484–494.

Flynn, J. C., Conaway, D. H., Cobbold, S., Waldmann, H., and Kong, Y. M. (1989). *Cell. Immunol.* **122**, 377–390.

Fuller, B. E., Okayasu, I., Simon, L. L., Giraldo, A. A., and Kong, Y. M. (1993). *Clin. Immunol. Immunopathol.* **69**, 60–68.

Hajdu, A., and Rona, G. (1969). *Experientia* **25**, 1325–1327.

Hirose, W., and Davies, T. F. (1988). *Immunology* **64**, 107–112.

Hutchings, P. R., Cooke, A., Dawe, K., Champion, B. R., Geysen, M., Valerio, R., and Roitt, I. M. (1992). *J. Exp. Med.* **175**, 869–872.

Imahori, S. C., and Vladutiu, A. O. (1983). *Proc. Soc. Exp. Biol. Med.* **173**, 408–416.

Imahori, S. C., and Vladutiu, A. O. (1984). *Clin. Immunol. Immunopathol.* **33**, 87–98.

Jones, H. E. H., and Roitt, I. M. (1961). *Br. J. Exp. Pathol.* **42**, 546–557.

Kojima, A., Tanaka-Kojima, Y., Sakakura, T., and Nishizuka, Y. (1976). *Lab. Invest.* **34**, 550–557.

Kong, Y. M. (1986). *In* "Immunology of Endocrine Diseases" (A. M. McGregor, Ed.), pp. 1–24. MTP Press Ltd., Lancaster, UK.

Kong, Y. M., David, C. S., Giraldo, A. A., ElRehewy, M., and Rose, N. R. (1979). *J. Immunol.* **123**, 15–18.

Kong, Y. M., Rose, N. R., ElRehewy, M., Michaels, R., Giraldo, A. A., Accavitti, M. A., and Leon, M. A. (1980). *Transpl. Proc.* **12** (Suppl. 1), 129–134.

Kong, Y. M., Okayasu, I., Giraldo, A. A., Beisel, K. W., Sundick, R. S., Rose, N. R., David, C. S., Audibert, F., and Chedid, L. (1982). *Ann. N. Y. Acad. Sci.* **392**, 191–209.

Kong, Y. M., Audibert, F., Giraldo, A. A., Rose, N. R., and Chedid, L. (1985). *Infect. Immun.* **49**, 40–45.

Kong, Y. M., Giraldo, A. A., Justen, J. M., Simon, L. L., and Fuller, B. E. (1986). *In* "The Thyroid and Autoimmunity" (H. A. Drexhage and W. M. Wiersinga, Eds.), pp. 151–152. Elsevier Science Publishers B.V. (Biomedical Division), Amsterdam.

Kong, Y. M., Giraldo, A. A., Waldmann, H., Cobbold, S. P., and Fuller, B. E. (1989a). *Clin. Immunol. Immunopathol.* **51**, 38–54.

Kong, Y. M., Waldmann, H., Cobbold, S., Giraldo, A. A., Fuller, B. E., and Simon, L. L. (1989b). *Clin. Exp. Immunol.* **77**, 428–433.

Kong, Y. M., Fuller, B. E., Giraldo, A. A., David, C. S., Krco, C. J., and Beito, T. G. (1992). *8th Int. Congr. Immunol.* 611.

Kotani, T., Umeki, K., Yagihashi, S., Hirai, K., and Ohtaki, S. (1992). *J. Immunol.* **148**, 2084–2089.

Krco, C. J., Gores, A., David, C. S., and Kong, Y. M. (1990). *J. Immunogenet.* **17**, 361–370.

Lewis, M., Giraldo, A. A., and Kong, Y. M. (1987). *Clin. Immunol. Immunopathol.* **45**, 92–104.

Lewis, M., Fuller, B. E., Giraldo, A. A., and Kong, Y. M. (1992). *Clin. Immunol. Immunopathol.* **64**, 197–204.

Lillehoj, H. S., and Rose, N. R. (1982). *Clin. Exp. Immunol.* **47**, 661–669.

Lillehoj, H. S., Beisel, K., and Rose, N. R. (1981). *J. Immunol.* **127**, 654–659.

Mackenzie, W. A., Schwartz, A. E., Friedman, E. W., and Davies, T. F. (1987). *J. Clin. Endocrinol. Metab.* **64**, 818–824.

Maron, R., Zerubavel, R., Friedman, A., and Cohen, I. R. (1983). *J. Immunol.* **131**, 2316–2322.

McKeever, U., Mordes, J. P., Greiner, D. L., Appel, M. C., Rozing, J., Handler, E. S., and Rossini, A. A. (1990). *Proc. Natl. Acad. Sci. USA* **87**, 7618–7622.

Nabozny, G. H., and Kong, Y. M. (1992). *J. Immunol.* **149**, 1086–1092.

Nabozny, G. H., Simon, L. L., and Kong, Y. M. (1990). *Cell. Immunol.* **131**, 140–149.

Nabozny, G. H., Flynn, J. C., and Kong, Y. M. (1991). *Cell. Immunol.* **136**, 340–348.

Okayasu, I. (1985). *Clin. Immunol. Immunopathol.* **36**, 101–109.

Okayasu, I., and Hatakeyama, S. (1983). *Clin. Immunol. Immunopathol.* **29**, 51–57.

Okayasu, I., Kong, Y. M., David, C. S., and Rose, N. R. (1981a). *Cell. Immunol.* **61**, 32–39.

Okayasu, I., Kong, Y. M., and Rose, N. R. (1981b). *Clin. Immunol. Immunopathol.* **20**, 240–245.

Okayasu, I., Hatakeyama, S., and Kong, Y. M. (1989). *Clin. Immunol. Immunopathol.* **53**, 254–267.

Parish, N. M., Roitt, I. M., and Cooke, A. (1988). *Eur. J. Immunol.* **18**, 1463–1467.

Paterson, P. Y., and Drobish, D. G. (1968). *J. Immunol.* **101**, 1098–1101.

Penhale, W. J., Farmer, A., and Irvine, W. J. (1975a). *Clin. Exp. Immunol.* **21**, 362–375.

Penhale, W. J., Farmer, A., Urbaniak, S. J., and Irvine, W. J. (1975b). *Clin. Exp. Immunol.* **19**, 179–191.

Penhale, W. J., Irvine, W. J., Inglis, J. R., and Farmer, A. (1976). *Clin. Exp. Immunol.* **25**, 6–16.

Poston, R. N. (1974). *J. Immunol. Methods* **5**, 91–96.

Rajatanavin, R., Appel, M. C., Reinhardt, W., Alex, S., Yang, Y.-N., and Braverman, L. E. (1991). *Endocrinology* **128**, 153–157.

Remy, J.-J., Texier, B., Chiocchia, G., and Charreire, J. (1989). *J. Immunol.* **142**, 1129–1133.

Romball, C. G., and Weigle, W. O. (1987). *J. Immunol.* **138**, 1092–1098.

Rose, N. R. (1975). *Cell. Immunol.* **18**, 360–364.

Rose, N. R. (1976). *In* "Textbook of Immunopathology" (P. A. Miescher and H. J. Muller-Eberhard, Eds.), pp. 215–229. Grune & Stratton, New York.

Rose, N. R., Twarog, F. J., and Crowle, A. J. (1971). *J. Immunol.* **106**, 698–704.

Rose, N. R., Molotchnikoff, M.-F., and Twarog, F. J. (1973). *Immunology* **24**, 859–870.

Rose, N. R., Bacon, L. D., Sundick, R. S., Kong, Y. M., Esquivel, P., and Bigazzi, P. E. (1977). *In* "Autoimmunity: Genetic, Immunologic, Virologic, and Clinical Aspects" (N. Talal, Ed.), pp. 63–87. Academic Press, New York.

Roubaty, C., Bedin, C., and Charreire, J. (1990). *J. Immunol.* **144**, 2167–2172.

Sakaguchi, S., and Sakaguchi, N. (1990). *J. Exp. Med.* **172**, 537–545.

Sakaguchi, S., Fukuma, K., Kuribayashi, K., and Masuda, T. (1985). *J. Exp. Med.* **161**, 72–87.

Salamero, J., and Charreire, J. (1985). *Cell. Immunol.* **91**, 111–118.

Silverman, D. A., and Rose, N. R. (1978). *J. Clin. Lab. Immunol.* **1**, 51–54.

Simon, L. L., Krco, C. J., David, C. S., and Kong, Y. M. (1985). *Cell. Immunol.* **94**, 243–253.

Simon, L. L., Justen, J. M., Giraldo, A. A., Krco, C. J., and Kong, Y. M. (1986). *Clin. Immunol. Immunopathol.* **39**, 345–356.

Sternthal, E., Like, A. A., Sarantis, K., and Braverman, L. E. (1981). *Diabetes* **30**, 1058–1061.

Stull, S. J., Kyriakos, M., Sharp, G. C., and Braley-Mullen, H. (1988). *Cell. Immunol.* **117**, 188–198.

Stull, S. J., Sharp, G. C., Kyriakos, M., Bickel, J. T., and Braley-Mullen, H. (1992). *J. Immunol.* **149**, 2219–2226.

Sugihara, S., Izumi, Y., Yoshioka, T., Yagi, H., Tsujimura, T., Tarutani, O., Kohno, Y., Murakami, S., Hamaoka, T., and Fujiwara, H. (1988). *J. Immunol.* **141**, 105–113.

Sugihara, S., Fujiwara, H., and Shearer, G. M. (1993). *J. Immunol.* **150**, 683–694.

Tang, H., Bedin, C., Texier, B., and Charreire, J. (1990). *Eur. J. Immunol.* **20**, 1535–1539.

Texier, B., Bedin, C., Roubaty, C., Brezin, C., and Charreire, J. (1992a). *J. Immunol.* **148**, 439–444.

Texier, B., Bédin, C., Tang, H., Camoin, L., Laurent-Winter, C., and Charreire, J. (1992b). *J. Immunol.* **148**, 3405–3411.

Tomazic, V., and Rose, N. R. (1976). *Immunology* **30**, 63–68.

Twarog, F. J., and Rose, N. R. (1969). *Proc. Soc. Exp. Biol. Med.* **130**, 434–439.

Vladutiu, A. O. (1982). *Clin. Exp. Immunol.* **47**, 683–688.

Vladutiu, A. O., and Rose, N. R. (1971). *Science* **174**, 1137–1139.

Vladutiu, A. O., and Rose, N. R. (1972). *Clin. Exp. Immunol.* **11**, 245–254.

Vladutiu, A. O., and Rose, N. R. (1975). *Cell. Immunol.* **17**, 106–113.

Weetman, A. P., McGregor, A. M., Rennie, D. P., and Hall, R. (1982a). *Immunology* **46**, 465–472.

Weetman, A. P., McGregor, A. M., Rennie, D. P., and Hall, R. (1982b). *Clin. Exp. Immunol.* **50**, 51–54.

Weetman, A. P., Gunn, C., Hall, R., and McGregor, A. M. (1985). *J. Clin. Lab. Immunol.* **17**, 1–6.

Williams, W. V., Kyriakos, M., Sharp, G. C., and Braley-Mullen, H. (1987). *Cell. Immunol.* **109**, 397–406.

Chapter 9

The NOD Mouse: A Model for Autoimmune Insulin-Dependent Diabetes

Dana Elias

Department of Cell Biology, The Weizmann Institute of Science, Rehovot 76100, Israel

I. History of the Model

The nonobese diabetic (NOD) mouse, which serves today as one of the best-characterized and most widely used models of autoimmune diabetes, was established serendipitously at the Shianogi Laboratories, Japan. An inbreeding program, whose goal was to derive a mouse strain with a high incidence of cataracts (CTs) from outbred ICR/Clea mice, produced a female with hyperglycemia among normal glycemic littermates. Interestingly, the progeny of this female fixed genes resistant to diabetes, and was called nonobese-normal (NON). In the future it served as a control strain for the diabetic line because it was derived from the same genetic pool. The second line, which originally had normal fasting blood glucose, fixed the genes that predispose for diabetes, resulting in mice that developed elevated fasting blood glucose due to autoimmune β cell destruction: the NOD mouse (Makino *et al.*, 1985).

II. The Animal

The original NOD/Shi mouse had a relatively low incidence of diabetes, and when some breeding pairs reached the Jackson Laboratory at Bar Harbor, Maine, a higher incidence of the disease was established in the NOD/Lt mice. Although this is a spontaneous-disease model, penetrance is usually not full, but is influenced by several environmental factors.

A. Gender

In colonies where the incidence of diabetes is less than 100%, onset is earlier and the incidence is higher in female than in male mice. Often, female NOD mice demonstrate overt diabetes by 3–6 months, with a cumulative incidence reaching 80–100%, while males develop overt diabetes at 5–8 months, with a cumulative incidence of 30–50%.

B. Colony

As a rule, the freer the colony from infections in general, the higher the incidence of diabetes (Leiter *et al.*, 1990). If the colony carries viral or bacterial infections, the incidence of diabetes is lower. In order to reach an incidence of 100%, the colony has to be maintained pathogen free. However, regardless of environmental factors, two NOD lines differ in their diabetic incidence: the NOD/Wehi line in which females have an incidence of less than 10% and males less than 1%, and the NOD/Lt line in which most females and many males develop diabetes. An immune mechanism of active suppression probably prevents NOD/Wehi from overt diabetes since treatment with cyclophosphamide (CY) induces diabetes in the NOD/Wehi mice.

C. Food

The composition of the food pellets also influences the level of diabetes in the colony. Food containing casein-hydrolysate or hypoallergenic baby formula will decrease the incidence of diabetes compared with casein, meat-meal, or other complex protein-containing chow (Elliott *et al.*, 1988).

D. Maintenance

Crowding the mice and frequent handling elevates the incidence of diabetes, probably by inducing stress. NOD mice, even before the onset of diabetes, were found to have both higher basal and stress-induced levels of corticosteroid hormones compared with other mouse strains. Moreover, the corticosteroid level in female NOD mice is higher than in males, a sexual dimorphism that fits the difference in incidence of diabetes. However, it is not clear whether the elevated corticosteroid level precedes or results from the diabetogenic process.

III. The Disease

Diabetes can be viewed in two ways. The clinical view traditionally was centered on the consequences of insufficient insulin. Clinically, diabetes is then an endocrine disease, marked principally by hyperglycemia. The immunological view of diabetes relates to the autoimmune process of β cell destruction that terminates in the endocrine disease. The immunological disease thus precedes the clinical disease. It is marked by insulitis and immunological reactivities.

A. Detection of Hyperglycemia

The NOD mouse is a model for insulin-dependent diabetes melitus (IDDM), a disease whose main feature is elevated blood glucose levels (hyperglycemia). Therefore, the easiest and most reliable way to detect the onset of diabetes in these mice is to test for glucose levels in the blood. Since the disease usually does not become manifest before the age of 3 months, that is probably the most productive age to start screening for hyperglycemia. A small sample of blood can be obtained either from the orbital sinus or from the tail. The level of glucose in whole blood can be determined by a variety of portable glucose detectors which are used primarily by diabetic patients to monitor their blood glucose levels. These glucose detectors are cheap, simple to use, require one drop of blood, and produce results in 30–90 s. However, for more reliable measurement, a laboratory-type glucose analyzer should be used; it requires separation of serum from blood and is more expensive. Hyperglycemia in mice is usually determined as glucose levels higher than 200 mg/dl or 11.1 mmol/liter.

Although NOD diabetes is thought to be a chronic, nonrelapsing disease, some mice may occasionally demonstrate transient hyperglycemia followed by a spell of normal blood glucose (normal glycemia). Therefore, to ascertain the onset of diabetes, it is important to recheck any hyperglycemic mouse a few days later. Only if two consecutive measurements demonstrate hyperglycemia, can we safely call the mouse sick.

Hyperglycemia results in glucose being secreted in the urine (glycosuria). Therefore, to avoid bleeding the mice too many times, it is possible to monitor the progression of diabetes by checking the appearance of glucose in the urine using diagnostic urine sticks, and only when persistent glycosuria is observed, measure blood glucose. Once a mouse is overtly diabetic, glucose levels will continue rising and within 3–5 weeks will reach levels of 500–700 mg/dl or 30–40 mmol/liter. At this point the mouse will die unless it is treated with exogenous insulin.

B. Immunological Lesions

The autoimmune destruction of the insulin-producing β cells in the pancreatic islets is accompanied by massive cellular infiltration surrounding and penetrating the islets—insulitis (Miyazaki *et al.*, 1985). The degree of infiltration can be monitored by surgically removing the pancreas and putting it into a fixative Bouin's solution for 24 hr, followed by washing in water and transferring the tissue to a 70% ethanol solution. The fixed pancreas can now be embedded in paraffin and cut by standard procedures. Hematoxylin-eosin stains the exocrine accini of the pancreas dark purple; the endocrine islets stain pink. The infiltrating cells stain purple.

A typical longitudinal histological examination of the NOD pancreas demonstrates the following: at 3–4 weeks of age, infiltrating cells surround the blood vessels (perivascular infiltration) but the islets are still clear. At 6–7 weeks, the infiltrating cells reach the islets, either surrounding them or accumulating at one pole. This is called peri-islet infiltration. Between 10 and 12 weeks, the infiltrating cells penetrate into the islets (intraislet infiltration) and the islets become swollen with lymphocytes. Following the onset of overt diabetes at 14–20 weeks, the infiltrate disappears, leaving the islets much shrunken in size. It is important to note that those NOD mice that escape clinical diabetes may still have severe insulitis. Thus, severe insulitis may exist with or without an overt loss of β cell function.

NOD mice also develop infiltrations of the salivary gland (sialitis) and at 6–8 months of age, some develop autoimmune lesions of the thyroid gland (thyroiditis). The subsets of cells in the infiltrate have been studied using frozen sections of the pancreas and immunohistochemistry (O'Reilley *et al.*, 1991). By staining with antibodies directed at markers of T cells, B cells, and macrophages, it was shown that macrophages predominate among the cells first infiltrating, followed by CD4+ T cells, then by CD8+ T cells and B cells.

C. Quantitation

Scoring the diabetes of NOD mice is based mainly on the development of hyperglycemia; insulitis may also be recorded. Several ways of defining the level of diabetes are used.

1. Incidence

The cumulative incidence of diabetes by the age of 7 or 8 months. By this age, any mouse that is going to develop the disease has already manifested overt diabetes. Incidence is described separately for females and males because in most colonies incidence varies with gender.

2. Age of Onset

The age at which 50 or 100% of the mice develop overt diabetes gives a good indication of how aggressive the disease is.

3. Blood Glucose

The above parameters consider all mice that have blood glucose levels above a certain point to be equivalent. However, different manipulations of the disease can result in clear differences in the mean blood glucose level, above and beyond the observed difference in onset and incidence. Therefore, the actual blood glucose concentration may be more revealing than incidence or the age of onset of hyperglycemia.

4. Insulitis

Although mice develop insulitis long before the onset of overt diabetes, and some mice will develop insulitis only, the histology of the pancreas can provide added information on the state of the disease. It is important to score as many islets as possible for no infiltrate and peri- or intraislet infiltrate; preferably, several sections should be scored from each pancreas.

D. Immune Reactivities

1. T Cells

Diabetes is caused in NOD mice by T cells, although macrophages also play an important role in the pathogenesis of the disease. This was demonstrated by adoptive transfer by splenic T cells from overtly diabetic NOD mice into young female or male irradiated NOD recipients (Wicker et al., 1986). Studies of the subpopulations transferring disease revealed that both

CD4+ and CD8+ T cells (Miller *et al.*, 1988), but not B cells, are necessary for diabetogenesis.

To elucidate the role of both CD4+ and CD8+ T cells in NOD mouse diabetes without the interference of endogenously recruited T cells, adoptive transfer experiments have been performed in which T cells were transferred from NOD females into NOD severe combined immunodeficiency (*scid/scid*) mice (Christianson *et al.*, 1993) or NOD athymic mice (Yagi *et al.*, 1992). Similar results were obtained by different investigators: CD4+ T cells from prediabetic NOD mice produced insulitis, but no islet destruction was observed and hyperglycemia did not develop. CD8+ T cells did not produce insulitis or hyperglycemia. However, when CD8+ T cells were transferred together with, or after CD4+ T cells, autoimmune diabetes developed. Taken together with the data from the immunohistochemical analysis of the lesions, it seems that CD4+ T cells home to the islets, attach themselves and proliferate, and enable the later-arriving CD8+ T cells to reach the islets and actually kill the β cells (Bedossa *et al.*, 1991). However, there is a contradictory report, in which CD4+ T cells could destroy islets in the absence of CD8+ cells *in vitro* (Bradley *et al.*, 1992). It is also conceivable that a state of hyperglycemia might be caused by a functional impairment of insulin secretion by existing β cells, in the absence of overt killing.

Thymocytes and splenic T cells of NOD mice produce lower than normal levels of interleukin-2 (IL-2) in response to concanavalin A (ConA). NOD T cells also demonstrate a reduced syngeneic mixed lymphocyte reaction (SMLR). NOD peritoneal exudate cells have lowered lipopolysaccharide (LPS)-induced IL-1 release (Serreze and Leiter, 1988). These phenomena can result in or reflect a defect in suppressor cell activation, which may be linked to the disease.

Several attempts to demonstrate limited T-cell receptor (TCR) *V*β use in NOD diabetes have produced conflicting results. Although some early reports stressed the role of *V*β*8*+ or *V*β*5*+ *T cells, later work demonstrated no V*β prefer-ences. Genetic elimination of *V*β*8*+ and *V*β*5*+ *T cells by introducing a mutant TCR V*β gene had no effect on insulitis and diabetes (McDuffie, 1991). More-over, analysis of TCR *V*β use, either by polymerase chain reaction (PCR) amplification with a panel of *V*β primers or by TCR analysis of a series of T-cell lines generated against islets revealed multiple TCR *V*β usage by infil-trating T cells (Candeias *et al.*, 1991; Walters *et al.*, 1992).

T-cell lines specific to undefined islet antigens were derived by several investigators either from peripheral (Haskins *et al.*, 1988) or from infiltrating T cells (Nagata and Yoon, 1992). Some of these lines could adoptively transfer insulitis and diabetes into young nonirradiated NOD recipients, or could mediate rejection of grafted islets. The fine antigen specificities of these undefined diabetogenic T cell lines have yet to be determined. However,

NOD diabetes has also been associated with T cells specific for certain defined antigens (see Section III,D,3).

2. Antibodies

Antibodies appear to play no role in the pathogenesis of diabetes in either humans or mice. However, since antibody responses are easier to measure than T-cell responses, screening for anti-β-cell autoantibodies in diabetes as a possible diagnostic method is worthwhile. The presence of several autoantibodies to various antigens has been detected before the onset of overt diabetes: insulin (Michel *et al.*, 1988), cytoplasmic-islet cell (Reddy *et al.*, 1988), glutamic acid decarboxylase (GAD) (Atkinson and Maclaren, 1988) and the 60-kDa heat shock protein (hsp 60) (Elias *et al.*, 1990). Autoantibodies to undefined antigens could be demonstrated by Western blotting NOD sera with islet extracts (Karounos and Thomas, 1990). Binding of antibodies to an islet-specific antigen of 52 kDa was demonstrated.

3. Antigens

Several studies demonstrated that the NOD mouse has no special β-cell antigen(s) not present in standard mice that could account for autoimmune reactivity. In these experiments, radiation chimeras were prepared from NOD F_1 progeny and a normal mouse strain, and the mice were reconstituted with bone marrow cells of either the NOD (Yasunami and Bach, 1988), the normal mouse strain, or the F_1 (Wicker *et al.*, 1988). Only irradiated F_1 mice reconstituted with NOD bone marrow cells developed insulitis. Therefore the information necessary for the propagation of β-cell autoimmunity is contained in the immune system and not in the β cell.

Some defined antigens were demonstrated to be self-antigens for NOD T cells:

a. The 60-kDa heat shock protein. This is a ubiquitous immunogenic protein. Hsp 60 can be located in the mitochondria of all cells. However, hsp 60 was also found to be part of the insulin-containing secretory granules of the β cell (Brudzynski *et al.*, 1992a,b). Whether hsp 60 has some special role relevant to insulin storage and/or secretion is unknown. Both healthy mice and humans have T cells which recognize the hsp 60 antigen. However, prediabetic NOD mice show augmented T-cell proliferative responses to this antigen, and to a defined epitope—a peptide corresponding to positions 437–460 of the human hsp 60 molecule. T-cell lines derived from prediabetic NOD splenocytes could adoptively transfer insulitis and early-onset hyperglycemia to nonirradiated 4- to 5-week-old NOD mice (Elias *et al.*, 1990). Thus, hsp 60 autoimmunity may have a functional role in causing diabetes in NOD mice.

b. Glutamic acid decarboxylase. Glutamic acid decarboxylase is an enzyme that is involved in the synthesis of the neurotransmitter γ-aminobutyric acid (GABA). Two variants of GAD exist, with molecular weights of 65 kDa and 67 kDa. Both exist in neural tissue and in the β cell. NOD mice manifest spontaneous T-cell responses to recombinants GAD_{65} and GAD_{67} from the age of 4 weeks, peaking around 8 weeks and diminishing as diabetes becomes overt (Tisch *et al.*, 1993). T-cell epitopes were found to be present at positions 509–528, 524–543, and 247–266 in the GAD_{65} sequence (Kaufman *et al.*, 1993). The functional relevance of GAD autoimmunity to the initiation and progression of diabetes has yet to be demonstrated.

c. Carboxypeptidase H. Carboxypeptidase H (CPH) is a 53 to 57-kDa enzyme, expressed in both α- and β-cell secretory granules (Guest *et al.*, 1991) and in neuroendocrine cells. This antigen is recognized by NOD T cells from the age of 6 weeks and onward (Tisch *et al.*, 1993).

Other β-cell antigens, such as islet cell antibody (ICA) 69 (Pietropaolo *et al.*, 1993) and the 38-kDa antigen (Roep *et al.*, 1990), have been detected in human patients. However, the role of these antigens in NOD diabetes remains to be determined.

IV. Genetics

In IDDM, genes in linkage disequilibrium with immune response genes in the major histocompatibility complex (MHC) or the immune response genes themselves seem to influence susceptibility. The NOD model is interesting since it clearly demonstrates the complex interaction between heredity and environment. NOD mice possess several special genetic traits, reviewed by Leiter (1989). Phenotypically, NOD mice are characterized by the following:

1. The lymphoid organs contain an unusually high number of T cells.
2. The lymphocytic infiltrations affect the pancreatic islets, the submandibular and lacrimal glands, and the thyroid.
3. Macrophage presentation of self-MHC to T cells in SMLR is deficient, and is linked to defective cytokine signaling between macrophages and T cells.
4. The CD8+/CD4+ ratio is abnormally elevated.

At least ten genes contribute to the susceptibility of NOD mice to diabetes. We discuss the MHC and non-MHC genes separately.

A. MHC Molecules

The NOD mouse MHC class I haplotypes are K^d and D^b in that they do not differ from other normal mouse strains. However, the susceptibility gene *Idd-*

I is located in the murine MHC on chromosome 17, and is a gene complex with two susceptibility loci, the class II genes *I-Aβ* and *I-Eα*. The *I-Aα* gene of NOD is the unexceptional *I-A^d*. However, the 5' portion of the *I-Aβ* gene is unique. It is homologous to the human HLA-DQB1*0302 IDDM-associated allele in having serine instead of aspartate at position 57 (Acha-Orbea and McDevitt, 1987). This NOD-specific *I-Aβ* allele was first designated *I-A^{nod}*, but its proper name is *I-Ag^7*. NOD mice do not express the other MHC class II product, *I-E* (Hattory *et al.*, 1986), owing to a mutation in the *I-Eα* gene. Indeed, the absence of the *I-E* product is crucial for NOD diabetes: introducing a normal *I-Eα* gene as a transgene completely abolished diabetes (Lund *et al.*, 1990). To summarize, the expression of *I-Ag^7* is essential, though not sufficient in itself, for both insulitis and diabetes. The absence of *I-E* is permissive for the development of autoimmunity.

B. Non-MHC Genes

The non-MHC genes that play a role in NOD diabetes are less well defined in their effect on the disease:

1. The *Thy-1* locus-linked *Idd-2* gene controls the initiation of insulitis and maps to chromosome 9 (Prochazka *et al.*, 1987).

2. The *Idd-3* locus, mapped to chromosome 3, may contribute to the development and severity of insulitis. Since it is essential for insulitis, it is also important for diabetes (Todd *et al.*, 1991).

3. The *Idd-4* locus on chromosome 11 shows no association with insulitis in nondiabetic progeny, but it may influence the frequency of insulitis, and perhaps controls the progression of severe insulitis to overt diabetes (Todd *et al.*, 1991).

4. The proximal region of chromosome 1 contains a few candidate genes. The genes responsible for the diabetogenic effect of cyclophosphamide on NOD mice include two separate loci: *IL-1r1** and *Lsh/Ity/Bcg* (Cornall *et al.*, 1991; Garchon *et al.*, 1991). The *bcg* gene is interesting since it determines host resistance or sensitivity to infectious disease. *Il-1r1* encodes the receptor of interleukin-1, which is a key cytokine in diabetes, since it is a cofactor in T-cell activation and is also cytotoxic to β cells *in vitro*. *Cd-28*, which is a T-cell activation molecule, also maps to this region. A gene controlling peri-islet insulitis and sialitis is found at the *Bcl-2* locus on chromosome 1 (Garchon *et al.*, 1991). Transgenic mice that express this gene in B cells have prolonged antibody production and develop a lupus-like disease.

5. A new gene, *tap1*, found in the MHC class II region is a transporter associated with antigen processing and is reviewed by Faustman (1993). Functional TAP1 is required for normal expression of MHC class I and is dependent on peptide loading.

Altogether, these findings shed a new light on experimental diabetes by demonstrating the association of specific genes with successive steps of the autoimmune process.

V. Treatment and Prevention

Prevention usually refers to treatment administered before the onset of disease. Since insulitis precedes the onset of overt diabetes by months, the terminology is somewhat confusing and different investigators will refer to interference at 1–3 months of age, before overt hyperglycemia, as either prevention or treatment. Generally speaking, treatment of NOD diabetes can be divided into immunological treatment, in which antibodies or reagents that directly influence the immune system are administered, and pharmacological treatment, in which the disease is not affected through immunomodulation.

A. Immunological Treatment

Some of the first observations demonstrating the immunological nature of NOD diabetes were based on immunomodulation of the disease. Administration of antilymphocytic serum or anti-CD3 antibodies to young NOD mice prevented both insulitis and diabetes (Kelley *et al.*, 1988). Moreover, administration of antibodies to the IL-2 receptor (IL-2R) coupled to diphtheria toxin, targeted the toxin to activated T cells that express the IL-2R, resulting in a block of diabetes development (Kelley, 1988). As the roles of CD4+ and CD8+ T cells in the pathogenesis of diabetes were being defined, specific monoclonal antibodies were used to block the respective T-cell subset. Accordingly, it could be demonstrated that both anti-CD4 and anti-CD8 antibodies, if administered at 5 weeks of age, could decrease insulitis and prevent diabetes (Hayward *et al.*, 1988). If the combined antibodies were administered after the onset of insulitis, partial clearing of the islet infiltrate could be achieved, but not total reversal of the disease.

Treatments directed against macrophages were also effective. Long-term administration of anti-I-A antibodies could abolish diabetes (Boitard *et al.*, 1988). Also, administration of silica particles, which affects phagocytic cells, blocks diabetes (Charlton *et al.*, 1988). Moreover, 5C6, a monoclonal antibody that blocks the adhesion-promoting receptor on macrophages, prevents the transfer of diabetes (Hutchings *et al.*, 1990).

A contrasting type of treatment sets out not to delete or block a certain cellular subtype, but rather to induce preventive mechanisms by immunostimulation. NOD mice are particularly sensitive to this type of modulation:

1. Cytokine Modulation

The following treatments have been reported to reduce insulitis and effectively block diabetes (Serreze et al., 1989):

1. Administration of poly I:C, an inducer of interferon-α/β.
2. Treatment with recombinant IL-2, which resulted in elevated IL-1 production by peritoneal macrophages.
3. Administration of tumor necrosis factor-α.

2. Immunostimulatory Treatment

Vaccination of young NOD mice with complete Freund's adjuvant (CFA) has a marked inhibitory effect on NOD diabetes (McInerney et al., 1991), and the protective effect can be transferred by T cells into naive NOD mice. CFA can also prevent rejection of syngeneic islet grafts when administered to already overtly diabetic mice.

Inoculation with live bacille Calmetti-Guiésin (BCG) vaccine prevents insulitis and overt diabetes, probably by inducing suppressor cells to inhibit lymphocyte functions (Yagi et al., 1991).

Induction of neonatal tolerance to allogeneic antigens in NOD mice resulted in a significant reduction of insulitis and diabetes. This was achieved by making the mice tolerant to either MHC antigens or minor histocompatibility antigens (Carnaud et al., 1992). The authors proposed that neonatal tolerance could induce polyclonal activation of the immune system, resulting in inactivation of diabetogenic T cells.

3. Antigen-Driven Immunomodulation

Oral administration of porcine insulin from the age of 5 weeks up to 1 year, in weekly doses of 1 mg, delayed the onset and reduced the incidence of diabetes (Zhang et al., 1991).

Intraperitoneal inoculation of hsp 60 in aqueous solution, at the age of 4–5 weeks ameliorated diabetes (Elias et al., 1991).

Intravenous injection of recombinant GAD_{65} in 3-week-old NOD mice reduced the insulitis score and prevented diabetes (Kaufman et al., 1993).

Intrathymic injection of recombinant GAD_{65} into 3-week-old NOD mice reduced insulitis and delayed the onset of diabetes (Tisch et al., 1993).

Intrathymic injection of β cells into 4-week-old NOD mice made them tolerant to islet cells and rendered them free of diabetes (Gerling et al., 1992).

A single subcutaneous injection of the 437–460 peptide of hsp 60 (p277) at 4 weeks of age prevented diabetes (Elias et al., 1991). Recently, the p277 peptide was found to be effective in treating the diabetogenic process just before (12–15 weeks) the appearance of overt diabetes (Elias and Cohen, 1994).

Genetic manipulation of the NOD MHC could also affect diabetes. NOD mice do not express I-E molecules, owing to a mutation in the α-chain. Transgenic NOD mice that express the I-E^d haplotype do not develop insulitis or diabetes (Hirofumi *et al.*, 1987), probably owing to modification of the T-cell repertoire in the I-E-expressing thymus. Moreover, specific removal of suppressor cells can result in a more aggressive type of diabetes. Administration of cyclophosphamide to young NOD mice, which affects suppressor T cells, induces massive insulitis and severe hyperglycemia 2 weeks later (Charlton *et al.*, 1989). The dose of CY required varies between 160 and 350 mg/kg, depending on the NOD colony. The more diabetes-resistant NOD colonies require higher doses. Administration of CY is especially helpful if the incidence of diabetes in the colony is low, or if a large number of diabetic mice are to be generated simultaneously. Male NOD mice, which in most colonies have at best a 50% incidence of diabetes with a delayed onset, can be induced by cyclophosphamide to develop aggressive diabetes.

B. Pharmacological Treatment

Free radicals and superoxides are suspected to be mediators of β-cell damage. Therefore, substances that act as free radical scavengers or antioxidants are plausible candidates for treatment.

Nicotinamide, a vitamin B-group substance, was administered in large doses before the onset of diabetes. The treated group had reduced levels of insulitis and maintained normal glycemia in comparison with the control group (Reddy *et al.*, 1990). When nicotinamide was administered immediately at the onset of diabetes, some drop in blood glucose levels was observed. However, administration of the drug 2 weeks after the onset of diabetes resulted in no effect.

Vitamin D, 1α,25-dihydroxyvitamin-D_3, administered to NOD mice could prevent the development of insulitis (Mathieu *et al.*, 1992).

Vitamin E treatment, given at 1000 IU/kg in the diet, resulted in no change in insulitis but reduce the incidence of diabetes. Therefore, these vitamins, if given early enough, could help block β-cell damage (Hayward *et al.*, 1992).

VI. Notes for the Beginner

As mentioned above, a clear diagnosis of the onset of diabetes can be tricky. It is extremely important to recheck any animal with signs of glycosuria and/

or hyperglycemia because NOD mice will occasionally have a short remission of clinical diabetes before the disease finally becomes irreversible.

If *in vitro* analysis of T-cell responses, or the propagation of T-cell lines is to be performed, the conventional use of syngeneic serum in the medium should not be applied here. NOD serum can be toxic to T cells possibly because of serum autoantibodies. Therefore, either heat-inactivated (56°C, 30 min) normal-strain mouse serum should be used, or one of the commercial defined culture media.

The *I-A* haplotype of the NOD mouse is distinct, yet resembles the *I-A^d* haplotype, so monoclonal antibodies to *I-A^d* can be used to stain NOD class II MHC.

Any experiment conducted to monitor the effect of a certain treatment on the incidence of diabetes should take into consideration how easy it is to prevent, or at least delay, NOD diabetes by immunostimulation.

VII. What the Model Has Taught Us about Human IDDM

The NOD mouse represents a model in which autoimmunity against β cells is the primary event in the development of insulin-dependent diabetes. Diabetogenesis is mediated through a multifactorial interaction between a unique MHC class II gene and multiple, unlinked, genetic loci. Moreover, the NOD mouse demonstrates beautifully the critical interaction between heredity and environment. The differences in disease incidence and age of onset among various colonies, depending on the cleanliness of the housing conditions, illustrates how environmental factors can affect the penetrance of diabetes-susceptible genes.

As for the autoimmunity recorded in NOD mice, most antigen-specific antibodies and T-cell responses were measured after these antigens were detected as self-antigens in diabetic patients. Still, the validation of the role these autoantigens play in NOD diabetes is extremely important, and may allow researchers to distinguish between pathogenic autoantigens and autoimmunity that is merely an epiphenomenon. Moreover, one should bear in mind that IDDM patients are genetically and probably pathogenically heterogeneous. Thus, NOD mice might represent only a part of the IDDM population. Use of an animal model to study a human disease always requires cautious interpretation, but the powerful tools it provides can be used effectively to learn about the etiology of the disease, and, it is hoped, to develop efficient interventions.

References

Acha-Orbea, H., and McDevitt, H. O. (1987). *Proc. Natl. Acad. Sci. USA* **84**, 2435–2439.
Atkinson, M. A., and Maclaren, N. K. (1988). *Diabetes* **37**, 1587–1590.

Bedossa, P., Thivolet, C., Bendelac, A., Bach, J. F., and Carnaud, C. (1991). *J. Immunol.* **146**, 85–88.

Boitard, C., Bendelac, A. Richard, M. F., Carnaud, C., and Bach, J. F. (1988). *Proc. Natl. Acad. Sci. USA* **85**, 9719–9723.

Bradley, B. J., Haskins, K., Larosa, F. G., and Lafferty, K. J. (1992). *Diabetes* **41**, 1603–1608.

Brudzynski, K., Martinez, V., and Gupta, R. S. (1992a). *J. Autoimmun.* **5**, 453–463.

Brudzynski, K., Martinez, V., and Gupta, R. S. (1992b). *Diabetologia* **35**, 316–324.

Candeias, S., Katz, J., Benoist, C., Mathis, D., and Haskins, K. (1991). *Proc. Natl. Acad. Sci. USA* **88**, 6167–6170.

Carnaud, C., Legrand, B., Olivi, M., Peterson, L. B., Wicker, L. S., and Bach, J. F. (1992). *J. Autoimmun.* **5**, 591–602.

Charlton, B., Bacelj, A., and Mandel, T. E. (1988). *Diabetes* **37**, 930–935.

Charlton, B., Bacelj, A., Slattery, R. M., and Mandel, T. E. (1989). *Diabetes* **38**, 441–447.

Christianson, S. W., Scultz, L. D., and Leiter, E. H. (1993). *Diabetes* **42**, 44–55.

Cornall, R. J., Prins, J. B., Todd, J. A., Pressey, A., DeLarato, N. H., Wicker, L. S., and Peterson, L. B. (1991). *Nature* **353**, 262–265.

Elias, D., and Cohen, I. R. *Lancet*, **343**, 704–706.

Elias, D., Markovits, D., Reshef, T., van-Der Zee, R., and Cohen, I. R. (1990). *Proc. Natl. Acad. Sci. USA* **87**, 1576–1580.

Elias, D., Reshef, T., Birk, O. S., van Der Zee, R., Walker, M. D., and Cohen, I. R. (1991). *Proc. Natl. Acad. Sci. USA* **88**, 3088–3091.

Elliott, R. B., Reddy, S. N., Bibby, N. J., and Kida, K. (1988). *Diabetologia* **31**, 62–64.

Faustman, D. L. (1993). *Biomed. Pharmacother.* **47**, 3–10.

Garchon, H. J., Bedossa, P., Eloy, L., and Bach, J. F. (1991). *Nature* **353**, 260–262.

Gerling, I. C., Serreze, D. V., Christianson, S. W., and Leiter, E. H. (1992). *Diabetes* **41**, 1672–1676.

Guest, P. C., Ravazzola, M., Davidson, H. W., Orci, L., and Hutton, J. C. (1991). *Endocrinology* **129**, 734–740.

Haskins, K., Portas, M., Wegmann, D., and Lafferty, K. J. (1988). *Diabetes* **37**, 1444–1448.

Hattory, M., Buse, J. B., Jackson, R. A., Glimcher, L., Dorf, M. E., Minami, M., Makino, S., Moriwaki, K., Kuzuya, H., Imura, H., Strauss, M. W., Seidman, J. G., and Eisenbarth, G. S. (1986). *Science* **231**, 733–735.

Hayward, A. R., Cobbold, S. P., Waldmann, H., Cooke, A., and Simpson, E. (1988). *Autoimmunity* **1**, 91–96.

Hayward, A. R. and Shreiber, M. (1989). *J. Immunol.* **143**, 1555–1559.

Hayward, A. R., Shriber, M., and Sokol, R. (1992). *J. Lab. Clin. Med.* **119**, 503–507.

Hirofumi, N., Kikutani, H., Yamamura, K., and Kishimoto, T. (1987). *Nature* **328**, 432–434.

Hutchings, P., Rosen, H., O'Reilley, L., Simpson, E., Gordon, S., and Cooke, A. (1990). *Nature* **348**, 639–642.

Karounos, D. G., and Thomas, J. W. (1990). *Diabetes* **39**, 1085–1090.

Kaufman, D. L., Clare-Salzer, M., Tian, J., Forsthuber, T., Ting, G. S. P., Robinson, P., Atkinson, M. A., Sercarz, E. E., Tobin, A. J., and Lehmann, P. V. (1993). *Nature* **366**, 69–72.

Kelley, V. E., Gaulton, G. N., Hattori, M., Ikegami, H., Eisenbarth, G. S., and Strom, T. P. (1988). *J. Immunol.* **140**, 59–61.

Leiter, E. H., Serreze, D. V., and Prochazka, M. (1990). Genetics and epidemiology of diabetes in NOD mice. *Immunol. Today* **11**, 147–149.

Leiter, E. H. (1989). *FASEB J* **3**, 2231–2241.

Lund, T., O'Reilly, L., Hutchings, P., Kanagawa, O., Simpson, E., Gravely, R., Chandler, P., Dyson, J., Picard, J. K., Edwards, A., Kioussis, D., and Cooke, A. (1990). I-E α-chain. *Nature* **345**, 727–729.

Makino, S., Hayashi, Y., Muraoka, Y., and Tochino, Y. (1985). *In*: "Current Topics in Clinical and Experimental Aspects of Diabetes Mellitus" (N., Sakamoto, H. K. Min, and S. Baba, Eds.), pp. 25–32. Elsevier, Amsterdam.

Mathieu, C., Laureys, J., Sobis, H., Vandeputte, M., Waer, M., and Bouillon, R. (1992). *Diabetes* **42**, 470–473.

McDuffie, M. (1991). *Diabetes* **40**, 1555–1559.

McInerney, M. F., Pek, S. B., and Thomas, D. W. (1991). *Diabetes* **40**, 715–725.

Michel, C., Boitard, C., and Bach, J. F. (1988). *Diabetologia* **31**, 322–328.

Miller, B. J., Appel, M. C., O'Neill, J. J., and Wicker, L. S. (1988). *J. Immunol.* **140**, 152–158.

Miyazaki, A., Hanafusa, T., Yamada, K., Miyagawa, J., Fujino-Kurihara, H., Nakajima, H., Nonaka, K., and Tami, S. (1985). *Clin. Exp. Immunol.* **60**, 622–630.

Nagata, M., and Yoon, J. W. (1992). *Diabetes* **41**, 998–1008.

O'Reilly, L. A., Hutchings, P. R., Crocker, P. R., Simpson, E., Lund, T., Kioussis, D., Takei, F., Baird, J., and Cooke, A. (1991). *Eur. J. Immunol.* **21**, 1171–1180.

Pietropaolo, M., Castano, L., Babu, S., Buelow, R., Kuo, Y. L. S., Martin, S., Martin, A., Powers, A. C., Prochazka, M., Naggert, J., Leiter, E. H., and Eisenbarth, G. S. (1993). *J. Clin. Invest.* **92**, 359–371.

Prochazka, M., Leiter, E. H., Serreze, D., and Coleman, D. L. (1987). *Science* **237**, 286–289.

Reddy, S., Bibby, N. J., and Elliott, R. B. (1988). *Diabetologia* **31**, 322–328.

Reddy, S., Bibby, N. J., and Elliott, R. B. (1990). *Diabetes Res.* **15**, 95–102.

Roep, B. O., Arden, S. D., de Vries, R. R. P., and Hutton, J. C. (1990). *Nature* **345**, 632–634.

Serreze, D. V., and Leiter, E. H. (1988). *J. Immunol.* **140**, 3801–3807.

Serreze, D. V., Hamaguchi, K., and Leiter, E. H. (1989). *J. Autoimmun.* **2**, 759–776.

Tisch, R., Xiao-Dong, Y., Singer, S. M., Liblau, R. S., Fugger, L., and McDevitt, H. O. (1993). *Nature* **366**, 72–75.

Todd, J. A., Aitman, T. J., Cornall, R. J., Ghosh, S., Hall, J. R. S., Hearne, C. M., Knight, A. M., Love, J. M., McAleer, M. A., Prins, J. B., Rodrigues, N., Lathrop, M., Pressey, A., DeLarato, N. H., Peterson, L. B., and Wicker, L. S. (1991). *Nature* **351**, 542–547.

Walters, S. H., O'Neill, J. J., Melican, D. T., and Appel, M. C. (1992). *Diabetes* **41**, 308–312.

Wicker, L. S., Miller, B. J., and Mullen, Y. (1986). *Diabetes* **35**, 855–860.

Wicker, L. S., Miller, B. J., Chai, J., Terada, M., and Mullen, Y. (1988). *J. Exp. Med.* **167**, 1801–1810.

Yagi, H., Matsumoto, M., Suzuki, S., Misaki, R., Suzuki, R., Makino, S., and Harada, M. (1992). *Cell. Immunol.* **138**, 130–141.

Yagi, H., Matsumoto, M., Kunomoto, K., Kawaguchi, J., Makino, S., and Harada, M. (1992). *Eur. J. Immunol.* **22**, 2387–2393.

Yasunami, R., and Bach, J. F. (1988). *Eur. J. Immunol.* **18**, 481–484.

Zhang, Z. J., Davidson, L., Eisenbarth, G. S., and Weiner, H. L. (1991). *Proc. Natl. Acad. Sci. USA* **88**, 10252–10256.

Chapter 10

The BB Rat Models of IDDM

Peter A. Gottlieb and Aldo A. Rossini

Division of Diabetes, Department of Medicine, University of Massachusetts Medical School, Worcester, Massachusetts 01655

I. History

The DP-BB and RT6-DR rat models of insulin-dependent diabetes mellitus (IDDM) have given us great insight into the pathogenesis and potential treatment of human IDDM (Parfrey *et al.*, 1989; Crisá *et al.*, 1992). In 1974, the Chappel brothers discovered the spontaneously diabetes-prone BB (DP-BB) rat in a colony of outbred Wistar rats at the BioBreeding Laboratories in Ottawa, Canada (Nakhooda *et al.*, 1977). The diabetes-resistant (DR) line was derived from DP-BB forebears in the fifth generation of inbreeding and has been continuously selected for resistance to the disease (Butler *et al.*, 1991).

II. Animals

To distinguish the various colonies of BB rats that have been established throughout the world, animals are designated BB/Wor for Worcester or BB/H for Hagedorn, for example (Marliss, 1983). Because each of these colonies was inbred separately, they have developed genetic polymorphisms that separate them into seven unique haplotypes (Prins *et al.*, 1991) (see Table I). Differing incidences of diabetes are noted not only in these different colonies, but also within the sublines maintained at the same colony (Butler *et al.*, 1991).

Table I
BB Rat Lines Grouped According to Allele Distribution at Nine Polymorphic Loci[a]

Haplotype	Line	Spontaneous diabetes	Colony
IA	DP-BB/Wor NB line	+	Worcester, USA
	DR-BB/Wor WA line	−	Worcester, USA
	DR-BB/Wor WB line	−	Worcester, USA
	DR-BB/Wor VB line	−	Worcester, USA
	BB/hooded	+	Toronto, Canada
	DR-BB/H	−	Gentofte, Denmark
	BB/Wor/Mol-WB	−	Ejby, Skensved, Denmark
IB	BB/Wor/Mol-BB	−	Ejby, Skensved, Denmark
IIA	DP-BB/Wor BA line	+	Worcester, USA
	DP-BB/B	+	Basel, Switzerland
	DP-BB/Hl (dp)	+	Dusseldorf, Germany
	BD/Ph	+	Philadelphia, USA
IIB	DP-BB/Wor BB line	+	Worcester, USA
	DP-BB/Wor PA line	+	Worcester, USA
	BB/OK	+	Karlsburg, Germany
	BB/Phi/K	+	Karlsburg, Germany
	DP-BB/H	+	Gentofte, Denmark
IIIA	BB/Hl (ndp)	−	Dusseldorf, Germany
IIIB	BC/Ph	−	Philadelphia, USA
IV	BA/Ph	+	Philadelphia, USA
	CD/Ph	+	Philadelphia, USA
	BB/D	+	Denver, USA
	BB/O	+	Oss, The Netherlands
	DP-BB/Wor BE line	+	Worcester, USA
	BBdp (outbred)	−	Ottawa, Canada
	BBn (outbred)	−	Ottawa, Canada

[a] Adapted from the data of Prins *et al.* (1991).

The University of Massachusetts Medical Center in Worcester houses the National Institutes of Health (NIH) breeding colony of BB rats. Six lines of DP-BB/Wor rats and two lines of DR-BB/Wor rats have been derived there from a specific breeding program of brother-sister mating. Animals for experimentation can be obtained from this colony in the United States. For other locations of BB rat colonies and suppliers, see Prins (1991).

Interventional studies involving either the DP- or DR-BB rat generally are begun at 30 days of age, which means that animals should be obtained at or shortly after weaning (21–23 days of age). Both male and female BB rats develop diabetes (DM) at similar frequencies. Experimental design dictates that groups be randomized according to both litter and sex.

Initially up to 10 weanlings can be placed in one cage, but by 45–50 days of age, a maximum of 4 animals of the same sex should be kept in one cage. Close attention must be paid to providing adequate water for diabetic animals to avoid death by dehydration.

Animals become capable of breeding at approximately 60 days of age. Ratios of one male to two female rats can maximize the number of litters obtained. Diabetic DP-BB rat females can have fewer litters and pups per litter. Careful control of blood glucose with daily insulin injections of PZI U-40 insulin (1 U/100 gBW) and urine testing for glucose and ketones can improve outcomes. An alternative approach that can be employed is to transfuse 30-day-old DP-BB rat females with virus-antibody-free (VAF) DR spleen cells (Burstein et al., 1989). This maneuver will protect most of the female recipients from developing DM and will allow for the production of more litters per animal.

Since DP-BB rats are lymphopenic and immunocompromised, it is recommended that they be housed under either VAF or specific-pathogen-free (SPF) conditions. Without these conditions, DP-BB rats will rapidly succumb to bacterial pathogens, most notably mycoplasma. Even when treated with agents to induce diabetes, DR-BB rats remain immunocompetent and can be maintained under less stringent circumstances.

Sterilized cages and bedding, cage hoods, autoclaved food (Purina 5010), and acid drinking water (or tetracycline water) should be employed in the care of these animals. Gowns, gloves, booties, and masks should be used by all animal caregivers. Microisolators and laminar flow units in clean rooms or biocontainment facilities can be used to establish VAF conditions. Sentinel animals must be kept and checked for the potential contaminations that regularly develop in these colonies.

Environmental factors have been found to affect the incidence and onset of diabetes in BB rats, as demonstrated by Like (1991). Placing DP-BB/Wor rats in a virus-free environment accelerates the age of onset of diabetes for all animals. In contrast, this same virus-free environment reduces the frequency of disease in DR-BB/Wor rats treated with anti-RT6.1 antibody. It should also be noted that special diets such as those that are casein free (Scott, 1988) or contain low essential fatty acids (Lefkowith *et al.*, 1990) have been shown to decrease the incidence of DM in these animals.

III. Genetics

The inheritance of diabetes in BB rats segregates with a gene associated with the rat major histocompatibility complex (MHC). Many studies have indicated that at least one RT1u class II allele must be present for diabetes susceptibility, as demonstrated by Colle (1990). A possible explanation for this association may be the uniqueness of the first external domains of the RT1B (DQ) and RT1D (DR) β-chains in both DP- and DR-BB rats in comparison with other rat or mouse class II sequences (Chao *et al.*, 1989). The protective effect of uncharged amino acids at position 57 of the DQ β-chain does not hold in the BB rat.

Table II
Characterization of BB Rat Models of IDDM

	Spontaneous		Induced	
	DP-BB rat	DR-BB rat	DR + aRT6	DR + aRT6 + Poly IC
Diabetes				
VAF	>85%	<1%	10%	95%
	(79 days)	(52 days)	(52 days)	(52 days)
CH	60–80%	<1%	50–60%	60–70%
	(91 days)	(52 days)	(52 days)	(52 days)
Resistance	No	Yes	Animals >60 days old	Animals >60 days old
Adoptive transfer of diabetes	Yes	No	Yes	Yes
Effect of KRV	None	Induces	Induces	?
Thyroiditis	25–90% >120 days (BA, NB sublines >50%)	<1%	40–50% (Only in CH rats <60 days)[a]	50–60% (Only in CH rats <60 days)[a]

Note. VAF, virus-antibody free; CH, conventionally housed.
[a] Thomas *et al.* (1991).

The principal non-MHC gene correlated with diabetes is one associated with lymphopenia. Lymphopenia is permissive for the development of diabetes in DP-BB rats, but it is not absolutely necessary in DR-BB rats, in whom diabetes can be found without lymphopenia being present (Like *et al.*, 1986; Guberski *et al.*, 1991; Sobel *et al.*, 1992). Recently, it was shown by Jacob (1992) that the lymphopenia gene is in tight linkage with neuropeptide Y (NPY), which is located on rat chromosome 4.

It has been theorized that the lymphopenia defect leads to the loss of the normal regulatory network that prevents autoreactive cells from initiating an autoimmune betacytotoxic response. Lymphopenia in the DP-BB rat appears to find its major expression in the loss of RT6+ T cells (Greiner *et al.*, 1986). RT6 is an alloantigen expressed on the surface of mature (postthymic) T cells. The gene coding for the RT6.1 alloantigen is found on chromosome 1 and appears to be structurally intact in the DP rat (Angelillo *et al.*, 1988). Furthermore, RT6.1+ cells can be found among the intraepithelial lymphocyte population (IEL) of the DP-BB rat (Edouard *et al.*, 1991; Waite *et al.*, 1993). Therefore, it appears that the lymphopenia gene defect leads to a shortened life span of thymus-derived T cells (apoptosis?) and so prevents the expression of the RT6 maturational antigen in most peripheral lymphoid tissues.

Finally, data from crosses between DP and Fischer rats have led to evidence of a third susceptibility gene, which is currently unmapped (Jacob *et al.*, 1992).

IV. The Disease

A. Diabetes-Prone BB Rat

The incidence of diabetes is 60–80% in both male and female diabetes-prone BB/Wor rats, although it can vary significantly by litter. Diabetes occurs spontaneously in DP-BB/Wor rats between 60 and 120 days of age (see Table II). The incidence of disease by 120 days of age in the virus-free environment of the NIH colony in Worcester averages 86% (Like *et al.*, 1991). The clinical onset is abrupt and characterized by hyperglycemia, weight loss, hypoinsulinemia, and ketonuria. In the absence of exogenous insulin therapy (PZI U-40 1.0 U/100 gBW/day), diabetic animals rapidly die.

Insulitis, a mononuclear cell infiltrate of the pancreatic islets, precedes the development of overt diabetes. Pathological studies have revealed that macrophages and/or dendritic cells are the first cells detected in islets and are followed by both CD4+ and CD8+ T cells, natural killer (NK) cells, and to a lesser extent, B cells (Parfrey *et al.*, 1989; Crisá *et al.*, 1992).

Interestingly, other autoimmune phenomena are seen in both DP- and RT6-DR-BB rats. Humoral autoimmunity in the form of antibodies to islet cells (ICA); glutamic acid decarboxylase (GAD); insulin; adrenal, ovary, and gastric parietal cells; and other antigens have been described. Thyroiditis—lymphocytic infiltration of the thyroid gland—is noted in over 50% of DP and anti-RT6-treated DR animals independent of the incidence of DM. Hypothyroidism is normally not seen unless both hemithyroidectomy and the administration of iodine are performed in certain sublines of the DP-BB/Wor rat (Rajatanavin *et al.*, 1991).

B. Induced Diabetes in the Diabetes-Resistant BB Rat

1. Anti-Rt6.1 Antibody

Diabetes can be induced in the normally diabetes-resistant BB rat by various regimens. The best-studied and characterized is the induction of diabetes by the depletion of RT6+ T cells (Greiner *et al.*, 1987). RT6.1 is an alloantigen expressed on the surface of mature (post-thymic) T cells. It is expressed on 60–80% of peripheral CD8+ T cells and 50% of peripheral CD4+ T cells. Depletion of these cells with rat antirat DS4.23 monoclonal antibody directed against RT6.1 beginning at the age of 30 days will induce diabetes in over 60% of conventionally housed (CH) DR-BB/Wor rats. VAF DR-BB rats do not develop insulitis, diabetes, or thyroiditis from anti-RT6 MAb alone (Thomas *et al.*, 1991) (see Table II).

The DS4.23 hybdridoma cell line can be grown under standard tissue culture conditions. Two milliliters of unconcentrated supernatant are administered intraperitoneally, beginning at 30 days of age, 5 times per week until the onset of DM, or through 60 days of age. Concentrating the supernatant will reduce the injection size and frequency.

2. PolyI:C

Polyinositol C (poly I:C), an inducer of gamma interferon, can accelerate disease development in DP-BB rats (Ewel *et al.*, 1992) and induce diabetes in DR-BB rats (Sobel *et al.*, 1992). It is available from Sigma Chemical Co. and it is mixed in phosphate-buffered saline (PBS). Poly IC is given three times a week intraperitoneally beginning at 30 days of age in both DP- and DR-BB rats. When this agent is used at a concentration of 5 μg/gBW, it accelerates diabetes in DP-BB rats and will induce insulitis or diabetes in 44% of virus-antibody-free rats and 71% of conventionally housed DR-BB rats. According to Sobel (1992), utilizing a dose of 10 μg/gBW of poly I:C can cause 100% of VAF DR-BB rats to become diabetic before 70 days of age.

3. Anti-Rt6.1 Antibody and Poly I:C

As noted above, VAF DR-BB rats treated with DS4.23 supernatant alone will not become diabetic. However, when DS4.23 Ab and poly I:C at a dose of 5 μg/gBW are used together, nearly 100% of treated animals can be made diabetic (Thomas *et al.*, 1991). Both agents are administered from 30 days of age and our experience has shown that treatment given for only 2 weeks is as effective as the recommended 30 days of therapy previously reported.

4. Killham's Rat Virus

It appears that Killham's rat virus (KRV) alone can induce spontaneous diabetes in DR-BB rats (Guberski *et al.*, 1991). A recent outbreak of spontaneous disease in a subcolony of DR-BB/Wor rats was correlated with the presence of KRV. Isolates of this virus were obtained from affected animals and found to transfer diabetes to naive DR-BB/Wor recipients. No abnormalities in T-cell function or RT6.1 cell number were detected, nor was the virus found to be directly betacytotoxic. This suggests that KRV in some as-yet-undefined way altered the balance between regulatory elements and autoreactive effector cells in favor of disease development.

Experiments using this virus must be done in a biocontainment facility in order to prevent spread of this pathogen. Thirty percent of 21- to 25-day-old DR-BB rats inoculated with 1×10^5 plaque-forming units (PFU/s) of KRV intravenously or intraperitoneally will develop disease by 60 days of age. This virus has no effect on the incidence or timing of DM development in DP-BB rats.

5. Alternative Modes of Disease Induction

Several other treatments can cause diabetes in DR-BB rats: (1) A single dose of irradiation (125–600 rads) given at 30 days of age will produce DM in about 25% of surviving DR-BB rats (Handler *et al.*, 1989). (2) Cyclophosphamide at a dose of 50 mg/ml given at 30 days of age can also induce disease (Like *et al.*, 1985). (3) Conditioned media, the supernatant of a 72-hr incubation of rat spleen cells with 5μg/ml concanavalin A (ConA), can cause 50% of DR-BB rats to become diabetic when 1 ml is given intraperitoneally five times a week from 30 days of age to 60 days of age (Handler *et al.*, 1984).

C. Adoptive Transfer of Disease

Recipients can be 30-day-old DP-BB rats, immunosuppressed MHC-matched (RT1u) rats (irradiated, young Wistar Furth rats), or an athymic MHC-compatible rat such as the Wag-*nu/nu*. Untreated DR-BB rats are resistant to adoptive transfer from either diabetic DP or RT6-treated-DR donors. Finally, the use of severe combined immunodeficiency (SCID) mice reconstituted with BB rat fetal liver may prove to be a novel and interesting system for more fully exploring the mechanisms leading to the development of DM (Greiner *et al.*, 1991).

Tissue culture medium is usually RPMI 1640 supplemented with 100 U/ml penicillin, 100 μg/ml streptomycin, 2 mM glutamine, $5 \times 10^{-5} M$ 2-mercaptoethanol, and 5–10% heat-inactivated fetal calf serum. After 72-hr incubation, cells are generally washed in RPMI1640 and injected in RPMI or PBS. The volume of injection should be kept at approximately 0.5 cc for intravenous administration.

1. DP-BB Rat

Lymphocytes from DP rats must be activated prior to adoptive transfer. Incubation of diabetic DP spleen cells (5×10^6 cells/ml) with concanavalin A at 5 μg/ml for 72 hr will render these cells capable of adoptive transfer, as first demonstrated by Koevary (1983). Stimulation with ionomycin (0.25 μM) and phorbol myristate acetate (PMA) at 20 ng/ml will allow diabetic DP spleen cells to transfer DM (Métroz-Dayer *et al.*, 1990). Isolated CD4+ T cells, when stimulated with these agents, but not by ConA, can also transfer disease. The intravenous dose needed for adoptive transfer is usually between 20 and 70×10^6 cells. In both DP-BB and DR-BB rat models, CD4+ and CD8+ T cells are required for the adoptive transfer of DM to naive, MHC-compatible recipients (Edouard *et al.*, 1993; Whalen *et al.*, 1993).

2. DR-BB Rat

Lymphocytes from CH anti-RT6.1 antibody-treated DR-BB/Wor rats can transfer disease with or without ConA activation to young DP and athymic MHC-matched Wag-*nu/nu* recipients (McKeever *et al.*, 1990). Activation with ConA or other agents may be necessary when VAF animals, rather than conventionally housed DR-BB rats, are employed. Inoculation with 100×10^6 nonactivated or fresh spleen cells has been shown to transfer diabetes. A lower dose (40×10^6) of ConA-activated spleen cells will cause disease. Nylon wool-purified T cells ($1–12 \times 10^6$) from either the spleen or lymph nodes of RT6-treated DR-BB/Wor rats can also transfer DM (Whalen *et al.*, 1993). Furthermore, spleen cells from RT6.1-depleted VAF DR-BB/Wor rats activated by specific staphylococcal enterotoxins can also transfer diabetes, as shown by Ellerman (1992).

D. Course of Disease

1. Onset

VAF DP-BB rats—mean age 76 days (range 55–120 days); VAF DR-BB rats—mean age 52 days (range 42–75 days) (see Table II).

2. Detection

Animals are screened by weight and urine glucose testing (Testape-Lilly) three times a week, beginning at least 10 days prior to the expected onset of DM. Blood glucose determinations are then used to confirm the diagnosis.

3. Duration

Permanent hyperglycemia occurs with development of ketosis if insulin is not administered, usually within several days of diagnosis.

IV. Quantitation

A. Insulitis

Mononuclear cell infiltrate of islets.

1. Mild—immune cells surrounding the islet, without invading the islet itself.
2. Moderate—immune cells invading the islet, but normal islet tissue still present.
3. Severe—immune cells totally engulf the islet and few if any normal islet cells are detectable.
4. End-stage—no beta cells, few immune cells, only remaining cells are alpha and delta cells. Very small, atrophic in appearance.

B. Diabetes

Blood glucose determinations >200 mg/dl (11 mM) performed on two separate days. Glucose analyzers are the gold standard, although many labs now use home blood glucose monitors as an alternative method.

V. Resistance

Kuttler (1991) has suggested that the few DP-BB rats who do not become diabetic by 120 days of age may have developed resistance to diabetes that can be transferred to naive recipients. Transfusions of DR-BB rat spleen cells will protect young DP-BB rats from the subsequent development of DM (Burstein *et al.*, 1989). This beneficial effect is correlated with the engraftment of RT6.1+ T cells.

DR-BB rats appear to be susceptible to the induction of diabetes prior to 60 days of age, but become quite resistant to disease development by these same agents after 60 days of age (Greiner *et al.*, 1987). The reason for this finding is not known.

VI. Expert Experience

As discussed previously, the incidence of disease in both models will be affected by the environment the animals are exposed to. To minimize the variability of both *in vivo* and especially *in vitro* studies, it may be prudent to perform most experiments in VAF conditions. In the DP-BB rat, approaches such as T-cell vaccination, which rely on the animal's ability to generate an appropriate antibody or T-cell response to an immunologic challenge, may not succeed owing to the dysregulated immune system of the DP-BB rat. Interpretation of transplantation experiments in the DP-BB rat must be balanced by the prolonged survival of any allograft in comparison with MHC-matched immunocompetent control strains. In contrast, the RT6-DR-BB rat, even while being treated with a cytotoxic antibody, continues to be an immunologically competent animal, unlike the DP-BB rat. Therefore, we feel that immunomodulatory experiments or transplantation studies can be successfully undertaken and reliably interpreted in this model.

VII. Lessons

It is much easier to prevent the initial development of diabetes than to avert the recurrence of autoimmune disease in both BB rat models of IDDM. Furthermore, it is more difficult to block autoimmune recurrence than allograft rejection.

Since prevention of diabetes development and even autoimmune recurrence appears to be so relatively easy to attain in the immunocompromised DP-BB rat, one must be cautious in generalizing these findings to immunocompetent human IDDM patients. Furthermore, one should note that since so many diverse therapies appear to prevent DM in the NOD mouse, the interpretation of prevention experiments in this animal model is also plagued by this concern.

In our experience, it is much more difficult to prevent both the initial development of diabetes (Mordes *et al.*, 1991) and the recurrence of autoimmunity in islet transplantation experiments in the RT6-DR-BB rat model (Gottlieb *et al.*, 1990). This animal appears to be more immunocompetent than either the DP-BB rat or the NOD mouse. Therefore, in our view, studies which can prevent or reverse DM in the RT6-DR model may hold the most promise as potential therapies for human IDDM patients.

References

Angelillo, M., Greiner, D. L., Mordes, J. P., Handler, E. S., Nakamura, N., McKeever, U., and Rossini, A. A. (1988). *J. Immunol.* **141**, 4146–4151.

Burstein, D., Mordes, J. P., Greiner, D. L., Stein, D., Nakamura, N., Handler, E. S., and Rossini, A. A. (1989). *Diabetes* **38**, 24–30.

Butler, L., Guberski, D. L., and Like, A. A. (1991). In "Frontiers in Diabetes Research. Lessons from Animal Diabetes III" (E. Shafrir, Ed.), pp. 50–53. Smith-Gordon, London.

Chao, N. J., Timmerman, L., McDevitt, H. O., and Jacob, C. O. (1989). *Immunogenetics* **29**, 231–234.

Colle, E. (1990). *Clin. Immunol. Immunopathol.* **57**, 1–9.

Crisá, L., Mordes, J. P., and Rossini, A. A. (1992). *Diabetes/Metab. Rev.* **8**, 9–37.

Edouard, P., Arnaoutlis, R., and Poussier, P. (1991). *Diabetes* **40** (Suppl. 1), 54A. (Abstract)

Edouard, P., Hiserodt, J. C., Plamondon, C., and Poussier, P. (1993). *Diabetes* **42**, 390–397.

Ellerman, K. E., and Like, A. A. (1992). *Diabetes* **41**, 527–532.

Ewel, C. H., Sobel, D. O., Zeligs, B. J., and Bellanti, J. A. (1992). *Diabetes* **41**, 1016–1021.

Gottlieb, P. A., Berrios, J. P., Mariani, G., Handler, E. S., Greiner, D., Mordes, J. P., and Rossini, A. A. (1990). *Diabetes* **39**, 643–645.

Greiner, D. L., Handler, E. S., Nakano, K., Mordes, J. P., and Rossini, A. A. (1986). *J. Immunol.* **136**, 148–151.

Greiner, D. L., Mordes, J. P., Handler, E. S., Angelillo, M., Nakamura, N., and Rossini, A. A. (1987). *J. Exp. Med.* **166**, 461–475.

Greiner, D. L., Shultz, L. D., Rossini, A. A., Mordes, J. P., Handler, E. S., and Rajan, T. V. (1991). *J. Clin. Invest.* **88**, 717–719.

Guberski, D. L., Thomas, V. A., Shek, W. R., Like, A. A., Handler, E. S., Rossini, A. A., Wallace, J. E., and Welsh, R. M. (1991). *Science* **254**, 1010–1013.

Handler, E. S., Mordes, J. P., and Rossini, A. A. (1984). *Diabetologia* **27**, 284A. (Abstract)

Handler, E. S., Mordes, J. P., McKeever, U., Nakamura, N., Bernhard, J., Greiner, D. L., and Rossini, A. A. (1989). *Autoimmunity* **4**, 21–30.

Jacob, H. J., Pettersson, A., Wilson, D., Mao, Y., Lernmark, °., and Lander, E. S. (1992). *Nat. Genet.* **2**, 56–60.

Koevary, S., Rossini, A. A., Stoller, W., Chick, W., and Williams, R. M. (1983). *Science* **220**, 727–728.

Kuttler, B., Dunger, A., Volk, H. D., Diamantstein, T., and Hahn, H. J. (1991). *Diabetologia* **34**, 74–77.

Lefkowith, J., Schreiner, G., Cormier, J., Handler, E. S., Driscoll, H. K., Greiner, D., Mordes, J. P., and Rossini, A. A. (1990). *J. Exp. Med.* **171**, 729–743.

Like, A. A., Weringer, E. J., Holdash, A., McGill, P., Atkinson, D., and Rossini, A. A. (1985). *J. Immunol.* **134**, 1583–1587.

Like, A. A., Guberski, D. L., and Butler, L. (1986). *J. Immunol.* **136**, 3254–3258.

Like, A. A., Guberski, D. L., and Butler, L. (1991). *Diabetes* **40**, 259–262.

Marliss, E. B. (1983). *Metabolism* **32** (Suppl. 1), 6–7.

McKeever, U., Mordes, J. P., Greiner, D. L., Appel, M. C., Rozing, J., Handler, E. S., and Rossini, A. A. (1990). *Proc. Natl. Acad. Sci. USA* **87**, 7718–7722.

Métroz-Dayer, M.-D., Mouland, A., Brideau, C., Duhamel, D., and Poussier, P. (1990). *Diabetes* **39**, 928–932.

Mordes, J. P., Handler, E. S., Greiner, D. L., Gottlieb, P. A., McKeever, U., Tafuri, A., Thomas, V. A., and Rossini, A. A. (1991). In "Frontiers in Diabetes Research. Lessons from Animal Diabetes III" (E. Shafrir, Ed.), pp. 106–113. Smith-Gordon, London.

Nakhooda, A. F., Like, A. A., Chappel, C. I., Murray, F. T., and Marliss, E. B. (1977). *Diabetes* **26**, 100–112.

Parfrey, N. A., Prud'homme, G. J., Colle, E., Fuks, A., Seemayer, T. A., and Guttmann, R. D. (1989). *CRC Crit. Rev. Immunol.* **9**, 45–65.

Prins, J.-B., Herberg, L., Den Bieman, M., and Van Zutphen, B. F. M. (1991). *In* "Frontiers in Diabetes Research. Lessons from Animal Diabetes III" (E. Shafrir, Ed.), pp. 19–24. Smith-Gordon, London.

Rajatanavin, R., Appel, M. C., Reinhardt, W., Alex, S., Yang, Y.-N., and Braverman, L. E. (1991). *Endocrinology* **128**, 153–157.

Scott, F. W. (1988). *In* "Frontiers in Diabetes Research: Lessons from Animal Diabetes II" (E. Shafrir and A. E. Renold, Eds.), pp. 34–39. John Libbey, London.

Sobel, D. O., Newsome, J., Ewel, C. H., Bellanti, J. A., Abbassi, V., Creswell, K., and Blair, O. (1992). *Diabetes* **41**, 515–520.

Thomas, V. A., Woda, B. A., Handler, E. S., Greiner, D. L., Mordes, J. P., and Rossini, A. A. (1991). *Diabetes* **40**, 255–258.

Waite, D. J., Handler, E. S., Mordes, J. P., Rossini, A. A., and Greiner, D. L. (1993). *Cell. Immunol.*, **152**, 82–95.

Whalen, B., McKeever, U., Mordes, J. P., Handler, E. S., Greiner, D. L., and Rossini, A. A. (1993). *12th International Immunology and Diabetes Workshop, Orlando, FL* 43. (Abstract)

Chapter 11

Experimental Myocarditis

Noel R. Rose,[1] Susan L. Hill,[1] and David A. Neumann[2]

[1]Department of Immunology and Infectious Diseases, The John Hopkins University, Baltimore, Maryland 21205

[2]Risk Science Institute, International Life Sciences Institute, Washington DC 20036

I. The Models

Our research team has developed two models of experimental myocarditis in mice. The first was produced by infecting inbred strains with a cardiotropic strain of coxsackievirus B3 (CB3). The model was designed to simulate the broad spectrum of pathological changes seen in humans with virus-induced myocarditis (Herskowitz *et al.*, 1985). By detailed analysis, we were able to discern two distinct pathological processes (Rose *et al.*, 1986). The initial phase of myocarditis is associated with the presence of infectious virus and is characterized by focal necrosis and infiltrates of polymorphonuclear and mononuclear inflammatory cells. During the later phase of disease, there is a diffuse mononuclear cell infiltrate and evidence of myocyte injury without significant myocyte necrosis. It is this later phase that we attribute to an autoimmune response instigated by the initial viral infection of the heart.

A feature of the second, autoimmune phase of CB3-induced myocarditis is the production of autoantibodies to the heavy chain of cardiac myosin (Wolfgram *et al.*, 1985; Alvarez *et al.*, 1987; Neu *et al.*, 1987). We subsequently developed a second model of experimental myocarditis by immunizing mice with purified mouse cardiac myosin (Neu *et al.*, 1987). The immune response and the histopathological changes resulting from myosin immunization closely simulated the later phase of CB3-induced myocarditis.

Susceptibility to experimental myocarditis is genetically determined, but genetic control of early disease differs from susceptibility to the late phase (Rose *et al.*, 1988) (Table I). Susceptibility to the later phase of disease is especially pronounced among inbred strains of mice with an "A" background; that is, A/J or its congenics such as A.SW, A.CA, or A.BY. The severity of disease depends upon the *H-2* haplotype of these strains, being most severe in A.SW and least marked in A.CA animals. Susceptibility to myosin-induced myocarditis is also genetically determined and is most prominent in A/J and

Table I
Responses of Inbred Mouse Strains to Coxsackievirus-B3 Infection[a]

Strain	*H-2*	Early (viral) myocarditis[b]	Late (autoimmune) myocarditis
A/J	a	++	++
A.BY/SnJ	b	++	++
A.CA/SnJ	f	+	+
A.SW/SnJ	g	++	+
BALB/CByJ	d	+	++
BALB.B/Kh	b	+	+
BALB.K/Kh	k	++	+
C3H/HeSn	k	+	−
C3H.SW/SnJ	b	++	++
C3HJK/SnJ	j	+	++
C3H.NB/SnJ	p	++	−
B10.A/Sg	a	+	−
B10.D2/SnJ	d	++	−
B10.M/SnJ	f	++	−
B10.WB/Sn	j	++	−
B10.BR.Sg	k	++	−
B10.Q/SgSf	g	++	−
B10.RIII/Sg	r	+	−
B10.S/SgSf	s	+	−
B10.PL/SgSf	u	+	−
B10.SM/SfSf	v	+	−

[a] Data from Rose *et al.* (1988).
[b] ++ = severe, + = mild, − = negative.

congenic strains. Conversely, strains such as C57B6, C57B10, and the congenics B10.A and B10.S, are resistant to the development of autoimmune myocarditis.

In our model of virus-induced myocarditis, the early phase of disease begins on day 3 postinfection, reaches a peak on day 7, declines perceptibly by day 15, and essentially resolves completely by day 21 (Rose *et al.*, 1987, 1988). The diffuse infiltration associated with the later phase of disease is first seen on day 9 after infection, the same time that myosin-specific, immunoglobulin G (IgG) class antibodies start to increase in the serum. (A low level of myosin-specific IgM and IgG antibodies is present in the sera of many normal mice.) The pathological changes of late-phase disease are maximal on days 15 to 21, but persist in most animals for as long as 60 days postinfection.

Myosin-induced myocarditis is elicited by giving two subcutaneous injections 1 week apart. Lesions are usually obvious 7 days after the second injection and persist at least until day 28. Both injections are given with complete Freund's adjuvant (CFA). Smith and Allen (1991) have used pertussis vaccine as a coadjuvant for myosin immunization.

In recent experiments, we have found that "nonresponder" B10.A mice produce the later, autoimmune phase of myocarditis if the CB3 infection is accompanied by an injection of bacterial lipopolysaccharide (LPS) (Lane *et al.*, 1991). The cytokines, interleukin-1 (IL-1) and tumor necrosing factor (TNF), are also capable of converting "nonresponder" to "responder" status (Lane *et al.*, 1992). Similarly, LPS, IL-1, or TNF given with myosin to "nonresponders" induced myocarditis and myosin-specific antibodies. Thus cytokines play a critical role in susceptibility to autoimmune myocarditis. The following sections present general methods for producing autoimmune myocarditis; the reader is referred to the published papers, which indicate how the general methods have been modified to achieve specific goals.

II. Production of Virus-Induced Myocarditis[1]

A. Animals

The inbred strains of mice are purchased from the Jackson Laboratories, Bar Harbor, Maine, or raised in our own animal facilities. The animals are infected with virus propagated in Vero cell cultures (see later discussion) at 3 weeks of age. Control mice are inoculated with uninfected Vero cell lysates at 3 weeks of age.

[1]See Wolfgram *et al.*, (1986).

B. Vero Cell Culture

Vero, a continuous line of African green monkey kidney cells (Flow Laboratories, McLean, Virginia), is maintained in Dulbecco's modified Eagle's medium (DMEM; Sigma Chemical, St. Louis, Missouri) which is supplemented with 10% fetal calf serum (FCS; Gibco, Grand Island, New York), 0.2 mM glutamine (Gibco) 50 μg/ml gentamicin (MA Bioproducts, Walkersville, Maryland) and 25 mM N-(2-hydroxyethyl)piperazine-N'-ethanesulfonic acid (HEPES; Sigma). The cells are grown in 25-cm^2 tissue culture flasks (T-25; Corning Glass, Corning, New York) in a humidified 37°C incubator containing a 5% CO atmosphere. Once the monolayers have become confluent, they are rinsed with Dulbecco's phosphate-buffered saline (PBS), and 2 ml of a 0.25% trypsin (1:250; Difco, Detroit, Michigan)–0.02% disodium ethylenediaminetetraacetate (EDTA; Sigma) solution is added. The excess solution is poured off and the flask is placed in the 37°C incubator until the cells are dislodged (approximately 3–5 min). Following the trypsin-EDTA treatment, the Vero cells are resuspended in 6 ml DMEM–10% fetal calf serum (FCS) and a total of 4×10^5 cells are added to a new T-25 flask containing 7 ml of fresh DMEM–10% FCS medium.

For virus titration or virus neutralization assays, Vero cells are suspended in supplemented DMEM containing 2% gamma-globulin-free FCS (GG-free FCS; GIBCO) and 3×10^3 to 5×10^3 cells/100 μl are plated into the wells of a 96-well microtiter plate (Costar, Cambridge, Massachusetts) and sealed with plate sealers (Costar). The plates are then placed at 37°C in a humidified CO$_2$ incubator. These Vero cell cultures are used after reaching 70–80% confluence 1 or 2 days later.

C. Virus Preparation

The original stock of coxsackievirus B3 (Nancy strain) used in our studies was obtained from Drs. A. M. Lerner and R. Khatib, Wayne State University, School of Medicine, Detroit, Michigan. Their virus had been given to them by Dr. I. Grodums, University of Saskatchewan, Saskatoon, Canada. The original prototype CB3 (Nancy) was isolated by Dr. Joseph Melnick of Houston, Texas, from a patient with a minor febrile illness.

A stock virus is prepared by adding 0.1–0.2 ml CB3 to confluent Vero cell monolayers in T-25 flasks containing 7 ml supplemented DMEM with 2% GG-free FCS. The flasks are incubated in a 37°C incubator overnight or until 95–100% of the cells exhibit cytopathic effects (CPEs). When the maximal CPE is reached, the cells are dislodged with a rubber policeman and the resulting cell suspension subjected to three freeze-thaw cycles. The virus-cell lysates are then centrifuged for 10 min at 10,000g at 4°C to remove the cellular debris. The supernatant is divided into aliquots, frozen, and stored at −70°C until used.

D. Virus Titration

The virus titration is carried out by diluting 20 μl of the virus pool in 180 μl of supplemented DMEM with 2% GG-free FCS, followed by four or more tenfold serial dilutions. Each dilution is then plated in triplicate wells of a microtiter plate containing Vero cells that are 70–80% confluent. The plates are sealed and incubated for 3 days at 37°C. The CPE is determined for each well. When any virus-induced cytopathology is observed in the Vero cell monolayer, a well is designated as positive. The 50% tissue culture infective dose ($TCID_{50}$) is determined. The equation for calculating the proportionate distance of the 50% end point above the dilution giving the next percent below 50% CPE is

$$\frac{(\% \text{ CPE at dilution above } 50\%) - (50\%)}{(\% \text{ CPE at next dilution above } 50\%) - (\% \text{ CPE at next dilution below})} = \frac{\text{Proportional}}{\text{distance}}$$

This method allows for the exact calculation of the 50% end point. The same procedure is used for the titration of the virus content of serum or of various organs removed at necropsy. For the heart, a 1% (w/v) suspension of the tissue is made in DMEM–2% FCS. For the other organs—spleen, thymus, and pancreas—a 10% tissue suspension is made. The organs are homogenized individually in ground-glass tissue grinders. Each organ suspension is frozen and thawed three times and then centrifuged at 13,000g for 10 min in a microfuge (Eppendorf, Brinkman Instruments, Westbury, New York). The resulting supernatant is then assayed for virus titer.

In each assay, a previously titered stock virus pool is included to assess interassay variation. In addition, each plate has three wells that receive 100 μl of fresh medium and three wells that receive 150 μl of medium containing 100 $TCID_{50}$ CB3. These two intra-assay controls allow for a comparison of 100% CPE and the appearance of uninfected Vero cell monolayers. The three wells containing virus also serve as the end point for the assay. When these wells reach 100% CPE, generally after 3 days, the assay is read. These six control wells are also included in the virus neutralization assay.

E. Virus Neutralization

Mouse serum samples are diluted 1:8 followed by twofold serial dilutions in DMEM-2% GG-free FCS to a total volume of 100 μl per dilution. The initial dilution of the serum of 1:8 reduces the sensitivity of this assay in that extremely low levels of antibody may be undetectable. However, it was necessary in order to prevent serum-induced cytotoxicity in the Vero cell culture. A standard quantity (2×10^3 $TCID_{50}$/ml) of CB3 is added to the equivalent volume of each serum dilution. The virus-serum mixture was then incubated at 37°C for 45 min to allow for neutralization. In addition to the experimental sera, a serum with a known neutralizing titer is included as an internal assay control. Following incubation, the mixtures are plated onto Vero cells in triplicate wells. The microtiter plate is sealed and incubated at 37°C for 3 days. After 3 days, the wells are examined for the absence of CPE as evidence of virus neutralization. The serum neutralizing titer is defined as the reciprocal of the greatest dilution of serum showing 100% viral inhibition compared with the uninfected Vero cell controls.

F. Infection and Necropsy

Three-week-old mice are inoculated intraperitoneally (ip) with 0.1 ml of a 5 $TCID_{50}$ CB3 suspension in DMEM. The mice are weighed and bled at various times by retroorbital bleeding. Mouse sera are individually collected and frozen at -70°C until viral and antibody assays can be performed. At the end of the experiment, the mice are anesthetized and sacrificed by cervical dislocation, the heart apex is removed and frozen for later virological determination. In some studies, the spleen, thymus, and pancreas are also removed and frozen for later virus titration. The remainder of the heart is fixed in 10% formalin in phosphate-buffered saline for histological examination. The heart weight is also determined for calculation of heart-to-body weight ratios.

The high mutability of the CB3 virus necessitates frequent passaging. The virus is annually passaged through mice. CB3 is inoculated at a dosage of 0.1 ml of a 5 $TCID_{50}$ CB3 suspension in DMEM and recovered from the heart. This is repeated 6 to 10 times. Final virus recovery is followed by $TCID_{50}$ determination and a small pilot study to determine the appropriate dose of virus for the development of optimal early- and late-stage cardiac lesions.

G. Lipopolysaccharide Treatment

CB3 infection of A/J mice and congenics on the A background results in autoimmune myocarditis. CB3-infected resistant mice, such as B10.A, which have been identically treated, are resistant to the autoimmune disease. LPS treatment of resistant B10.A mice renders them susceptible to the autoimmune sequela of CB3 infection (Lane *et al.*, 1991). In these experiments B10.A mice, 14 to 20 days of age, are inoculated intraperitoneally with a 1:3 dilution of 0.1 ml of 5 TCID of CB3 and with 25 μg LPS (from *Salmonella*

Minnesota Re 595 Sigma) in 0.1 ml sterile saline intraperitoneally. A second injection of LPS is given on day 4. Similar results are obtained when CB3-infected mice are treated with 100 mg of IL-1 synthetic peptide 163–171 (Sigma) or 250 ng of TNF synthetic peptide 114–130 (ICN Biochemicals, Costa Mesa, CA) (Lane *et al.*, 1992).

III. Production of Myosin-Induced Myocarditis

A. Antigen Preparations

Cardiac and skeletal muscle preparations are produced using two different protocols (Neu *et al.*, 1987a). These include whole-muscle extraction and purification of myosin. A cocktail of protease inhibitors (leupeptin, 1 mg/ml; antipapain 2 mg/ml; benzamidine, 10 mg/ml; Trasylol 10,000 units; in 0.9% w/v sodium chloride (NaCl), pH 7.0) is used during the course of the myocardial and skeletal muscle extractions. It consists of 1 mg/ml leupeptin, 2 mg/ml antipapain, 10 mg/ml benzamidine, and 10,000 units of Trasylol, all dissolved in 0.9% w/v sodium chloride (NaCl), pH 7.0. All procedures are carried out at 4°C. Immediately after removal hearts are submerged in a cold solution of 30 mM KCl in PBS (pH 7.2) to induce diastolic arrest.

1. Whole Muscle Extracts

Muscles of the limbs and back are quickly removed and rinsed in cold PBS, pH 7.2. The heart is submitted to diastolic arrest in 30 mM KCl followed by addition of the protease inhibitor cocktail. Once the muscles are isolated and washed, the excess buffer is removed and the tissue minced. Each tissue is homogenized in a low salt buffer [1% Triton X-100, 0.1 M KCl, 2 mM MgCL$_2$, 2 mM ethyleneglycol-*bis*-(β-aminoethylether)N, N,N',N'-tetraacetic acid (EGTA), 0.5 mM dithiothreitol (DTT), 10 mM Tris–HCl, pH 7] by using a conical glass homogenizer. After obtaining a fine suspension, a 2× sample buffer [0.5 M Tris–HCl, 25% v/v glycerol, 10% w/v sodium dodecyl sulfate (SDS), 0.5% w/v bromophenol blue and DTT, pH 6.8] is added. The homogenate is then boiled for 5 min and centrifuged using an airfuge (Beckman) at 20 psi for 5 min. This preparation is prepared fresh each time.

2. Purified Myosin

Hearts or skeletal muscle from 40 mice are quickly removed, rinsed in cold PBS, and placed in a cold PBS or 30 mM KCl solution as described above. An approximate organ weight is determined, the tissue minced with scissors and homogenized in a conical ground-glass homogenizer with 10 ml/gm tissue of precooled modified Hasselbach-Schneider solution at 4°C (0.3 M KCl,

0.15 M K$_2$HPO$_4$, 0.01 M Na$_4$P$_2$O$_7$, 1 mM MgCl$_2$, pH 6.8) containing 20 μl of protease inhibitors. The suspension is then extracted with mixing at 4°C for 90 min.

B. Immunization

Three-to-six-week-old mice of either sex are immunized with cardiac or skeletal muscle myosin. Briefly, the myosin preparations are diluted in 50 mM sodium pyrophosphate, pH 7.0, to the working concentration, usually 1.0 mg/ ml. The antigens are then mixed with an equal volume of complete Freund's adjuvant containing *Mycobacterium tuberculosis* H37Ra (Difco). A total of 200 μl of the emulsion is injected subcutaneously (s.c.) into right and left inguinal and the thoracic regions. Seven days later, the mice are reinjected using the same protocol. Sham immunizations are performed with sodium pyrophosphate in CFA. Sera are obtained by retroorbital bleeding on days 7, 14, 21, and 28 after the first immunization. The samples are stored individually at −70°C for future evaluation. B10.A mice, which are normally resistant to autoimmune myocarditis, develop the disease if they are immunized with cardiac myosin emulsified in complete Freund's adjuvant and cotreated with LPS, IL-1, or TNF, as described in Section II,G.

IV. Evaluation

A. Histology

The 10% formalin-fixed heart is imbedded in paraffin according to standard procedures. Transverse sections of the hearts are cut at two levels to ensure adequate representation of the heart pathology. Ten serial sections, 5–6 microns thick, are cut at each level and then stained with hematoxylin-eosin. The stained sections are evaluated by two independent observers. Areas of necrosis, mononuclear cell infiltration, fibrosis, and mineralization are located anatomically, described, and quantitated using a 0–4 scale. Grade 0 indicates that there are no detectable lesions in the tissue sections examined, while grades 2, 3, and 4 represent 1–10%, 10–25%, and >25% of the myocardium in tissue sections examined affected, respectively.

B. Indirect Immunofluorescence Assay

The heart, kidney, liver, skeletal muscle (gastrocnemius), stomach, submaxillary salivary gland, and pancreas from normal syngeneic mice are used in this assay. The organs are rinsed in PBS, frozen, and then mounted in orthinine carbamoyl transferase (OCT) medium (Miles Labs, Elkhart, Indiana). Four-micron-thick sections are cut and placed onto ethanol-cleaned microscope slides. The tissue sections are then air dried for 1–1.5 hr and used immediately in an indirect immunofluorescence assay (IIF) or frozen at −70°C until needed.

Each section is washed in PBS for 5 min. This is followed by blocking with 3% bovine serum albumin (BSA) in PBS for 30 min in a humidified chamber. The section is then overlaid with 50 μl of the appropriate dilution of mouse serum in blocking solution (PBS/3% BSA). Each serum is initially tested at a 1:50 dilution. If the serum is being titrated, five twofold serial dilutions are made following an initial 1:10 dilution. The sections are incubated with the serum dilutions in a humidified chamber for 30 min, after which the slides are rinsed three times in PBS and then washed in PBS for 30 min. Next, the sections are overlaid with 50 μl of fluorescein isothiocyanate (FITC)-conjugated goat antimouse immunoglobulins containing rhodamine B counterstain, 15 μl/ml (Difco). The appropriate dilution of FITC-labeled immunoglobulins is determined by titrating the conjugate 1:50, 1:100, and 1:200 in blocking solution (PBS/3% BSA). These dilutions are assayed on tissue sections treated with a serum that had previously been demonstrated to react with striated muscle and nuclei. The dilution used in further assays is the dilution which had the greatest reactivity with minimal background fluorescence. The FITC conjugates include goat antimouse immunoglobulins (Organon-Technics, West Chester, PA), goat antimouse IgG (Tago, Burlingame, California) and goat antimouse IgM (Organon-Technics).

The sections with the conjugate counterstain are incubated in the humidified chamber for 30 min. This is followed with a triple rinse and 30-min wash in PBS. After the final wash, excess PBS is blotted off the slide and each section is mounted in a drop of glycerol–PBS (9:1) and a coverslip added. The entire assay is performed at room temperature. The sections are observed for reactivity using a Zeiss fluorescent microscope. The slides are stored in folders at 4°C if future analysis is required.

A 0 to 4+ grading scale is used to identify the intensity of the reaction of the sera with the various mouse tissues. The grading scheme is as follows: 0 is no reaction above background; +/− is a questionable reaction in which there was a low level of green fluorescence in some cells, which faded rapidly upon observation; 1+ is a definite reaction but it is difficult to identify specific areas of reaction since the dull green color is generally quite diffuse; 2+ is a moderate reaction in which it is possible to define reactivities throughout the tissue, which does not fade during the period of observation; 3+ is a strong reaction which allows for multiple observations before the fluorescence fades significantly and is due to nearly all of the tissue reacting with the serum being tested; and 4+ is an intense reaction that does not fade rapidly. However, the 4+ reaction is often so bright that there is distortion owing to the high level of fluorescence, which makes it difficult to delineate the amount of tissue reactivity.

Four controls are included in each assay. A PBS–PBS control, which uses PBS as the initial overlay and in place of the conjugate overlay, is done to detect the presence of autofluorescence in the tissue. A PBS–conjugate control, in which PBS replaces the serum overlay, allows for the visualization of any nonspecific binding of the conjugate with the normal tissue. The final two controls are a proven negative serum, usually a normal mouse serum of the strain being tested and a positive serum which has a 3+ reaction.

C. Absorption Studies

The heart, kidneys, livers, and skeletal muscle (gastrocnemius) are removed from 30–50 mice. The organs are rinsed free of blood in cold borate-buffered saline (BBS; 0.17 M borate, 0.12 M NaCl, pH 8.0) and minced with scalpels. The organs are then homogenized in BBS and centrifuged at 2000g at 4°C for 10 min. The pellet is then washed until the supernatant clarifies and is saved as the insoluble fraction. The original supernatant and subsequent washings are pooled and centrifuged at 16,300g at 4°C for 1 hr. The resulting pellet is saved as the microsomal fraction and the resulting supernatant is designated as the soluble fraction. Each of the three fractions from the four organs is dialyzed against 1200 volumes of distilled water and then lyophilized.

The lyophilized organ extracts are used to absorb the serum samples which were positive for autoantibodies in order to determine their specificity. Four milligrams of any individual fraction are combined with 0.1 ml of diluted (1:10) serum. The mixture is then placed on a rocker panel for 1 hr at room temperature. Following this incubation, the slurry is centrifuged for 10 min in a microcentrifuge. The supernatant is removed and used in an indirect immunofluorescence assay.

D. Western Immunoblotting

Different antigenic preparations are loaded on a 3–16% gradient SDS–polyacrylamide gel. The gels are subjected to electrophoresis at 55 V for 2–3 hr using a mini-slab gel electrophoresis apparatus (Hoeffer Sci. Inst., San Francisco, California). Next, the proteins are electrophoretically transferred onto 0.45 μm Immunobilon polyvinylidene-difluoride (PVDF) (Millipore Corp., Bedford, Massachusetts) in a buffer containing 25 mM Tris base (Sigma) and 192 mM glycine, pH 8.1, at 250 mA in 4°C for 2 hr in a circulating bath. The strips are air-dried and used immediately or stored at room temperature until used. For immunodetection, the PVDF strips are prewetted with 100 percent methanol and placed into individual troughs in plastic lid boxes (Hoeffer Scientific) for 1 hr at room temperature in 2 ml of 50 mM Tris, containing 0.15 M NaCl, 0.05% Tween-20, 5% nonfat dry milk (Carnation Co., Los Angeles, California). Sera are diluted in 50 mM Tris, 0.5 m NaCl, 0.05% Tween-20, pH 7.4, Tris-buffered saline with Tween (TBS-T), sealed and allowed to incubate with constant rocking for 2 hr at room temperature. After removal of the antiserum, the strips are washed three times (15 min each) in TBS-T. The strips are overlaid with 2 ml of goat F(ab)'2 antimouse F_cIgG (Jackson Immuno Research Laboratories, Inc., Westgrove, PA), and diluted at 1:2000 in TBS-T. The strips are allowed to incubate 1 hr at room temperature, washed three times (15 min) in TBS-T, and 2 ml of avidin-peroxidase diluted 1:50,000 in TBS-T are placed on the strips and allowed to incubate at room temperature for 1 hr. The strips are again washed three times in TBS-T and developed with 2.2 mM 3,3-diaminobenzidine solution (Sigma) made up in 100 mM Tris, pH 7.0 containing 1.7 mM NiCl$_2$, 0.03% v/v, 30% H_2O_2. The strips are allowed to develop 5 min at room temperature or until the desired intensity is reached. The reaction is stopped by washing the strips three to five times in dH_2O. The strips are air dried and reactivity is assessed by correlation with molecular weight standards.

E. Enzyme-Linked Immunosorbent Assay

Individual wells in polystyrene microtiter plates (Dynatech Laboratories, Inc., Alexandria, VA) are coated with 0.5 μg myosin in 100 μl 0.15 M carbonate–bicarbonate buffer, pH 9.6. Fifty millimolar sodium pyrophosphate is added to the carbonate buffer to maintain myosin in its soluble state. After 1 hr at 37°C, the plates are washed with PBS containing 0.1% Tween-20 (PBS-T), and the excess binding sites are blocked with 2% bovine serum albumin (BSA) in PBS-T for 30 min at 37°C. Sera are diluted in PBS-T containing 1% BSA, and 100 μl of the dilution added to the wells and incubated for 1 hr at 37°C. One hundred microliters of sera diluted in PBS-T containing 1% BSA are added to the wells and incubated for 1 hr at 37°C. After three washes with PBS-T, 0.5 μg of peroxidase-labeled goat antimouse Ig, IgG, and IgM (Organon-Technics) are added to the wells and incubated for 30 min at 37°C. After 3 washes in PBS-T, the plates are incubated for 30 min with 100 μl/well of Extravidin peroxidase (1/40,000). They are then washed three times in PBS-T followed by the addition of 150 μl of substrate solution (80 mg o-phenylenediamine in 20 ml citrate buffer and 8 μl 30% H_2O_2, pH 5). After 30 min at 37°C the optical density (OD) is measured at 450 nm. The reaction is then stopped by adding 50 μl of 3 M H_2SO_4. The OD is measured at 490 nm if the reaction has been stopped.

F. Immunoglobulin Elution

Hearts from treated or control animals are pooled and minced in 40 ml of RPMI 1640 under aseptic conditions. The minced tissue is transferred to sterile tubes and centrifuged for 10 min at 850g at room temperature. After three additional washes in RPMI, the tissue is resuspended in 11 ml of RPMI containing 160 U/ml of collagenase (Sigma). The suspension is incubated at 37°C for 1 hr with constant rocking, and decanted into a petri plate, where the residual tissue is ground between the frosted ends of sterile microscope slides. The preparation is centrifuged for 5 min at 50g at room temperature.

The digested tissue is washed with RPMI containing 1 mM phenylmethylsulfonylfluoride (PMSF) and twice with RPMI alone. The pellet is resuspended in 20 ml of 0–02 M citric acid in phosphate-buffered saline, pH 3.2, and incubated for 3 hr at 37°C with constant rocking. Insoluble material is pelleted by centrifugation at room temperature for 10 min at 1200g. The supernatant is neutralized with 20 ml of 1 M Tris-base and dialyzed in the cold against several changes of PBS containing 0.02% sodium azide. The protein concentration of the dialyzed eluates is determined by the bicinchoinic acid (Pierce Chemical Co., Rockford, Illinois) procedure. Dialyzed eluates are tested for the presence of heart-reactive antibodies.

G. Immunohistochemistry

A direct immunohistochemistry procedure is used to detect the *in situ* deposition of IgG in the hearts of the treated animals. An indirect immunohistochemistry procedure is used for detecting serum autoantibodies to normal heart, brain, thyroid, stomach, pancreas, intestine, and kidney tissue; for the detection of MHC class I and class II antigens on heart tissue; for the identification of inflammatory cells in the heart; and for the detection of IL-1- and TNF-secreting cells. Frozen tissue sections (5 microns) are placed onto Histostik (Accurate Antibodies, Westbury, New York)-coated slides and acetone fixed for 10 min. Slides are washed in two changes in Tris-buffered saline (TBS) followed by incubation with 1% avidin in TBS for 20 min in a humidified chamber. The slides are then washed in TBS for 5 min and incubated with 0.5% biotin (10 mg/ml) in TBS for 20 min in a humidified chamber. They are again washed in fresh TBS for 20 min. Endogenous peroxidase is inactivated by a 30-min incubation with 0.5% hydrogen peroxide in TBS–milk and 1% normal rabbit serum (NRS). Sections are blocked in TBS–milk and 1% NRS for 10 min. This and all subsequent incubations are performed at room temperature with TBS–milk washes following each incubation period.

For the determination of serum autoantibodies reactive to normal tissues, sera are diluted 1:100 in TBS–milk with 1% normal goat serum and incubated for 1 hr with sections from normal heparinized-saline perfused mouse tissues. Heart-bound IgG and serum IgG autoantibody in the treated mice are detected by a 30-min incubation with biotin-conjugated goat F(ab)'2 antimouse IgG (Fc-specific) (Jackson Immunoresearch).

MHC class I and class II antigens are detected by using tissue culture supernatants from the mouse hybridoma clones 11-4.1 and 11-5.2.1.9 (American Type Culture Collection, ATCC, Rockville, Maryland), respectively, followed by a 1-hr incubation with biotin-conjugated goat antimouse IgG2a (Southern Biotechnology Assoc., Birmingham, Alabama) for class I and goat antimouse IgG2b (Southern Biotechnology) for class II.

Heart inflammatory cells are identified by using tissue culture supernatants from the rat hybridoma clones M1/9.3.4.HL.2 (anticommon leukocyte antigen), 30-H12 (anti-Thy 1.2), GK1.5 (anti-L3T4), 53-6.72 (anti-Lyt 2), and M3/84.6.34 (anti-MAC-3) from the ATCC followed by a 1-hr incubation with biotin-conjugated rabbit antirat IgG (Vector Laboratories, Burlingame, California). IL-1- and TNF-secreting cells are identified by using a rabbit anti-murine IL-1 reagent (Genzyme, Boston, Massachusetts) and rabbit anti-TNF (Endogen, Boston, Massachusetts) followed by a 1-hr incubation with biotin-conjugated goat antirabbit IgG (Vector). Tissues are incubated for 1 hr with avidin and biotinylated horseradish peroxidase complex (Vectastain ABC, Vector Laboratories), and with diaminobenzidene substrate for 8 min. The slides are immersed in copper sulfate solution (0.5% copper sulfate in 0.15 M NaCl) for 2 min, followed by counterstaining with Mayer's modified hematoxylin (Polyscientific, Bay Shore, New York).

H. Isolation of Heart Inflammatory Cells

Inflammatory cells are obtained from the heart tissue of treated mice. Briefly, ten hearts from virus-infected or myosin-immunized mice are placed into RPMI 1640 medium (Sigma) and minced under sterile conditions. The tissue debris is pelleted by centrifugation and washed in RPMI 1640. The tissue is resuspended in collagenase/RPMI 1640 medium and incubated for 1 hr at 37°C with gentle rocking. The tissue suspension is centrifuged (50g for 5 min) and the supernatant layered onto Ficoll–Hypaque for inflammatory cell recovery. Inflammatory cells (2 × 10^5 per well) are placed into 24-well tissue culture plates suspended in 1 ml of RPMI 1640 medium containing 5% fetal calf serum for further testing.

I. Adoptive Transfer of Lymphoid Cells

Spleens are aseptically removed from mice at various times following treatment. Single-cell suspensions are prepared in RPMI 1640 (Sigma) by disrupting the spleens from three animals on a stainless steel mesh. The cells are sedimented by centrifugation and resuspended in 0.83% ammonium chloride to lyse contaminating erythrocytes. After three washes in RPMI 1640, the cells were resuspended at a density of 1×10^8 cells/ml in RPMI 1640 containing 1% normal rat serum, 1% L-glutamine, 0.02 mM 2-mercaptoethanol, 5 mM HEPES, and gentamicin (50 µl/100 ml). Myocarditis is adoptively transferred to 1-week-old syngeneic mice treated with LPS (as described earlier) on days 0 and 4 if the cells are administered intraperitoneally on day 3.

In another experimental approach, heart inflammatory cells are obtained by mincing the hearts from 10 mice treated with myosin, as described above. The minced tissue is washed three times in RPMI 1640 and incubated overnight at 37°C on a petri plate containing 10 ml of medium. The cells are recovered by repeated aspiration, pelleted by centrifugation, and treated as described earlier to eliminate erythrocytes. The cells are resuspended at 5.5×10^6 cells/ml. Myocarditis is observed when 0.1 ml of this preparation is administered intraperitoneally to 1–2-week-old syngeneic mice that were pretreated with LPS.

Acknowledgment

We thank our many colleagues who developed the methods described. They include Drs. Ahvie Herskowitz, Kirk Beisel, Luanne Wolfgram, Nikolas Neu, Susan Craig, Floria Alvarez, Monica Traystman, and James Lane. Our research is supported by National Institutes of Health grant HL33878. Dr. Susan Hill is supported by National Institutes of Health Research training Grant RRO 07002.

References

Alvarez, F. L., Neu, N., Rose, N. R., Craig, S. W., and Beisel, K. W. (1987). *Clin. Immunol. Immunopathol.* **43**, 129–139.

Herskowitz, A., Beisel, K. W., Wolfgram, L. J., and Rose, N. R. (1985). *Hum. Pathol.* **16**, 671–673.

Lane, J. R., Neumann, D. A., Lafond-Walker, A., Herskowitz, A., and Rose, N. R. (1991). *Cell. Immunol.* **136**, 219–233.

Lane, J. R., Neumann, D. A., Lafond-Walker, A., Herskowitz, A., and Rose, N. R. (1992). *J. Exp. Med.* **175**, 1123–1129.

Neu, N., Beisel, K. W., Traystman, M. D., Rose, N. R., and Craig, S. W. (1987a). *J. Immunol.* **138**, 2488–2492.

Neu, N., Craig, S. W., Rose, N. R., Alvarez, F., and Beisel, K. W. (1987b). *Clin. Exp. Immunol.* **69**, 566–574.

Neu, N., Rose, N. R., Beisel, K. W., Herskowitz, A., Gurri-Glass, G., and Craig, S. W. (1987c). *J. Immunol.* **139**, 3630–3636.

Rose, N. R., Wolfgram, L. J., Herskowitz, A., and Beisel, K. W. (1986). *Ann. N.Y. Acad. Sci.* **475**, 146–156.

Rose, N. R., Beisel, K. W., Herskowitz, A., Neu, N., Wolfgram, L. J., Alvarez, F. L., Traystman, M. D., and Craig, S. W. (1987). *In* "Autoimmunity and Autoimmune Disease" (D. Evered, Ed.), pp. 3–24. Wiley, Chichester, UK.

Rose, N. R., Herskowitz, A., Neumann, D. A., and Neu, N. (1988a). *Immunol. Today* **9**, 117–119.

Rose, N. R., Neumann, D. A., Herskowitz, A., Beisel, K., and Traystman, M. (1988b). *Pathol. Immunopathol. Res.* **7**, 266–278.

Smith, S. C., and Allen, P. M. (1991). *J. Immunol.* **147**, 2141–2147.

Wolfgram, L. J., Beisel, K. W., and Rose, N. R. (1985). *J. Exp. Med.* **161**, 1112–1121.

Wolfgram, L. J., Beisel, K. W., Herskowitz, A., and Rose, N. R. (1986). *J. Immunol.* **136**, 1846–1852.

Chapter 12

Experimental Hepatitis

Ansgar W. Lohse and Karl-Hermann Meyer zum Büschenfelde

Department of Medicine, Johannes Gutenberg-University, D-6500 Mainz , Germany

I. History of Experimental Autoimmune Hepatitis

The first attempts to induce an experimental hepatitis in animals go back to the beginning of the century. A summary of the various models published is given in Table I. This list does not claim to be exhaustive. It does not include some of the studies performed without adequate controls. Some minor variations of the models described have also been omitted. For many years chronic active hepatitis in rabbits induced by immunization of heterologous (human) liver antigens in adjuvant was the standard animal model of hepatitis (Meyer zum Büschenfelde *et al.*, 1972). This model was very helpful in earlier studies on the role of humoral immune responses to liver antigen, but the lack of inbred strains for study of T cell responses, and the difficulties of keeping rabbits as laboratory animals, led to the abandonment of this model.

More recently, murine experimental autoimmune hepatitis (EAH) has been established in various laboratories (Kuriki *et al.*, 1983; Mori *et al.*, 1984; Watanabe *et al.*, 1987; Lohse *et al.*, 1990a). Protocols and animal strains differ somewhat in different labs, but the systems used are becoming increasingly

Table I

Animal Models of Autoimmune Hepatitis[a]

Year	First author	Species	Antigen	Adjuvant	Injections	Results
1908	Fiessinger	Rabbit	Nuclear proteins	—	$3–8 \times$ i.p.	Biliary cirrhosis in 3 out of 7 animals; negative results in dogs and guinea pigs
1946	Casals	Mouse	Homo.LH	—	$10 \times$ i.p.	Periportal inflammation and necroses in 4/10 mice
1959	Behar	Guinea pig Hamster	Homo.LH	CFA	$1 \times$ i.m.	Early focal necroses in 11/31 animals (days 3–4) Focal necroses in only 3/16 hamsters
1962	Dodd	Rabbit	Rat LH	CFA	$6 \times$ s.c. $1 \times$ i.m.	Periportal infiltrations after 1 week
1963	Iliesco	Rabbit	Homo.LH	CFA	$9 \times$ s.c.	Hepatocellular necroses
1964	Coppo	Rat	Syng.LH	CFA	at least $12 \times$ s.c.	Focal inflammatory changes and necroses
1965	Scheiffarth	Rabbit	Homo.LH	CFA	$9 \times$ s.c.	Periportal infiltrations and necroses (in some animals)
1967	Scheiffarth	Mouse	Homo.LH	CFA	$6 \times$ i.m. + i.p.	Periportal infiltrations and necroses, no lesions with kidney antigen, successful passive transfer
1968	Kössling	Rabbit	Hum.LSP	CFA	$11–40 \times$ i.p.	Chronic hepatitis, no hepatitis following immunization with rabbit LSP
1983	Kuriki	Mouse	Syng.LH	Klebsiella	$3–11 \times$ i.m.	Frequent immunizations more effective, passive transfer of disease possible
1984	Mori	Mouse	Syng. S-100	CFA	$6 \times$ i.m.	Passive transfer possible, T-cell-mediated disease, specific cytotoxicity
1987	Watanabe	Mouse	Syng. S-100	CFA	$8 \times$ s.c.	Thymectomy facilitated disease induction and prolonged disease duration
1990	Lohse	Mouse	Syng. S-100	CFA	$1(–3) \times$ i.p.	Subacute T-cell-mediated hepatitis, specific T-cell reactivity, autoantibodies follow disease

[a]This table includes the earliest studies of experimental hepatitis and all those studies showing significant disease that were induced with relevant control antigens. LH = liver homogenate, LSP = liver-specific protein, S-100 = 100,000g supernatant of liver homogenate, homo. = homologous, syn = syngeneic, CFA = complete Freund's adjuvant, i.p. = intraperitoneally, i.m. = intramuscularly, s.c. = subcutaneously.

similar. We therefore concentrate our discussion on the most recent and reliable model of EAH.

II. Animals

EAH can be induced in a number of mouse strains. Most experiments were done in 5- to 7-week-old male C57 BL/6 mice, which get the most severe disease (Lohse *et al.*, 1990b). However, we have found this to differ a little in different substrains and different environments. Here in Mainz we get equally severe disease in female BALB/c mice from the colony in Hannover (Zentralinstitut für Versuchstierkunde, Hannover, Germany). Female C57BL/6 are a little less susceptible than male C57BL/6 mice, while female BALB/C mice get more severe disease than male BALB/C mice. C3H mice do not get severe disease. Earlier murine models of EAH used different mouse strains, namely SMA mice (Kuriki *et al.*, 1983), B10.A(5R) mice (Araki *et al.*, 1987), and A/J mice (Watanabe *et al.*, 1987), but none of these studies compared various strains. Lewis rats are not susceptible to EAH (Lohse *et al.*, 1990a). While some of the earlier models required neonatal thymectomy or irradiation, EAH in C57BL/6 or BALB/C mice can be induced without any pretreatment.

The effect of the cage environment has not been investigated. We have the impression that the cleaner the environment of the mice, the more severe the disease. Animals thus far have all been kept on a standard diet, but again the best results were achieved in animals receiving autoclaved food.

III. Genetic Background

As summarized in the previous section, the genetic background for induction of EAH is uncertain (Lohse *et al.*, 1990b). Data are not sufficient to allow speculation about susceptibility genes. It has been observed that the susceptible strains are low-responder strains to F-protein, a liver-specific antigen and a component of the antigen preparation used for immunization.

IV. Induction and Time Course

A. Antigen Preparation

EAH is induced by immunization with syngeneic liver antigens. The immunogen used is the 100,000g supernatant of liver homogenates and has been labeled S-100 (Mori *et al.*, 1984; Lohse *et al.*, 1990a). In antigen preparation, the liver is first flushed with cold phosphate-buffered saline (PBS) before taking it out of the animal. This procedure removes much of the enormous blood pool of the liver. After the abdomen is opened, the vena cava is cut to allow blood to run off. The portal vein is then cannulated with a fine needle and PBS is slowly injected. Cannulating the portal vein in the mouse after bleeding the animal from its caval vein requires some practice. Correct positioning and successful flushing of the liver are easily seen because the liver immediately pales as one injects the PBS. The gallbladder is removed, the liver cut into pieces, and homogenized in a homogenizer. After 10-min of centrifugation at 150g to remove whole cells and the nuclear fraction, the supernatants are centrifuged for 1 hr at 100,000g. All steps are performed at 4°C. It appears important that freshly isolated S-100 antigen be used. S-100 antigen does not store well—both freezing and refrigeration appear to decrease the immunogenicity. The use of proteinase inhibitors in antigen preparation has not been investigated. The S-100 preparation is likely to include all soluble liver proteins and is thus very crude. The membrane fractions and nuclear fraction, however, do not induce significant hepatitis.

B. Adjuvant and Immunization

All successful models of autoimmune hepatitis have used complete Freund's adjuvant (CFA) except one study using polysaccharides of *Klebsiella pneumoniae* (Kuriki *et al.*, 1983). We have not tried to vary the content of *Mycobacterium tuberculosis* in Freund's adjuvant, as has been done in experimental autoimmune encephalomyelitis. S-100 antigen (possibly diluted in PBS) and CFA have to be well emulsified, as in other models. We have always used two interconnected glass syringes for preparation of the emulsion and pushed the mixture through the connection as fast as possible and as often as necessary. It usually takes 10 min to make a good emulsion, and this is determined by an increase in the resistance when the glass syringe is pushed. The dose of S-100 antigens used for immunization seems to be of little significance (Lohse *et al.*, 1990a). We have mostly used 2.5 mg S-100 proteins in 0.5 ml of PBS mixed with 0.5 ml of CFA per animal. A tenfold lower dose (250 µg) is still effective. Lower doses have not been tested. The route of administration is intraperitoneal. When intraperitoneal immunization is used, a single injection is sufficient to induce moderate to severe disease. Adding one or two injections at weekly intervals increases maximum disease activity only slightly. EAH can also be induced by intramuscular injections, but this induces milder disease, and usually three weekly injections are required for induction (Mori *et al.*, 1985; Lohse *et al.*, 1990a). Subcutaneous immunization, even when repeated frequently, only induces very mild disease, and after immunization in the footpads, no disease has been observed.

C. Passive Transfer

EAH can be passively transferred by activated T cells from diseased animals (Mori *et al.*, 1985; Lohse *et al.*, 1990a). These experiments were done with splenocytes of animals at the peak of histological disease activity. Activation *in vitro* was undertaken in a 48-hr culture period with the T-cell mitogen concanavalin A (ConA) and 10^7 activated T cells injected into naive 6-week-old recipients. Passively induced disease was observed 1 week after transfer; it was mild and of markedly shorter duration than actively induced disease. Passive transfer of splenocytes without activation *in vitro* does not induce significant disease. The reasons why passively transferred disease is milder than actively transferred disease are not clear. Spleens of animals at the peak of the disease have now been shown to contain both antigen-specific and nonspecific suppressor activity (Lohse and Meyer zum Büschenfelde, 1993). Thus protective cells are transferred together with pathogenic cells, and this might explain the milder disease. In earlier models of experimental hepatitis, passive transfer could only be induced in irradiated recipients, which has not been tested in the present model.

D. Time Course

EAH runs a subacute to chronic course. Biochemical and histological evidence of disease activity can be seen 1 week after a single immunization with S-100 antigens in CFA (Lohse, 1991). Disease activity peaks between 3 and 4 weeks and subsides thereafter. Biochemical evidence of hepatocyte necroses (raised transaminase levels) normalizes within the next 4–8 weeks, but the histological severity of the disease regresses more slowly, with inflammatory infiltrates still present after 6 months. However, hepatocyte necroses are no longer observed histologically at these later stages of the disease. When three weekly immunizations are given instead of one, disease severity peaks about 1 week later and regression of the severity is a little slower than after a single injection. Relapses have not been observed and reinduction of the disease has not been tried.

E. Concanavalin A-Induced Liver Injury

We would like to mention in this context a recently published new model of experimental hepatitis in mice induced by injection of concanavalin A (Tiegs *et al.*, 1992). Although not an autoimmune disease, it is a T-cell-mediated liver injury that promises to be an important model for the study of toxic as well as immune-mediated liver disease. The model was described by Tiegs *et al.*, 1992. Injection of more than 1.5 mg/kg concanavalin A intravenously into male NMRI or BALB/C mice induced liver injury with transaminase release within 8 hr. Depending on the dose injected, animals die within about 24 hr, or otherwise recover uneventfully. Disease could not be induced in T-cell deficient mice (severe combined immunodeficiency—SCID mice or nude mice), and was prevented by dexamethasone, cyclosporin, FK 506, and anti-CD4 monoclonal antibody (pre-)treatment. Pretreatment of mice with silica particles that destroyed Kupffer cells and hepatic endothelial cells also prevented ConA-induced liver injury. Lymphocyte adherence to sinusoidal endothelial cells and hepatocyte bled formation have been histologically described (Tiegs et al., 1992). Since this is a very new model, little detail can be reported, and many questions remain. The authors tell us that NMRI mice are more susceptible than BALB/C, and we have personally found that at least in BALB/C mice, doses of more than 10 mg/kg are required to induce liver injury reliably. In addition, when injecting lower doses of ConA, it is better to measure transaminases 16 hr after injection rather than the 8 hr reported in the paper, at which time levels may still be normal, while at higher doses animals may often be dead by 16 hr.

V. Quantitation

Scoring of hepatitis is generally done histologically. This applies not only to models of autoimmune hepatitis. We have also found biochemical evidence of hepatitis in the form of raised alanine aminotransferase (ALT) levels helpful in characterizing the time course of experimental autoimmune hepatitis, but would not recommend it for routine use. The ConA model is an exception, as the massive acute liver cell necrosis leads to very high transaminase levels, which are more impressive and more informative than the histological picture (Tiegs et al., 1992). In experimental autoimmune hepatitis, however, ALT levels never rise very high and quantitation of disease severity may be more difficult. ALT levels in mice seem to be a little erratic, so that at every stage of the disease there is considerable overlap. Although the disadvantage of histology is that it requires some experience to perform, the techniques can be learned fairly easily, if two caveats are observed:

1. The animal colony must be free of mouse hepatitis virus, and this should be checked regularly (a routine in most animal facilities).

2. Injection of CFA alone induces some histological changes that need to be distinguished. CFA characteristically induces small granulomas, but only very rarely periportal infiltration.

Histological grading is done on a scale of 0 to 3 (Lohse et al., 1990a): grade 0, normal appearance; grade 1, minor inflammatory infiltrates; grade 2, moderate liver damage with inflammatory infiltrates; and grade 3, extensive infiltrates in portal tracts and lobules. Inflammatory changes in grades 1 and 2 are normally confined to the periportal region. Hepatocyte necroses are usually associated with more pronounced infiltrates, and thus are found in grades 2 and 3.

VI. Resistance

Resistance has not received any attention in the model of EAH. Earlier experiments in rabbits have shown that continued immunizations result in chronic hepatitis and prevent recovery. Similar experiments in the murine model have not been performed.

VII. Expert Experience

Preparation of fresh antigen and a good emulsion of the antigen in CFA seem critical in inducing disease successfully. When this is attended to, a single immunization is sufficient to induce moderate to severe disease. As for some reason or other the antigen preparations or immunizations may sometimes be suboptimal, we often do two immunizations at weekly intervals when we want to be sure to induce disease, although this is not an established protocol.

For reasons that we do not know, some animals may die the first day after the immunization. This happens only rarely after a single immunization, but can be observed more often after repeated injections. The intraperitoneal application of CFA leads to diffuse peritonitis and adhesions. Death is presumably caused by inadvertent injection into a blood vessel or perforation of a bowel wall. When planning an experiment with repeated injections, we always start with more animals than the minimum required for the final data analysis in order to be sure to have large enough groups at the end of the experiment. Because of variability in the severity of disease among individual animals, we always use a minimum of five animals per group and often ten animals per group.

CFA-induced peritonitis makes the sterile preparation of intraabdominal organs a little difficult. When sterile organs are required, one should dissect very slowly and carefully, using blunt instruments whenever possible. The spleen is markedly enlarged in EAH, containing on average of 300×10^6 cells. As it is usually the spleen that one wants as a sterile intraabdominal organ, and as the spleen is so large, one may choose to remove just part of the spleen. This procedure is not what is generally advised for sterile removal of the spleen, but in practice it is much easier in EAH to remove about two thirds of the spleen by bluntly dissecting its ventral part and then cutting it. When taking liver for histology, sterility is not important, but an unruptured segment is needed. Again, we cut a ventral segment rather than trying to remove the whole liver.

VIII. Lessons

EAH was developed as a model of human autoimmune hepatitis (AIH). Autoimmune hepatitis in humans is a heterogeneous disease, which most often occurs in young females and generally responds very well to immunosuppressive therapy (Maddrey, 1991). AIH is often not recognized or is misdiagnosed as chronic non-A, non-B (non-C) viral hepatitis. Even when thus left untreated for considerable time periods, the disease in some patients is moderate to mild, and transient spontaneous remissions can be observed. EAH in many ways reflects this disease process. EAH also is often mild to moderate, and spontaneous remission occurs. We have recently found antigen-specific and nonspecific suppression to be associated with recovery (Lohse and Meyer zum Büschenfelde, 1993). The maximum of suppression is observed at the peak of biochemical and histological disease activity, that is, around week 4. As remission is achieved, suppressor activity regresses.

Autoantibodies are critical in diagnosing AIH in patients, but their role in pathogenesis appears tenuous. Histologically one sees predominantly T-cell infiltrates, and autoantibody levels correlate very poorly with disease activity. EAH supports the concept of a T-cell-mediated disease and can be transferred by T cells. In addition, autoantibodies in EAH appear only after the peak of disease and are associated with recovery rather than pathogenesis (Lohse et al., 1992). It is intriguing that the titers of these liver autoantibodies in EAH continue to rise during recovery. Autoantibodies may be an expression of a T-helper (Th2 cell) response, which is often considered protective, while the original pathogenic T-cell response is likely to be Th1 mediated. These aspects require further study. Murine EAH has not been around for long, so much still needs to be done.

References

Araki, K., Yamamoto, H., and Fujimoto, S. (1987). *Clin. Exp. Immunol.* **67**, 326–334.
Behar, A. J., and Tal, C. (1959). *J. Path. Bacterial.* **77**, 591–596.
Casals, J., and Olitsky, P. K. (1946). *Proc. Soc. Exp. Biol.* **63**, 383–389.
Coppo, G. C., and Tedeschi, G. (1964). *Gastroenterologia* **7**, 39–54.
Dodd, M. C., Bigley, N. J., Geyer, V. B., *et al.* (1962). *Science* **137**, 688–689.
Fiessinger, N. (1908). *In* (A. Maloine, Ed.): Etude histologique epérimentale et pathologique. Paris, Thesis, 1908.

Hopf, U., and Meyer zum Büschenfelde, K. H. (1974). *Br. J. Exp. Path.* **55**, 509–513.
Hopf, U., Meyer zum Büschenfelde, K. H., and Hütteroth, T. H. (1976). *Klin. Weschr.* **54**, 591–598.
Iliesco, M., Berceanu, S., Radu, I., and Hergot, L. (1963). *Arch. Roum. Path. Exp.* **22**, 41–47.
Kössling, F. K., Meyer zum Büschenfelde, K. H. (1968). *Virch. Arch. Path. Anat.* **345**, 365–376.
Kuriki, J., Murakami, H., Kakumu, S., Sakamoto, N., Yokoshi, T., Nakashima, I., and Kato, N. (1983). *Gastroenterology* **84**, 596–603.
Lohse, A. W. (1991). *Semin. Liver Dis.* **11**, 241–247.
Lohse, A. W., Manns, M., Dienes, H. P., Meyer zum Büschenfelde, K. H., and Cohen, I. R. (1990a). *Hepatology* **11**, 24–30.
Lohse, A. W., Manns, M., Meyer zum Büschenfelde, K.-H. (1990b). *Hepatology* **12**, 627–628.
Lohse, A. W., Brunner, S., Kyriatsoulis, A., Manns, M., and Meyer zum Büschenfelde, K. H. (1992). *J. Hepatol.* **14**, 48–53.
Lohse, A. W., and Meyer zum Büschenfelde, K. H. (1993). *Clin. Exp. Immunol.* **94**, 163–173.
Maddrey, W. C., and Combes, B. (1991). *Semin. Liver Dis.* **11**, 248–255.
Meyer zum Büschenfelde, K. H., and Hopf, U. (1974). *Br. J. Exp. Path.* **55**, –508.
Meyer zum Büschenfelde, K. H., Kössling, F. K., and Miescher, P. A. (1972). *Clin. Exp. Immunol.* **10**, 99–108.
Mori, Y., Mori, T., Ueda, S., Yoshida, H., Iesato, K., Wakashin, Y., Wakashin, M., and Okuda, K. (1984). *Clin. Exp. Immunol.* **57**, 85–92.
Mori, Y., Mori, T., Ueda, S., Yoshida, H., Iesato, K., Wakashin, Y., Wakashin, M., and Okuda, K. (1985a). *Clin. Exp. Immunol.* **61**, 577–584.
Mori, T., Mori, Y., Yoshida, H., Ueda, S., Ogawa, M., Iesato, K., Wakashin, Y., Wakashin, M., and Okuda, K. (1985b). *Hepatology* **5**, 770–777.
Ogawa, M., Mori, Y., Mori, T., Ueda, S., Yoshida, H., Kato, I., Iesato, K., Wakashin, Y., Azemoto, R., Wakashin, M., Okuda, K., and Ohto, M. (1988). *Clin. Exp. Immunol.* **73**, 276–282.
Scheiffarth, F., Warnatz, H., and Niederer, W. (1965). *Virch. Arch. Path. Anat.* **339**, 358–365.
Scheiffarth, F., Warnatz, H., and Mayer, K. (1967). *J. Immunol.* **98**, 396–401.
Tiegs, G., Hentschel, J., and Wendel, A. (1992). *J. Clin. Invest.* **90**, 196–203.
Watanabe, Y., Kawakami, H., Kawamoto, H., Ikemoto, Y., Masuda, K., Takezaki, E., Nakanishi, T., Kajiyama, G., and Takeno, H. (1987). *Clin. Exp. Immunol.* **67**, 105–113.
Watanabe, Y., Masuda, K., Ikemoto, Y., Kikkawa, M., Nakanishi, T., Kawakami, H., and Kajiyama, G. (1988). *J. Gastroenterol. Hepatol.* **3**, 361–371.

Chapter 13

Adjuvant Arthritis

Marca H. M. Wauben, Josée P. A. Wagenaar-Hilbers, and
Willem van Eden

*Utrecht University, Faculty of Veterinary Science, Institute of Infectious Diseases and
Immunology, Department of Immunology, Utrecht, The Netherlands*

I. History of the Model

Adjuvant arthritis was described first by Pearson (1956) as a disease inducible in genetically susceptible rats by a single intracutaneous inoculation of killed mycobacteria suspended in oil, a substance known as complete Freund's adjuvant (CFA). Evidence for the T-cell-mediated autoimmune nature of the disease was obtained in subsequent studies, which demonstrated successful adoptive transfer of the disease by using thoracic-duct lymphocytes (Whitehouse *et al.*, 1969) or induction of the disease with *in vitro*-selected, mycobacteria-reactive, T-cell lines (Holoshitz *et al.*, 1983). More recent studies have shown the suppression of clinical disease with the use of antibody infusion specifically targeted at T cells, demonstrating the T-cell nature of the disease (Yoshino and Cleland, 1992).

II. Animals

The disease is inducible in rats, and wide variations in frequency and severity of lesions are observed in different strains (Table I). Mice are in general not susceptible to adjuvant arthritis as induced in rats. It was seen that bacillus Calmette-Guérin (BCG) cell walls emulsified in different adjuvants injected into one hind paw led in some mice to a migratory polyarthritis that also affected the noninjected hind paw and resembled a transient adjuvant disease as normally seen in rats. The incidence was 20–40% and the mice tested were A/J, Balb/J, CBA/J, C57Bl/6J, and DBA/1J (Whitehouse *et al.*, 1974).

In a (too?) small series of rhesus monkeys tested, no adjuvant disease was seen and the animals experienced severe local ulcerations owing to the intradermal inoculation (Bakker *et al.*, 1990).

Although some reports do mention relative sex preferences in susceptible rats, overall there does not seem to be a serious sex restriction in susceptibility. Young rats, 1 or 7 days after birth, seem to be not susceptible, while from 21 days onward rats were found susceptible. Old animals, at the age of 9

Table I

Rat Strains (Weight 150–300 g)[a]

Strain	Rat major histocompatibility complex (RT1)	Incidence (%)
Outbred		
Sprague-Dawley (SD)		± 60
Wistar CFN and HLW		± 40
Inbred		
Lewis (Lew)	l	90–100
Fisher (F344)	lvl	20
Buffalo (Buf)	b	50[a]
Brown Norway (BN)	n	100[b]
Lew. 1N	nvl	66
WF. 1N	n	100
MAXX	n	100
Dark Agouti (DA)	avl	100
Wistar King Aptekman (WKA)	k	75
Wistar Furth (WF)	u	<10

[a] Data were taken from Brito *et al.* (1988); Carlson *et al.* (1985); Crowe *et al.* (1985); Glenn and Gray (1969); Griffiths (1988); Hogervorst *et al.* (1991); Kayashima *et al.* (1978); Kohashi *et al.* (1979); Ramos-Ruiz *et al.* (1991); Waksman *et al.* (1960).

[b] For Buffalo and brown Norway, sex differences in incidence are known. In brown Norway, females are resistant and incidence percentage is based on male incidence, whereas in Buffalo, males are resistant and incidence percentage is based on female incidence.

months, were found to be relatively resistant (Glenn and Gray, 1965). In general it can be said that optimal susceptibility is present in the age period from 6 to 12 weeks after birth.

The possible influence of major histocompatibility complex (MHC) genes on susceptibility has been suggested from a small study using a limited number of rat strains (Battisto *et al.*, 1982). The microbiological environment seems to influence susceptibility. In Fisher rats it was shown that germ-free animals were susceptible, whereas conventionally kept animals were resistant (Kohashi *et al.*, 1979). Selective recolonization of the germ-free Fisher rats with *Escherichia coli* bacteria was shown to induce resistance (Kohashi *et al.*, 1986). Also, the acquired resistance following remission of actively induced disease seems to be positively influenced by microbial environment (I. R. Cohen, personal communication).

Treatment with low doses of cyclophosphamide given 2–3 days prior to disease induction may lead to a more severe arthritis. Larger doses seem less effective. Cyclophosphamide treatment after disease induction did not enhance but instead slightly decreased the incidence of arthritis (Kayashima *et al.*, 1978). Pretreatment with hydrocortisone may lead to more severe arthritis in a dose-dependent manner similar to that of cyclophosphamide (Kayashima *et al.*, 1978).

Thymectomy or splenectomy does not inhibit adjuvant arthritis (Glen and Gray, 1965) and may lead to more severe disease (Kayashima *et al.*, 1976). Also, low-dose (200 rad) total body irradiation may increase susceptibility to arthritis (Kayashima *et al.*, 1976).

III. Induction of the Disease

A. Active Induction

The disease is induced with mycobacteria in a suitable oily adjuvant. Various different mycobacterial substances have been held responsible for disease induction and no autoantigen has been defined with certainty. The presence of mycobacterial antigens as an essential constituent for disease induction in most instances has made adjuvant arthritis into an interesting model for studying the capacity of microbial antigens to influence tolerance for self-antigens. Through an analysis of mycobacteria-specific T-cell clones that transferred disease into naive irradiated recipients (Holoshitz *et al.*, 1983, 1984), it was found that the epitope recognized by these T-cell clones was the 180–186 sequence of the mycobacterial 65-kDa heat-shock protein (a member of the hsp 60 family) (Van Eden *et al.*, 1988). No disease is induced by peptide 180–186 without the addition of Freund's complete adjuvant. The definition of hsp 60 as a critical antigen in adjuvant arthritis has been an impetus for further studies in the area of bacterial heat-shock proteins and their role in the breaking or maintenance of self-tolerance, not only in arthritis, but also in other autoimmune diseases.

B. Antigen Used

Various mycobacterial preparations are used. The use of heat-killed *Mycobacterium tuberculosis* (Mt) strain H37Ra (Difco Laboratories, Detroit, Michigan) is recommended. The particle size of the mycobacteria in oil may influence the induction of disease. Therefore, adequate grinding of mycobacteria is advised. This can be done by using pestle and mortar. Dried mycobacteria are put into a roughened glass mortar and 3 drops of oil are added. The mixture is ground to a paste over 120 s. The rest of the oil is added with continuous grinding over a further 30 s. The preparation can be kept at 4°C and will remain stable, as far as biological properties are concerned, on prolonged storage. Sedimented material can be redispersed by shaking. Preparations failing to meet this criterion should be discarded. The preferred concentration of mycobacteria in oil is 10 mg/ml and 0.1 ml of the suspension is inoculated intracutaneously. Mineral oil can be used (incomplete Freund's adjuvant, Difco). Less severe disease may be obtained with lower concentration of mycobacteria in oil (1–5 mg/ml). As an alternative to *M. tuberculosis*, *M. butyricum* or a mixture of three strains of *M. tuberculosis* (C, DT, PN) can be used to induce disease in certain rat strains. The relative efficiencies of various sorts of oily vehicles have been studied by Whitehouse, who tested over 100 distinct adjuvants. Squalene, pristane, hexadecane, and 1-octadecane proved to be excellent substitutes for mineral oil (Whitehouse *et al.*, 1974).

That the role of the oily adjuvant may be critical to the adjuvant arthritis model is indicated by the fact that in some strains of rats adjuvant (like?) disease is induced by the oily component itself. This is seen in DA rats with mineral oil (Kleinau *et al.*, 1991) or with pristane in mice (Thompson *et al.*, 1990). Mycobacteria administered in a saline suspension fail to induce arthritis (Ward and Jones, 1962), except for intraperitoneal inoculation following prior induction of peritonitis (Levine and Saltzman, 1991). Other mycobacterial substances with known arthritogenic capacities include the Wax D derived from mycobacterial cell walls. Wax D isolated from *M. tuberculosis* H37Rv, H37Ra, C, DT, or PN, emulsified in an appropriate adjuvant was seen to induce arthritis (Koga and Pearson, 1973; Koga *et al.*, 1976; Kayashima *et al.*, 1976). Further studies have indicated that the peptidoglycan moiety of Wax D is the critical substance (Jolles *et al.*, 1960; Asselineau *et al.*, 1958). Also, isolated cell walls of *M. bovis* BCG emulsified in adjuvant may be used (Whitehouse *et al.*, 1974).

If needed, coimmunization of other antigens in the disease inducing-preparation is possible: Equal volumes of the antigen in phosphate-buffered saline (PBS) or water can be added drop after drop during constant vortexing of the disease-inducing preparation (mycobacteria suspended in oil). Alternatively, the antigen in PBS or water can be mixed at room temperature by vortexing and then by forcing it repeatedly through a 30-gauge stainless steel double-headed needle inserted between 1-ml syringes. This process is continued for at least 5 min, until a uniformly white emulsion is obtained.

C. Route of Immunization

The preferred route of administration is intracutaneous into the base of the tail. The advantage of tail immunization, in contrast to footpad immunization, is that all four paws can be used to evaluate the development of arthritis. The tail injection is given mostly in the dorsal side of the base of the tail, although some studies have stated that subcutaneous injections in the third distal part of the tail (Kapusta et al., 1972) or at 1 inch distal to the base may be successful (Cozine et al., 1973). However, in general, subcutaneous, intraperitoneal, intramuscular, and intravenous inoculations of the adjuvant did not produce arthritis or produced it less frequently. After intracutaneous immunization of the tail, the inoculation site becomes necrotic in 3–7 days after immunization.

Another conventional route of administration is intracutaneous injection of 50 μl into one hind footpad (Iigo et al., 1991; Lopez-Bote et al., 1988; Best et al., 1984). The latter procedure is likely to affect proper macroscopic scoring of joint inflammation at the ipsilateral side.

For Wax D immunization, a frequently used procedure was direct inoculation of 5 μl of disease-inducing preparation into the inguinal lymph nodes via a 20-gauge, 1-inch needle. Rats were anesthetized and lymph nodes preexposed. Injection was continued until the emulsion could be seen to be leaving the node and moving up the draining lymphatic vessel. The incision was closed with wound clips (Newbould, 1965).

D. Transfer of the Disease

1. Antibodies

It was not possible to transfer the disease when sizable amounts of either acute phase or convalescent serum (up to 15 ml i.v.) were transferred from arthritic into normal recipients (Waksman et al., 1960). Furthermore, there is no evidence indicating a role for autoantibodies in disease induction. However, it appeared that both in patients suffering from rheumatoid arthritis

(RA) and in Lewis rats with adjuvant arthritis (AA), the glycosylation pattern of immunoglobulin G (IgG) was changed. The IgG heavy chains lack terminal galactose from the biantennary oligosaccharide on the conserved N-glycosylation site on the CH2 domain, resulting in an increased level of agalactosyl IgG (Rook, 1988; Parekh *et al.*, 1985).

2. T Lymphocytes

Transfer of the disease process was not successful when living sensitized lymph node cells (LNCs) were passed from donors sensitized with mycobacteria/adjuvant into noninbred recipients, even though the recipient was previously given whole-body irradiation or had been rendered tolerant to the donor cells (Waksman *et al.*, 1960). However, it is possible to transfer the arthritic disease passively from sensitized donors to normal recipients under certain conditions, namely (1) use of viable lymph node or spleen cells, (2) utilization of a highly inbred strain of rats, (3) harvesting cells from donors during certain time intervals after adjuvant injection, and (4) transfer via an appropriate route of sufficient viable cell numbers from sensitized lymph nodes or spleen, but not from the thymus (Carl *et al.*, 1964).

There are two protocols for transferring T lymphocytes: passive transfer with spleen or lymph node cells, and passive transfer with T-cell lines or clones.

a. Transfer with spleen or lymph node cells. The protocols used in the first reports on the successful transfer of the disease with spleen or lymph node cells were as follows (Carl *et al.*, 1964; Glenn *et al.*, 1977; Waksman and Wennersten, 1963):

1. Lewis rats were immunized in the skin of the superscapular area in multiple deposit sites (total amount of 0.4 ml) and 0.1–0.2 ml into two footpads with Wax D of the human Canetti strain emulsified in light mineral oil.

2. Lymphoid cells were collected at days 9–11 postinoculation from the axillary, olecranon, submaxillary, superficial, and deep cervical, inguinal, and popliteal lymph nodes; harvested, and pooled from several donors. The same was done for the spleens.

3. Two to 2.3×10^8 sensitized viable lymph node cells or 2.7×10^8 viable sensitized spleen cells were necessary to transfer the disease when injected in the tail vein of the recipient rat. (Because of the high dose of cells, the inoculation was usually given over a period of 3–10 min!). Other immunization routes were not successful.

A critical time period was documented after adjuvant injection, during which lymph node or spleen cells have the capacity to transfer arthritis to normal recipients. This was between 9 and 11 days after administration of adjuvant, when sometimes a mild arthritis was already seen in donor rats. At day 14, it is no longer possible to transfer the disease. (By that time all donor rats have a flourishing and severe polyarthritis.) The onset of passively induced arthritis is 3–6 days after inoculation of the sensitized cells. Lesions which developed in the recipients were identical in type and form to those observed after adjuvant-induced disease (Carl *et al.*, 1964; Pearson, 1959; Pearson and Wood, 1952), but generally they were not as severe or extensive (Carl *et al.*, 1964).

Although passive transfer of adjuvant arthritis to normal recipient rats was well documented in the 1960s (Waksman and Wennersten, 1963; Carl *et al.*, 1964; Whitehouse *et al.*, 1969), within the past decade the experiments have appeared to be difficult to reproduce. Investigators attempting direct cell-mediated passive transfer of AA to normal rats reported failures or the induction of only very mild forms of the disease (Taurog *et al.*, 1983a; Waksman and Wennersten, 1963). However, after T-cell depletion (thymectomy and whole-body irradiation) of the recipients, as few as 6×10^7 cells successfully transferred the disease (Taurog *et al.*, 1983a). It appeared that whereas immunosuppression of the recipients was necessary in these studies for the induction of arthritis by direct transfer of adjuvant-sensitized cells, in contrast, severe arthritis could be induced in either immunosuppressed or normal recipients by transfer of adjuvant-sensitized cells that had been incubated *in vitro* with concanavalin A (ConA) (Taurog *et al.*, 1983a).

The revised transfer protocol was as follows:

• Lewis rats were immunized in all four footpads and in six intradermal sites along the trunk with 1 ml of 3 mg/ml *Mycobacterium butyricum* in light mineral oil.

• Eleven days later, cervical, axillary, olecranon, inguinal, and popliteal lymph nodes and spleen were harvested and passed over a Ficoll gradient or through a nylon wool column.

• Lymph node cells were cultured for 48–72 hr with $3 \mu g/ml$ of ConA.

• One and two-tenths to 2.6×10^8 lymph node cells or $0.2–1.9 \times 10^8$ spleen cells were transferred i.v. into the recipient.

The mean day of disease onset was day 4 or 5 after cell transfer.

The passively transferred adjuvant arthritis was not merely due to passenger adjuvant associated with the transferred cells because irradiation of the cells just before transfer did not result in disease (Taurog *et al.*, 1983a). After characterization of the cell population that transferred the disease, it appeared that the cells were Ig$^-$ CD8$^-$, esterase negative, CD4$^+$ nonadherent cells (Taurog *et al.*, 1983b). It appeared that the arthritogenicity, that is, the capacity to transfer arthritis of the adjuvant-sensitized, mitogen-stimulated cells, correlated with the magnitude of interleukin-2 (IL-2) production and not with the degree of [^{3}H] thymidine incorporation. (high IL-2 results in better transfer) (Taurog et al., 1983b). Furthermore, phytohemagglutinin (PHA) stimulated much lower levels of IL-2 in the adjuvant-sensitized cells, and these cells could not transfer the disease! Therefore, it is possible that the difference in the lymphokine secretion triggered by the two mitogens explained the difference in efficacy in transferring the disease (Taurog et al., 1983b). This is further supported by the findings that T-helper cells belonging to the TH1 subset play an important role in AA.

In some fluorescence studies using fluorescein isothiocyanate (FITC)-labeled, ConA-activated, adjuvant-sensitized T lymphocytes, it has been found that part of the injected activated lymphocytes migrate to the synovium and that proliferative responses of lymphocytes from knee synovial tissue of rats with passively induced AA showed dose-dependent proliferative responses to Mt (Quinn Dejoy et al., 1990).

    b. Transfer with T-cell line or clone. Passive transfer of AA with a well-defined T-cell line or clone has only been described in the Lewis rat. A CD4$^+$ T-cell line (line A2) was generated from a rat immunized with CFA. At day 9, draining LNCs were isolated and cyclically restimulated with Mt and expanded on growth medium containing IL-2 (Holoshitz et al., 1983). To transfer the disease by this A2 cell line, the T cells were restimulated in vitro with the specific antigen (Mt) or with the mitogen ConA in the presence of accessory cells for 3 days. Cells were washed twice with PBS and 2×10^7 cells in 1 ml PBS were injected into the tail vein of Lewis rats which were irradiated 2 hr earlier with 750 rad by a ^{60}Co gamma-ray source (Holoshitz et al., 1983, 1984). The mean day of disease onset, between days 6 and 12, was earlier than by actively induced disease, between days 14 and 15. However, the passively induced arthritis was less severe than the actively induced disease.

After subcloning of the A2 T-cell line, a CD4$^+$ T-cell clone, clone A2b, was generated which recognized, besides the 180–188 amino acid sequence of the mycobacterial 65-kDa heat-shock protein (van Eden et al., 1988), parts of a proteoglycan molecule on cartilage (van Eden et al., 1985). To transfer the disease by this T-cell clone A2b, the same protocol can be used as for the A2 cell line (Holoshitz et al., 1984). However, compared with the passive disease induction with the parental cell line A2, the mean day of disease onset after transfer of activated A2b cells was somewhat earlier, day 5, and the disease was also more severe. Neither A2 nor A2b induced AA in nonirradiated rats. Furthermore, irradiation of A2 or A2b with 1500 rads abrogated their ability to cause disease in irradiated Lewis rats.

IV. Course of the Disease

After active induction of disease with mycobacterial antigens, clinical disease, which can be seen macroscopically by inspection of the joints, becomes overt around 14 days after injection. The severity is seen to increase over a period of 1–2 weeks and will gradually diminish during the subsequent 1–3 weeks. Although the active inflammatory responses gradually subside, the swelling and apparent anatomical deformities may last for a longer period. Especially in the ankle joints, anatomical deformations resulting in ankylosis are usually irreversible.

Passive disease, following transfer of lymphocytes, is usually seen to start earlier (on day 8 after inoculation of cells) and to develop into a less severe form of arthritis. Generally, spontaneous relapses do not occur. Upon rechallenge with mycobacterial antigens, animals usually have developed resistance to the disease and will not develop arthritis again. However, in some instances, arthritis may develop again. It is possible that previous exposure to bacterial antigens, before the initial induction of disease, contributes to the development of resistance subsequent to remission.

V. Quantitation of the Disease

The progress and severity of the disease may be quantified physically, histologically, radiographically, or by magnetic resonance imaging (MRI).

A. Physical Examination

Mercury or water plethysmography was used to measure the increase in hind paw volume (i.e., the volume of mercury or water displaced by the paw and the leg) (Francis et al., 1988; Winter et al., 1962; Rosenthale and Nagra, 1967). Swelling of hind paws was also quantitated by measuring the thickness of the ankle from the medial to the lateral malleolus with a constant-tension caliper (Trentham et al., 1977).

An arthritic index can be used to score the degree of periarticular erythema and edema, as well as deformity of the joints. The severity of involvement of each paw can be graded from 0 to 4 (Trentham et al., 1977; Wood et al., 1969) or, to quantitate the arthritis more accurately, each joint can be evaluated separately for swelling and erythema. (max. score of 156/rat) (Taurog et al., 1985). Nodules on ears or tails can be scored as well (Rosenthale, 1970). The knee is excluded because neither swelling nor erythema of the knee could be reliably quantitated by physical examination.

B. Histological Examination

Joints with early inflammation show discrete changes, such as vascular dilatation, mild mixed neutrophil and mononuclear infiltrates, early hyperplasia of synovial lining cells and focal granulation tissue. In joint spaces there is some mixed inflammatory exudate. At this stage the articular cartilage is intact (Terrier *et al.*, 1985). In severe AA, there are diffuse, intense, mixed, inflammatory cell infiltrates composed of mononuclear cells and neutrophils. The synovium and subsynovial connective tissues are markedly edematous, with focal areas of necrosis. The hyperplastic synovium encroaches into the joint space. Reactive granulation tissue extends into the periarticular soft tissues, as well as into subchondral bone, with destruction of the articular cartilage and invasion of the marrow space (Terrier *et al.*, 1985).

In late arthritis pannus extends across the surface of the articular cartilage, resulting in fibrous ankylosis. Bone remodeling and periosteal new bone formation is evident (Terrier *et al.*, 1985).

In disease transferred by cloned T cells (Stanescu *et al.*, 1987), the histological findings were similar, although less severe than in actively induced disease. Inflammatory signs were present already at day 4 after inoculation, when no joint edema was evident. In electron microscope studies, using large molecules of cationized ferritin, which were excluded from normal cartilage matrix, penetration of arthritic cartilage was seen, showing identical patterns in actively induced and passively induced disease. Also, transfer of antiovalbumin T lymphocytes followed by ovalbumin injection in the joints showed an identical histological pattern, an indication that the changes were attributable to the action of T lymphocytes irrespective of whether or not the target antigen was to the joint (Stanescu *et al.*, 1987).

C. Radiographical Examination

Hind paws and knees can be evaluated for the following alterations: soft-tissue swelling, osteoporosis, widening or narrowing of joint space, periosteal new bone formation, bone erosions, heterotopic ossification (Terrier *et al.*, 1985; Taurog *et al.*, 1985).

D. MRI Analysis

To score soft-tissue manifestations of arthritis, anatomic sections made transaxially through the hind paws and knees of the rats, using a one-dimensional MRI or double-spin echo technique (SE), can be used (Terrier *et al.*, 1985; Borah and Szeverenyi, 1990). In comparison with both conventional radiographs and physical evaluation, early inflammatory soft-tissue changes were detected more frequently by MRI. On the other hand, bony lesions were better evaluated by conventional radiography. A detailed analysis of bone demineralization, bone erosions, periosteal new bone formation, or joint space alterations was not possible owing to the limited spatial resolution of MRI (Terrier *et al.*, 1985).

VI. Resistance to the Disease

Different rat strains show wide variations in their resistance to adjuvant arthritis induction. The genetic factors determining these variations are mostly unknown. As an explanation for the marked difference in resistance between, for example, Lewis and Fisher rats, some authors have described a changed hormonal status due to differences in the hypophyseal–adrenal axis between these strains (Sternberg *et al.*, 1989).

More generally, it seems that differential resistance is due to a differential regulation of immunity to exogenous microbial antigens such as those present in the intestinal microflora. The example is given by Fisher rats, which are resistant in the conventional situation. However, when bred germ-free, they tend to be as susceptible as Lewis rats and after recolonization with certain bacterial organisms, their resistance seems to develop (Kohashi *et al.*, 1979). Acquired resistance is also observed after spontaneous remission of adjuvant disease in Lewis rats. A second challenge with mycobacteria in oil generally does not lead to disease. Thus, even in the susceptible rats, mechanisms contributing to resistance can be activated.

Preimmunization of animals with water-soluble fractions of mycobacteria or low doses of mycobacteria—10 μg of Mt given intradermally 3 and 5 weeks prior to disease induction—were seen to lead to a raised resistance against disease induction (Gery and Waksman, 1967; Larsson *et al.*, 1989). Furthermore, protocols seen to be ineffective in inducing adjuvant disease, such as administration of mycobacteria suspended in saline or alternative routes of administration, such as subcutaneous, intraperitoneal, intramuscular, and intravenous, were generally seen to enhance resistance (Glenn and Gray, 1965). Also, when susceptible rats do not develop disease for unknown reasons, resistance is seen to remain after subsequent intradermal inoculations (Glenn and Gray, 1965).

Immunization with mycobacterial hsp 65 has been found to raise resistance to subsequent induction of adjuvant arthritis (Van Eden *et al.*, 1988; Billingham *et al.*, 1990). Since similar observations have been made in models in which arthritis was induced with components such as pristane (Thompson *et al.*, 1990), streptococcal cell walls (Van den Broek *et al.*, 1989), and collagen type II (Ito *et al.*, 1991), it is possible that T-cell responses to (endogenous mammalian?) hsp 60 may confer resistance to arthritis irrespective of the nature of the trigger leading to arthritis (van Eden, 1991). This may also be relevant to the observed effects of preadministration of incomplete Freund's adjuvant (IFA) in reducing adjuvant arthritis (Cannon *et al.*, 1993), since IFA has been seen to induce responses to hsp 60 (Anderton *et al.*, 1993).

In some studies, infusion of T-cell clones has been shown to prevent active induction of adjuvant arthritis. This has been done by using both unmanipulated (Cohen *et al.*, 1985) and artificially attenuated (Lider *et al.*, 1987) antigen-specific T cells. The T cells used in these so-called T-cell vaccination approaches were specific for the 180–186 sequence of the mycobacterial hsp 65. Also, immunization with synthetic peptides comprising this sequence (Yang *et al.*, 1990) or peptide analogs with minor modifications, such as hsp 65 180–188 $L^{183} \rightarrow$ A (Wauben *et al.*, 1992), has been seen to enhance resistance to active induction of disease.

More generalized anti-T-cell interventions have been studied in adjuvant arthritis. Infusion of anti-pan T-cell monoclonal antibodies (W3/13) has been described as delaying disease development (Larsson *et al.*, 1985; Billingham *et al.*, 1989), whereas anti-CD8 (OX8) did not have such an effect (Larsson *et al.*, 1989). Anti-CD4 antibodies produced a dose-related inhibition of developing arthritis and anti-MHC class II antibodies also inhibited arthritis (Billingham *et al.*, 1989). Infusion of anti-T-cell receptor antibodies (R73) suppressed disease, and infusion from birth prevented disease completely (Yoshino and Cleland, 1992).

Antigen-specific manipulations of disease resistance have included studies on oral tolerance. Oral administration of collagen type II during the week before disease induction suppressed the development of disease. This was not seen after oral administration of mycobacteria (Zhang *et al.*, 1990). In another study, oral BCG but not purified protein derivative (PPD) inhibited disease in a susceptible strain of rats, whereas both BCG and PPD were seen to enhance disease in a relatively resistant strain of rats (Bersani-Amado *et al.*, 1990). Some studies have indicated the significance of diet and especially the presence in the food of trace elements with regard to disease resistance. Dietary absence of magnesium, copper, or zinc salts may promote disease resistance (Yiangou and Hadjipetrou-Kourounakis, 1989).

VII. Expert Experience

In the induction of active disease by immunization in the skin at the base of the tail, the success rate appears to be easily influenced by the technical aspects of the immunization procedures. Optimal results will be obtained when a local, circumscribed elevation of the skin surface remains after immunization. During the period prior to overt disease, the development of a skin ulceration at the same spot is predictive of good disease development. In the absence of ulceration, it is likely that the inoculation was not done in the optimal way, and no disease will develop.

Wide variations in success rates may be seen with changes in batches of mycobacteria used, the source of animals (commercial supplier), and housing (and food) conditions. The AA model seems particularly sensitive to changes in exogenous factors. In addition, the model is very sensitive to artifacts caused by handling. For example, in studies of resistance induction by immunological immunization, it seems essential to have control animals exposed to the same manipulation (sham inoculations, administration of same adjuvants, etc.) as the experimental group. Some adjuvants are inhibitory with respect to disease susceptibility, others have disease-potentiating abilities. Pretreatment protocols with the use of the adjuvant dimethyldioctadecylammonium bromide (DDA) (Snippe and Kraaieveld, 1989) will lead to very severe disease after mycobacterial immunization at a later time.

VIII. Lessons

Many investigators use adjuvant arthritis as a model for human rheumatoid arthritis because the peripheral joint lesions in the model have most of the features that characterize rheumatoid arthritis except for their relatively nonprogressive nature and some histological differences. The nature of the autoantigen in adjuvant arthritis is unknown. Indirect evidence suggests that cellular immunity directed against cartilage proteoglycans plays a role. An arthritogenic T-cell clone with specificity for the hsp 65 molecule of mycobacteria was seen to respond to proteoglycans (Van Eden et al., 1985), and preimmunization with proteoglycans has been seen to increase the incidence and severity of adjuvant arthritis (Van Vollenhove et al., 1988).

In many cases, however, the full picture of adjuvant arthritis includes other specific tissue lesions, such as iridocyclitis, nodular lesions of the skin, genitourinary lesions, and diarrhea. In some aspects, such a clinical syndrome with involvement of peripheral joints and spine, the eye, skin, and genitourinary tract may resemble Reiter syndrome, reactive forms of arthritis, or Behçet syndrome. Alternatively, the transient nodular lesions with spontaneously remitting arthritis may resemble rheumatic fever or erythema nodosum with arthritis. Finally, some authors have pointed out some similarities with ulcerative colitis or sarcoidosis (Pearson et al., 1961). In humans, exposure to high doses of mycobacteria, as in the case of adjuvant immunotherapy for cancer, may also lead to a transient arthritis (Torisu et al., 1978). This may be the direct counterpart of adjuvant arthritis in humans.

The model is frequently used to test anti-inflammatory drugs. Furthermore, the model seems very suitable for the study and development of T-cell-directed immunomanipulative strategies, since compared with other models, such as that of collagen-induced arthritis, adjuvant disease seems to be more prominently T-cell dependent (Yoshino and Cleland, 1992). However, since adjuvant arthritis is a nonprogressive disease, which spontaneously remits, the possibilities of using the model for therapeutic immunointervention are limited. As soon as disease has been established, immunoregulation is activated as part of the host's physiological response to suppress disease. The time interval suitable for additional artificial manipulative actions is therefore short at best. Furthermore, the insidiously aggressive nature of the disease, which leads to an almost complete destruction of joints and results in a bony ankylosis, is not always ideal for testing and evaluating subtle therapeutic interventions.

The model is unique in the sense that the induction of disease is *not* done with a defined self-antigen and may be done, depending on the circumstances, in the absence of any antigen, such as in the case of oily compounds. This situation may make the model scientifically attractive as a model for the various forms of human arthritis, which are also characterized by a lack of well-defined self-antigens.

Acknowledgment

We thank Mrs. Jona Gianotten for excellent editorial support.

References

Anderton, S. M., v.d. Zee, R., and Goodacre, J. A. (1993). *Eur. J. Immunol.* **23**, 33–38.

Asselineau, J., Buc, H., Jollies, P., and Lederer, E. (1958). *Bull. Soc. Chim. Biol.* **40**, 953.

Bakker, N. P. M., Van Erck, M. G. M., Zurcher, C., Faaber, P., Lemmens, A., Hazenberg, M., Bontrop, R. E., and Jonker, M. (1990). *Rheum. Int.* **10**, 21.

Bersani-Amado, C. A., Barbuto, J. A. M., and Jancar, S. (1990). *J. Rheumatol.* **17**, 738–742.

Battisto, J. R., Smith, R. N., Beckmann, K., Sternlicht, M., and Welles, W. L. (1982). *Arthr. Rheum.* **25**, 1194–1199.

Best, R., Christian, R., and Lewis, D. A. (1984). *Agents Action* **4**, 265–268.

Billingham, M. E. J., Fairchild, S., Griffin, E., Drayer, L., and Hicks, C. (1989). *In* "Therapeutic Control of Inflammatory Disease" (A. J. Lewis, Ed.), pp. 242–253. Elsevier, New York.

Billingham, M. E. J., Carney, S., Butler, R., and Colston, J. (1990). *J. Exp. Med.* **171**, 339–344.

Borah, B., and Szeverenyi, N. M. (1990). *Magn. Res. Med.* **15**, 246–259.

Cannon, G. W., Griffiths, M. M., and Woods, M. L. (1993). *Arthr. Rheum.* **36**, 126–131.

Carl, M., Pearson, M. D., Fae, D., and Wood, F. D. (1964). *J. Exp. Med.* **120**, 547–573.

Cohen, I. R., Holoshitz, J., v. Eden, W., and Frenkel, A. (1985). *Arthr. Rheum.* **8**, 841–845.

Cozine, W. S., Jr., Stanfield, A. B., Stephens, C. A. L., Jr., and Mazeur, M. T. (1973). *Proc. Soc. Exp. Biol.* **143**, 528–530.

Francis, M. D., Hovancik, K., and Boyce, R. W. (1988). *J. Bone Min. Res.* **3**, S135 (Suppl. 1).

Gery, I., and Waksman, B. H. (1967). *Int. Arch. Allergy* **31**, 57–68.

Glenn, E. M., and Gray, J. E. (1965). *Am. J. Vet. Res.* **26**, 114, 1180–1194.

Glenn, E. M., Bowman, B. J., Rohloff, N. A., and Seely, R. J. (1977). *Agents Action* **7**, 265.

Hogervorst, E. J. M., Boog, C. J. P., Wagenaar, J. P. A., Wauben, M. H. M., v.d. Zee, R., and v. Eden, W. (1991). *Eur. J. Immunol.* **21**, 1289–1296.

Holoshitz, J., Naparstek, Y., Ben-Nun, A., and Cohen, I. R. (1983). *Science* **219**, 56–58.

Holoshitz, J., Matitiau, A., and Cohen, I. R. (1984). *J. Clin. Invest.* **73**, 211–215.

Iigo, Y., Takashi, T., Tamatani, T., Miyasaka, M., Higashida, T., Yagita, H., Okumura, K., and Tsukado, W. (1991). *J. Immunol.* **147**, 4167–4171.

Ito, J., Krco, C. J., Ya, D., Lutra, H., and David, C. S. (1991). *J. Cell. Biochem.* 284–290.

Jolles, P., Nguyen-Trung-Luong-Cross, and Lederer, E. (1960). *Biochem. Biophys. Acta* **43**, 559.

Kapusta, N. A., Hadjipetrou-Kourounakis, L., and Rotenberg, A. D. (1972). *Immun. React. Exp. Mod. Rheum. Dis.* 203–207.

Kayashima, K., Koga, T., and Onoue, K. (1976). *J. Immunol.* **117**, 1878–1883.

Kayashima, K., Koga, T., and Onoue, K. (1978). *J. Immunol.* **120**, 1127–1131.

Kleinau, S., Erlandsson, H., Holmdahl, R., and Klareskog, L. (1991). *J. Autoimmun.* **4**, 871–880.

Koga, T., and Pearson, C. (1973). *J. Immunol.* **111**, 599–608.

Koga, T., Kato, K., Kotani, S., Tanaka, A., and Pearson, C. M. (1976). *Int. Arch. Allergy Appl. Immun.* **51**, 395–400.

Kohashi, O., Kuwata, J., Umehara, F., Takahashi, T., and Ozawa, A. (1979). *Infect. Immun.* **26**, 791–794.

Kohashi, O., Kohashi, Y., Takahashi, T., Ozawa, A., and Shigematsu, N. (1986). *Arth. Rheum.* **29**, 547–553.

Larsson, P., Holmdahl, R., Dencker, L., and Klareskog, L. (1985). *Immunology* **56**, 383–391.

Larsson, P., Holmdahl, R., and Klareskog, L. (1989). *J. Cell. Biochem.* **40**, 1–8.

Levine, S., and Saltzman, A. (1991). *Arthr. Rheum.* **34**, 1, 63–67.

Lider, O., Karin, N., Shinitzky, M., and Cohen, I. R. (1987). *Proc. Natl. Acad. Sci. USA* **84**, 4577–4580.

Lopez-Bote, J. P., Bernabeu, C., Marguet, A., Fernandez, J. M., and Larraga, V. (1988). *Arthr. Rheum.* **31**, 769–775.

Newbould, B. B. (1965). *Immunology* **9**, 613.

Parekh, R. B., Dwek, R. A., Sutton, B. J., Fernandez, D. L., Leung, A., Stanworth, D. R., Rademacher, T. W., Mizuochi, T., Taniguchi, T., Matsuta, K., Takeuchi, F., Nagano, Y., Miyamoto, T., and Kobata, A. (1985). *Nature* **316**, 452–457.

Pearson, C. M. (1956). *Proc. Soc. Exp. Biol. Med.* **112**, 95–101.

Pearson, C. M. (1959). *In* "Mechanisms in Hypersensitivity, International Symposium," Detroit, 1958.

Pearson, C. M., and Wood, F. D. (1952). *Arthr. Rheum.* **2**, 440.

Pearson, C. M., Waksman, B. H., and Sharp, J. T. (1961). *J. Exp. Med.* **113**, 485–510.

Quinn Dejoy, S., Ferguson-Chanowitz, K., Oronsky, A. L., Zabriskie, J. B., and Kerwar, S. S. (1990). *Cell. Immunol.* **130**, 195–203.

Rook, G. A. W. (1988). *J. Immunol. (Meeting review, Scand.)* **28**, 487–493.

Rook, G., Thompson, S., Buckley, M., Elson, C., Brealey, R., Lambert, C., White, T., and Rademaker, T. (1991). *Eur. J. Immunol.* **21**, 1027–1032.

Rosenthale, M. E. (1970). *Arch. Int. Pharmacoclyn.* **188**, 14–22.

Rosenthale, M. E., and Nagra, C. L. (1967). *Proc. Soc. Exp. Biol. N.Y.* **125**, 149.

Snippe, H., and Kraaieveld, C. H. (1989). *In* "Immunological Adjuvants and Vaccines" (G. Gregoriades, A. C. Allison, and G. Poste, Eds.), pp. 47–50. Plenum Press NI, London.

Stanescu, R., Lider, O., v. Eden, W., Holoshitz, J., and Cohen, I. R. (1987). *Arthr. Rheum.* **30**, 779–792.

Sternberg, E. N., Hill, J. M., Chrousos, G. P., Kamilaris, T., Listwak, S. J., Gold, P. W., and Wilder, R. L. (1989). *Proc. Natl. Acad. Sci. USA* **86**, 2374–2378.

Taurog, J. D., Sandberg, G. P., and Mahowald, M. L. (1983a). *Cell. Immunol.* **75**, 271–282.

Taurog, J. D., Sandberg, G. P., and Mahowald, M. L. (1983b). *Cell. Immunol.* **80**, 193–204.

Taurog, J. D., Kerwar, S. S., McReynolds, R. A., Sanberg, G. P., Leary, S. L., and Mahowald, M. L. (1985). *J. Exp. Med.* **162**, 962–978.

Terrier, F., Hricak, H. L., Revel, D., Alpers, C. E., Reinold, C. E., Levine, J., and Genant, H. K. (1985). *Invest. Radiology* **20**, 813–823.

Thompson, S. J., Rook, G. A. W., Brealey, R. J., v.d. Zee, R., and Elson, C. J. (1990). *Eur. J. Immunol.* **20**, 2479–2484.

Torisu, M., Miyahara, T., Shinohara, N., Ohsato, K., and Sonazaki, H. (1978). *Cancer Immunol. Immunother.* **5**, 77–83.

Trentham, D. E., Townes, A. S., and Kang, A. H. (1977). *J. Exp. Med.* **146**, 857–868.

Van den Broek, M. F., Hogervorst, E. J. M., v. Bruggen, M. C. J., v. Eden, W., v.d. Zee, R., and v.d. Berg, W. (1989). *J. Exp. Med.* **170**, 449–466.

Van Eden, W. (1991). *Immun. Rev.* **121**, 5–28.

Van Eden, W., Holoshitz, J., New, Z., Frenkel, A., Klajman, A., and Cohen, I. R. (1985). *Proc. Natl. Acad. Sci. USA* **82**, 5117–5120.

Van Eden, W., Thole, J. E. R., v.d. Zee, R., Noordzij, A., v. Embden, J. D. A., Hensen, E. J., and Cohen, I. R. (1988). *Nature* **331**, 171–173.

Van Vollenhoven, R. F., Soriano, A., McCarthy, P. E., Schwartz, R. L., Garbrecht, F. C., Thorbecke, G. J., and Siskind, G. W. (1988). *J. Immunol.* **141**, 1168–1173.

Waksman, B. H., and Wennersten, C. (1963). *Int. Arch. Allergy* **23**, 129.

Waksman, B. H., Pearson, C. M., and Sharp, J. T. (1960). *J. Immunol.* **85**, 403.

Ward, J. R., and Jones, R. S. (1962). *Arthr. Rheum.* **5**, 557–564.

Wauben, M. H. M., Boog, C. J. P., v.d. Zee, R., Joosten, I., Schlief, A., and v. Eden, W. (1992). *J. Exp. Med.* **176**, 667–677.

Whitehouse, D. J., Whitehouse, M. W., and Pearson, C. M. (1969). *Nature* **224**, 1322–1325.

Whitehouse, M. W., Orr, K. J., Beek, W. J., and Pearson, C. M. (1974). *Immunology* **27**, 311–330.

Winter, C. A., Risley, E. A., and Nuss, G. W. (1962). *Proc. Soc. Exp. Biol. Med.* **111**, 544–547.

Wood, F. D., Pearson, C. M., and Tanaka, A. (1969). *Int. Arch. Allergy Appl. Immunol.* **35**, 456.

Yang, X. D., Gasser, J., Riniker, B., and Feige, U. (1990). *Autoimmunity* **3**, 11–23.

Yiangou, M., and Hadjipetrou-Kourounakis, L. (1989). *Int. Allergy Appl. Immunol.* **89**, 217–221.

Yoshino, S., and Cleland, L. G. (1992). *J. Exp. Med.* **175**, 907–915.

Zhang, Z. Y., Lee, C. S., Lider, O., and Weiner, H. L. (1990). *J. Immunol.* **145**, 2489–2493.

Chapter 14

Murine Models of Spontaneous Systemic Lupus Erythematosus

Chaim Putterman[1,2] and Yaakov Naparstek[1]

[1]The Clinical Immunology and Allergy Unit, Department of Medicine,
Hadassah University Hospital, Jerusalem 91120, Israel
[2]Department of Microbiology and Immunology, Albert Einstein College of Medicine,
Bronx, New York 10461

I. Introduction

The first model of murine lupus was developed in the early 1960s, after the New Zealand Bielschowsky black (NZB/bl, or NZB) mouse bred by M. Bielschowsky died at an early age from immune hemolytic anemia. When the NZB was mated with the unrelated New Zealand white (NZW), the resultant female offspring died from immune glomerulonephritis with lupus erythematosus (LE) cells (Heyler and Howie, 1963), thus offering the first opportunity to study systemic lupus erythematosus (SLE) in the animal model. Since then, several animal (especially mice) strains have been developed which spontaneously develop a lupus-like illness remarkably similar to that

occurring in man. Murine models have been used to study etiology and pathogenesis, role of environmental factors and genetic predisposition, and the
response to different therapeutic modalities (Manolios and Schrieber, 1986).
Different clinical expressions of SLE arise in the models at predictable
ages, enabling comparison of the premorbid animal with the situation after
disease expression. It also enables study of the disease course, unaffected by
extrinsic intervention—which of course is not usually possible in the human
counterpart.

As we have mentioned, since 1960 several successful and reproducible
models of animal lupus have been developed (Hahn, 1987). Of these, specific
murine models have been particularly useful, and continue to serve in the
continuing investigation of this multisystem disease. Two forms of disease
develop in each mouse strain. Early in life, the mice develop multiple immunological aberrations, followed later by immune complex disease and other
autoimmune features (Wood and Zvaifler, 1989). We will focus our attention
on two of the murine lupus models in widespread investigational use, namely,
the NZB × NZW F_1 hybrid and the MRL-*lpr/lpr*. We discuss clinical features
and characteristics of each model, as well as molecular genetics, effects of
hormonal modulation, and important immunopathogenetic mechanisms.

II. (NZB × NZW) F_1

A. History

NZB mice are characterized by two major populations of autoantibodies:
natural thymocytotoxic antibodies (NTA), and high titers of antierythrocytic
antibodies. Most of the mice die from hemolytic anemia, although lymphoid
malignancies and kidney diseases may also at times be the cause of death.
Other clinical features include peptic ulcer, vasculitis, and infectious complications (Hahn, 1987; Bielschowsky and Goodall, 1970; Milich and Gershwin,
1980). By 1 month of age, immunoglobulin M (IgM) autoantibodies against
T cells begin to be detectable in NZB mice, while they are 100% present by
3 months. Prognosis is not markedly affected by sex, with mean survival
about 470 days in males and 425 days in females.

The F_1 hybrid (BW) mice are derived from breeding the NZB with the
phenotypically normal NZW, developed by W. H. Hall at the Otago Medical
School in Dunedin, New Zealand. In the resultant (NZB × NZW) F_1 hybrid
described by Heyler and Howie (1963), the dominant pattern of immune
hemolytic anemia in the NZB parent changes to a fatal immune nephritis
similar to the glomerulonephritis in human SLE. The short life span of the

BW female and the predictability of the pathological changes are additional features making this model particularly attractive for study and research.

B. General Features

The average body weight of the BW mouse at 5 months of age is 41 g. Disease is more severe and accelerated in females, with survival for only an average of 245 days, while in the males the course of the kidney disease is much slower, with death only after 406 days (Theofilopoulos and Dixon, 1985). BW mice carry the H-2^d/H-2^z at the H-2 locus, and the coat color is brown (Andrews et al., 1978).

C. The Disease

1. Autoantibodies

The level of immunoglobulins in the serum of a mature 7- to 12-month-old BW female is two to three times higher than in a nonautoimmune strain of mice. The main increase in immunoglobulins is found in the IgG 1 and IgG 2a subclasses (Theofilopoulos and Dixon, 1985).

The BW mouse inherits the early maturity and activation of its B cell from the NZB parent, with synthesis of immunoglobulins detectable by 1 month or even earlier. However, in contrast to NZB, early IgM (2 months) is specific for antinuclear antigens (ANA), rather than erythrocytes or T cells. The ANA are directed against double-stranded (ds) and single-stranded (ss) DNA (most closely associated with the development of nephritis), double-stranded RNA, histones, and tRNA. By 5–7 months of age, IgG anti-DNA increases and eventually dominates; subclasses IgG 2a and IgG 2b are the most frequent (Steward and Hay, 1976). The high levels of anti-DNA are associated with increased levels of circulating immune complexes and marked decreases in levels of complement (Andrews et al., 1978).

Other autoantibodies against nuclear antigens also appear in this model. Antihistone antibodies with very low titers are present before 4 months of age, progressively increasing to high levels in 100% of mice at 8 months, while concurrently maturing from IgM to IgG (Gioud et al., 1983). The histones against which the antibodies are predominantly directed are H2B and H3, while in humans, histones H1 and H2B are the major target antigens (Hardin and Thomas, 1983). Eilat et al. (1976) demonstrated the presence also of anti-RNA antibodies in BW mice, recognizing a trinucleotide sequence of single-stranded RNA (Eilat et al., 1980).

Other autoantibodies are present in BW sera, but probably are of less importance to the pathogenesis of lupus. Thirty-five to 78% of BW females develop antierythrocyte antibodies (Hahn, 1987) but anemia is more closely related to renal failure, and hemolysis is not prominent. In the male BW, the incidence of these antibodies is 20–40%, which is not significantly different from the normal mouse (Shirai and Mellors, 1972). As for NTA, 20% of BW mice are positive at 2 months, 50% by 6 months, and nearly 100% after 12 months of age. However, the presence of this autoantibody is probably of little clinicopathological consequence.

2. Clinical and Pathological Manifestations

a. Kidney. The leading cause of death in all the major murine lupus models is glomerulonephritis, which is subacute and proliferative in the MRL/lpr mouse (see later discussion), while in the BW female the histology is more chronic and obliterative (Theofilopoulos and Dixon, 1985). Other pathological features include mesangial and intravascular protein deposits, proliferation of all glomerular cellular elements, and crescent formation. Immunofluorescent studies (Dixon, 1981) reveal granular deposits of IgG and C3. Deposits are first found in the mesangium around 5 months of age. As the disease progresses, glomerular capillary wall deposits are also found. Outside the glomerulus, deposits can be found in the peritubular tissue and arterioles and increase in frequency with age. Antibodies eluted from the glomeruli are predominantly [50% (Lambert and Dixon, 1968) or up to 85% (Hahn, 1987)] IgG anti-DNA, with IgG 2a the dominant isotype in the deposits. Concentrations of ANA, anti-ds DNA, and anti-ss DNA are 2–10, 25–31, and 5–13 times higher, respectively, than their concentration in serum (Andrews *et al.*, 1978; Lambert and Dixon, 1968).

Areas are found in the glomerular basement membrane that have a high anionic charge. Another factor that might render anti-DNA nephritogenic is a cationic charge. IgGs eluted from BW kidneys were indeed found to be very cationic, with isoelectric focusing points of pH 8.5–9.0, while anionic anti-DNA antibodies were found not to adhere to BW glomeruli (Dang and Herbeck, 1984).

b. Thymus. Severe cortical thymic atrophy is characteristic of all murine SLE strains (Theofilopoulos and Dixon, 1981). The initial pathological lesion is cortical thymocyte loss, with or without cystic medullary degeneration. An overwhelming majority of mice show medullary atrophy, while 5–10% show medullary hyperplasia, which maintains thymic size despite the cortical loss. Thymic atrophy with abnormal fine structure appears by the fourth month in the female BW mouse, and by 6–7 months 70–90% of their cortexes are lost. The histologic lesions of the New Zealand (NZ) thymus consist of lymphoid hyperplasia in the medulla, infiltration with mast cells, and epithelial degeneration and vacuolization, correlating with a decrease in thymic hormone levels (Howie and Heyler, 1968; Bach *et al.*, 1973).

c. Cardiovascular disease.   Fifteen percent of BW mice show evidence of acute or healed myocardial infarction of either ventricle when examined at autopsy. On histological examination, small and medium arteries have focal degenerative lesions, with deposition of periodic acid Schiff (PAS)-positive material in the intima and media. The media can show degenerative changes without surrounding inflammation, while intimal cells occasionally proliferate or swell. These vascular lesions, with associated platelet aggregation, may occlude the arterial lumen. Immune deposits of IgG, C3, and viral envelope protein gp 70 (see later discussion) are present in the walls of myocardial vessels, both arterial and venous. Vascular occlusion and thrombosis seem to be mediated by immune complexes, resulting in decreased blood flow and ultimately infarction (Accinni and Dixon, 1979; Berden *et al.*, 1983; Pansky and Freimer, 1974).

d. Lymphoid hyperplasia.   Splenic and lymph node hyperplasia characterize all types of spontaneous murine SLE, but the degree varies greatly among different strains. In BW mice, this phenomenon is not prominent, and only mild lymphadenopathy (normal size to two to three times normal) and splenomegaly are present. Accordingly, lymphoid tumors are also very infrequent (<10%), and thymomas appear very rarely (Hahn *et al.*, 1975).

e. Miscellaneous.   Other extrarenal lesions can also occur in the BW model, but appear only in a low incidence or are clinically insignificant (Hahn, 1987; Theofilopoulos and Dixon, 1985). Lymphocytic infiltration of salivary glands, xerophthalmia, and immune complex deposits on oocytes, endometrium, dermal–epidermal junction, choroid, and ciliary process have all been reported.

D. Pathogenesis and Genetics

1. B and T Cells

Polyclonal B-cell hyperactivity is characteristic of all murine lupus models, with hyperglobulinemia and increased production of antibodies. It is thought that this activation in the New Zealand strains (NZB and (NZB × NZW) F_1) strains may be due to a primary B-cell abnormality. Marrow from NZB mice transferred into healthy, irradiated, histocompatible mice induces disease, while normal marrow grafted into irradiated NZB mice has a protective effect (Kincade *et al.*, 1982; Norton *et al.*, 1975).

The *xid* gene is an X-linked recessive immunodeficiency gene. In either the homozygous or the hemizygous state, this gene causes deletion or delays maturation of a subset of mature B cells (LyB 3^+, LyB 5^+), responsible for immune responses to polysaccharide antigens with repeating structures (Scher, 1982). Introduction of the *xid* gene into the BW mouse results in significantly decreased production of polyclonal immunoglobulins and auto-antibodies, and almost normal life spans (Steinberg et al., 1982). Marked attenuation in autoimmune manifestations with the insertion of the xid gene into BW and other lupus strains also points to a pivotal role for hyperactive B cells in murine SLE pathogenesis. Whether B cell hyperactivity results from stem cell defects or abnormal regulatory function is still unclear.

Cell transfer studies using NZB and nonautoimmune DBA/2 mice bearing the xid gene have shown that the phenotype of the excess number of auto-antibody-producing cells is associated with the environment of the recipient, rather than with the origin of the B cells. This indicates that at least some defects in the NZB mice that lead to B-cell hyperactivity reside, not in the B cells, but rather in the milieu in which they mature (Klinman et al., 1988).

Although the B-cell immune response of the BW mouse involves many different clones, it is by no means an unrestricted response. Hahn and her colleagues have described an idiotypic restriction on serum immunoglobulins of the BW mice. This restriction develops with age, with three public idio-types ultimately dominating the serum immunoglobulins. Two of these idio-types, Id GN1 and Id GN2, are found on approximately half of the glomerular immunoglobulins (Hahn and Ebling, 1987).

The relations between the immunoglobulin genes in lupus mice and their normal counterparts have been addressed by many researchers. Analysis of the immunoglobulin heavy-chain, variable-region haplotypes of NZB and NZW mice have shown that they are almost indistinguishable from those of nonautoimmune mice, suggesting that the germ-line gene repertoire of these lupus mice may be normal. Structural studies of the anti-DNA antibodies themselves produced by the BW mice indicate that the V_H and V_L sequences are closely related to V genes used in exogenous responses, or belong to known V-gene families. From this it can be concluded that these anti-DNA autoantibodies are encoded by the same germ-line gene repertoire used in the synthesis of antibodies to exogenous antigens (Theofilopoulos et al., 1989). A contrasting viewpoint was presented in a recent review by Eilat (1990), who argued that some BW anti-DNA antibodies are indeed encoded by unique "anti-DNA" germ-line genes.

Two opposing theories relating to somatic mutations and autoimmunity have been proposed: (1) Autoantibodies may be due to somatic mutation of normal antibodies that in lupus escape regulation or are generated at an abnormal rate (Davidson et al., 1987; Diamond and Scharff, 1984). (2) Un-mutated germ-line genes may encode anti-self autoantibodies, which are lost during the somatic mutation as part of the physiological response to inciting antigens (Naparstek et al., 1986).

Some IgG anti-DNA antibodies whose expressed V_H segments are encoded by germ-line genes were found to contain many somatic mutations (Eilat *et al.*, 1988). Behar and Scharff (1988), when analyzing anti-DNA antibodies from individual B-cell clones, also found a large number of somatic mutations. These antibodies have a high ratio of replacement mutations to silent mutations in the complementarity-determining regions (CDR). This ratio in the CDR is high when compared with that in the framework regions, indicating a positive selection of B cells by an antigen. These somatic mutations may result in affinity maturation of the antibody response to antigen, and in the case of anti-DNA antibodies, support the view that the autoimmune response to DNA is driven by the antigen.

T cells in the BW model may be responsible for regulating the pace of the disease (Smith and Steinberg, 1983). Neonatal thymectomy tends to accelerate the disease, although thymectomy at 6–10 weeks does not have this effect (Steinberg *et al.*, 1970). Therefore, this postulated "regulator" must work within the first few weeks of life. The role of T cells in the BW mouse strain is also suggested by studies of successful therapeutic interventions targeted exclusively against T cells. Treatment of BW mice with monoclonal anti-CD4 antibodies was found to retard the development of autoimmunity (Carteron *et al.*, 1990).

B-cell hyperfunction in BW mice may also result from a lack of, or deficiency in, suppressor T cells. Krakauer (1976) found that concanavalin A (ConA)-activated spleen cells of adult BW mice have decreased suppressor potential relative to controls. Furthermore, *in vivo* administration of supernatant from ConA-activated spleen cells from normal mice to BW mice resulted in attenuation of the autoimmune process (Krakauer *et al.*, 1977). However, Crieghton *et al.* (1979), looking at IgG and IgE responses to exogenous antigens, found no difference in suppressor T-cell function between lupus and normal mice.

Cytokines have also been implicated in pathogenesis of lupus in the BW mouse, although data is still preliminary. BW mice were found to produce reduced levels of tumoui necrosis factor-α, while replacement therapy with recombinant tumoui necrosis factor-α significantly delayed development of nephritis (Jacob and McDevitt, 1988).

2. Viruses

Many features of SLE, including fever, fatigue, and myalgia are also present in viral disease (Krieg, 1991). Recent reports of autoimmune features in patients with human immunodeficiency virus (HIV) infection (Krieg and Steinberg, 1990a) have rekindled interest in the role of viruses and retroviruses in the pathogenesis of murine and human SLE. Several lines of evidence were initially thought to support a viral role in pathogenesis. Murine leukemia virus antibodies were identified in the glomeruli and circulation of BW mice (Mellors *et al.*, 1969), while autoimmune disease was transferred to normal Swiss mice by filtrates of spleen from NZB mice (Mellors and Huang, 1967).

The second group of viruses implicated consisted of the C-type viruses, with major attention given to viral envelope gp 70 antigen. Both the viral antigen as well as the anti-gp 70 antibody are expressed in NZB and BW mice, with large amounts of antibody found in glomerular deposits (Levy and Pincus, 1970). These findings were contradicted, however, when circulating gp 70 was found in nearly all mouse strains tested (Levy, 1973). Therefore, it seems that viruses are probably not the primary pathogens in murine SLE, although a secondary role is envisioned by some authors (Woods and Zvaifler, 1989).

Recently, Krieg and Steinberg (1990b) demonstrated unusual endogenous retroviral expression in high levels in the thymuses of lupus-prone mice, which were undetectable in normal controls. Such endogenous retroviruses may play a role in regulating lymphocyte activation (Krieg et al., 1989). Epstein-Barr virus infection of human B cells prevents programmed cell death, otherwise known as apoptosis (Gregory et al., 1990). Steinberg (1992) postulated that endogenous retroviral expression may delay apoptosis in lupus thymocytes, which may allow the escape of self-reactive T cells, thereby initiating the autoimmune process.

3. Influence of Sex Hormones

Similar to the situation in human SLE, sex hormones significantly modulate disease in the BW lupus strain, much more than in any other murine lupus model. When castrated or treated with estrogens, male BW mice develop the "female" pattern of immune hyperactivity, namely, early IgM to IgG switch of anti-DNA production, and accelerated fatal immune nephritis (Roubinian et al., 1979). Conversely, female BW mice treated with castration and androgens or with antiestrogenic preparations, have marked suppression of IgG anti-DNA production and glomerulonephritis, with significantly prolonged survival (Roubinian et al., 1978). It is important to emphasize, however, that age is a critical factor in the influence of sex hormones, and studies in 5-week-old mice showed only partial effects of sex hormone reversal (Smith and Steinberg, 1983). Many other studies confirm these findings, and support the basic premise that androgens are protective and suppress autoantibody production in this model, while estrogens are permissive and enhance antibody production.

E. Summary

BW mice predictably develop an SLE-like disease, characterized by polyclonal B-cell hyperactivity and overproduction of autoantibodies, particularly IgG antibodies of anti-DNA specificity. Clinically, the major manifestation is immune complex deposition, including anti-DNA antibodies in the glomeruli, resulting in proteinuria, azotemia, and death from renal failure. Kidney disease begins earlier and is more fulminant in females, and survival is shortened accordingly. Other, less important, extrarenal immune manifestations may appear in the cardiovascular system and salivary glands. The most important parallels to the human disease are kidney involvement, anti-DNA autoantibody production, and the marked influence of sex hormones.

III. MRL-*lpr/lpr*

A. History

The MRL strains were developed in 1976 by E. D. Murphy and J. D. Roths at the Jackson Laboratory (Murphy and Roths, 1977). The strain was derived as a by-product from a series of crosses between LG/J mice and AKR/J, C3H/Di, and C57Bl/6J, intended to transfer a mutation for achondroplasia from the leukemic background of AKR/J to a background without an increased incidence of leukemia. A backcross to LG/J mice followed by inbreeding to eliminate dental malocclusion resulted in some offspring exhibiting massive lymphoid proliferation, high-titer anti-DNA, and early lethal immune nephritis. Further inbreeding allowed separation of two lines with over 95% genetic homology: MRL-*lpr/lpr* ("lpr" denoting lymphoproliferation) and MRL/n, lacking the lpr gene, and subsequently not expressing lymphadenopathy. Several features distinguish MRL-*lpr/lpr* (MRL/l) from other strains of murine lupus models: (1) massive lymphoproliferation, (2) a rheumatoid arthritis (RA)-like polyarthritis in certain mice colonies, with a high incidence and titer of rheumatoid factor (RF), (3) a high frequency of lupus-specific autoantibodies (such as anti-Sm), and (4) high levels of circulating immune complexes and cryoglobulins.

B. General Features

Mean body weight for MRL/l females at 5 months of age is 48 g, and for males 41 g. MRL/n mice average 43 g at this age. Survival of the MRL/n averages 476 days for females and 546 days for males, while in the lpr survival is markedly shortened to 143 days for females and 154 days for males. As in the BW, the usual cause of death is progressive renal failure and azotemia. In our own experience, mice can die even with only moderate kidney disease and mild azotemia. Death then is probably due to the massive lymphoproliferative process which infiltrates vital organs. In the MRL, the *H-2* locus is *H-2^k*, and the coat color is white (Andrews *et al.*, 1978).

C. The Disease

1. Autoantibodies

Among the murine lupus strains, the MRL/l is the highest producer of IgG, ANA, and antibodies to DNA. Serum IgG levels reach an extremely high level of 25 mg/ml at 5 months of age, with elevation of all IgG subclasses. This massive hyperglobulinemia is accompanied by high levels of cryoglobulin, the IgG 3 subclass in particular (Abdelmoula *et al.*, 1989). Monoclonal paraprotein is present in up to 43% of 5- to 6-month-old MRL/l female mice, versus only 17% of BW females. High levels of circulating immune complexes can be found in almost all old mice of this strain, and in high quantities. Antierythrocyte antibodies (7%) and NTA are of little practical importance in the MRL/l (Andrews *et al.*, 1978).

MRL/l mice produce a higher proportion of antibodies to ssDNA relative to dsDNA, compared with the BW. In MRL/l females, antibodies to DNA circulate by 6–8 weeks of age, followed by proteinuria at 2–3 months, and azotemia at 3–6 months. MRL/l males lag behind females by about 1 month. It is the positively charged IgG 2a and IgG 2b isotype autoantibodies that deposit in the glomeruli (Ebling and Hahn, 1980; Slack *et al.*, 1984).

Anti-DNA antibodies eluted from the kidneys of MRL/l mice differ from their serum counterparts, not only by their physicochemical properties, but also by their antigen specificities. A very large proportion of these antibodies express the H130 idiotype, which is a major idiotype of the MRL/l anti-DNA response (see later discussion), and they all cross-react with heparin. This suggests that kidney binding antibodies in MRL/l may be a subpopulation of the serum anti-DNA antibodies characterized by specificity for glycosaminoglycans (Naparstek *et al.*, 1990).

Anti-Sm antibodies (and other SLE-specific autoantibodies) are a unique feature of the MRL strain (both MRL/l and MRL/n), while NZB and BW are uniformly negative (Eisenberg *et al.*, 1978; Pisetsky *et al.*, 1980). Anti-Sm antibodies appear relatively late, and are found in MRL/l mice at 4 months of age in about 37% of females and 10% of males. In MRL/n mice, the incidence increases to 83% in females and 57% in males at 9–12 months of age (Theofilopoulos and Dixon, 1985). It is important to emphasize that despite similar levels of anti-DNA, anti-Sm-positive mice may exhibit large variation in anti-Sm levels. The antigen specificity of the murine anti-Sm of the MRL is for the same small nuclear ribonucleoproteins as in the human response. Another recently described SLE-specific autoantibody is antiribosomal P

(Bonfa *et al.*, 1988). Antiribosomal P and anti-Sm were found to correlate in the individual animal, as they do in human disease (Elkon *et al.*, 1989).

2. Clinical and Pathological Manifestations

a. Kidney. Immune glomerulonephritis in the MRL/l strain takes a subacute proliferative form. Histological examination reveals glomerular lesions involving accumulation of monocytes, proliferation of endothelial and mesangial cells, with occasional crescent formation and basement membrane thickening. The mice develop significant proteinuria, with urinary protein values ranging from 2.6 to 3.8 mg/day at 3–6 months, and a 20% incidence of advanced anasarca in the terminal stages of the disease. A common finding is infiltration of the interstitium, with lymphocytes as part of the generalized lymphoproliferation.

On immunofluorescence, renal deposits of IgG and C3 are already present in a granular pattern by 2 months of age, and continue to increase until 5 months. Deposits are found in the mesangium and particularly in the capillary wall (Theofilopoulos and Dixon, 1985).

Concentration of ANA and anti-dsDNA in immunoglobulins from renal eluates of MRL/l mice are two to six and one to six times higher, respectively, than those found in serum. As in BW mice, it is thought that the alkaline anti-DNAs are the more nephritogenic (Andrews *et al.*, 1978; Lambert and Dixon, 1968).

MRL/n also develop a chronic nephritis, but associated with much lower levels of autoantibodies than the MRL/l. Both males and females are similarly affected, and death usually occurs by 2 years of age (Murphy and Roths, 1977).

b. Thymus. In the MRL mice, thymic histological changes are similar to those described above for the BW strain, but appear earlier in the disease course. Thymic atrophy and cystic medullary necrosis appear by 2 months, and progress to a complete loss of cortical areas by 3.5 months (Theofilopoulos and Dixon, 1985).

c. Cardiovascular system. Involvement of the heart and vascular system is also characteristic of the MRL/l, with degenerative lesions in the coronary arteries and evidence of myocardial infarctions in 9 out of 41 mice studied by Andrews *et al.* (1978). Degenerative vascular lesions appear early in life, while an exudative vasculitis can appear later on. In about 75% of older MRL/l mice, a necrotizing polyarteritis of medium-sized arteries can be found. Involvement of the kidneys, mesentery, coronary circulation, and genital organs has been described (Berden *et al.*, 1983; Cohen and Eisenberg, 1991). Another related feature is the sudden development of high levels of autoantibodies and circulating immune complexes together with the onset of the vasculitis.

d. Lymphoid hyperplasia. The lymphoproliferative disorder of the MRL/l is the most exclusive abnormality of this lupus strain. Lymphoproliferation occurs in all mice of both sexes, and is manifest mainly as massive generalized lymphadenopathy. Cervical, axillary, and mesenteric lymph nodes are all involved and enlarged. This process begins as early as 8 weeks of age; lymph nodes are enlarged up to 100 times above normal by 16–18 weeks, compared with only two to three times normal in NZ mice (Hahn, 1987).

On histological examination, the predominant cells are lymphocytes, with small numbers of histiocytes, plasma cells, and immunoblasts. The massive proliferation of lymphocytes results in obliteration of the normal nodal architecture. The dominant population of T cells infiltrating the lymph nodes is of the double negative phenotype (see Section III,D,1). All murine isotypes and IgG subclasses are represented in the infiltrating plasma cells, with a predominance of IgG 1 and IgG 2a. In about one-third of old, terminally ill MRL/l mice, there is a paradoxical reduction in the size of the lymph nodes, owing to extensive hemorrhage and cystic necrosis in the larger lymph nodes.

Splenomegaly is also present in the MRL mice, but proportionately much less than the lymph node enlargement. Relative to the 145-mg spleen of age-matched MRL/n, old MRL/l have spleens with an average weight of 735 mg (about five times greater). Despite the massive lymphoproliferation, it is not thought to be a malignant state, although a prelymphomatous condition cannot be ruled out (Theofilopoulos and Dixon, 1985). Surprisingly perhaps, the incidence of true lymphoid neoplasia is low (<10%) in the MRL/l, while in the longer living MRL/n, the incidence rises to 40%.

e. Arthritis. Another exceptional manifestation in the MRL/l strain among the murine SLE models is a disease remarkably similar to human rheumatoid arthritis (Hang *et al.*, 1982). One-month-old mice have no significant synovial abnormalities. By 3–4 months of age, 45% of the mice show early synovial changes consisting of subsynovial mononuclear infiltration and synovial thickening. Periarticular vasculitis with pannus formation and early articular erosions can be seen at this stage. As the pathological process progresses, by 5–6 months 75% of the mice have significant articular damage. The synovium is thickened by synovial cell proliferation and cellular infiltration. Over 50% of affected joints show erosion and joint destruction. Perivascular infiltration is prominent and common (>80%), involving mononuclear and polymorphonuclear cells, with vascular destruction in periarticular regions. The periarticular tissues affected include muscles, fascia, tendons, and nerves (Hang *et al.*, 1982).

It is important to emphasize, however, that the incidence and extent of arthritis varies widely from colony to colony. In our experience, the arthritis is usually not detectable clinically, but only by the characteristic histopathological findings.

Together with the complete clinical and histological picture of RA in certain MRL/l colonies, this strain is also unique in the production of RF. IgM and IgG RFs can be found at 3–4 months of age. The polyclonal IgM RF reacts with all mouse IgG subclasses, but the majority react most strongly with murine IgG 2a (Theofilopoulos *et al.*, 1983). This may be explained by a larger representation of this subclass in the immune complexes present in MRL.

The clinical significance of the RF in the pathogenesis of the RA-like picture is uncertain. There is a clear and consistent correlation between the presence of IgM RF and joint pathology. Eighty percent of mice with arthritis have high levels of RF, while 95% of mice with IgM RF have synovitis or arthritis. Congenic MRL/n mice without the *lpr* gene do not have demonstrable RF or arthritic manifestations. Nevertheless, the presence of RF is probably not sufficient for the development of arthritis, as introduction of the *lpr* gene into normal mice strains results in very high levels of IgM RF, but no arthritis develops.

f. Miscellaneous. Hang *et al.* reported (1982) that about 60% of older MRL/l mice have salivary gland periductal mononuclear infiltrates, associated with acinar destruction. These findings suggested that MRL can also serve as an experimental model for Sjögren's disease. Eye abnormalities were found to be frequent in MRL mice. Hoffman and co-workers (1983, 1984) found an 85% incidence of conjunctivitis, and a 100% incidence of lacrimal gland mononuclear infiltrates in MRL/l mice. These findings were present in MRL/n and other lupus models, but not as frequently. Band keratopathy with bilateral calcium corneal deposits was seen in 90% of MRL/l mice, associated with hypercalcemia, increased serum PTH binding, and some histological changes in the parathyroid. Posterior uveitis was also noted in 35% (7/20 mice) of adult MRL/l mice.

Other rarer manifestations include pulmonary vasculitis and interstitial pneumonitis, infiltrative skin lesions with dermal-epidermal junction immunoglobulin deposition, myositis, and deafness (Cohen and Eisenberg, 1991).

D. Pathogenesis and Genetics

1. B and T Cells

B-cell activation is present in the MRL/l strain, as in all murine lupus models. MRL/l mice produce IgG 1 and IgG 2a in particular. Slack *et al.* found that MRL/l females from 2–5 months of age have an eight-fold increase in IgG 2a-producing cells, a sixfold increase in IgG 2b-producing cells, and smaller increases in IgG 1 and IgG 3-secreting cells (Slack *et al.*, 1984). Similarly, Raveche *et al.* (1982) using cell cycle analysis found that spleens of MRL/l mice had higher numbers (both absolute and relative) of spontaneously proliferating cells at disease onset relative to normal mice. This proliferation was not found in thymus or bone marrow. A previously held view is that murine SLE is a manifestation of polyclonal B-cell activation, with some B lymphocytes producing autoantibodies that lead to cell injury (Steinberg, 1984). However, it is thought that the immune defect resides proximally to the B cell, particularly in the MRL strain. Support for this concept lies in the ability of marrow stem cells (proximal to mature B cells) to transfer the disease to irradiated, histocompatible recipients (Akizuki *et al.*, 1978).

B cells in the lpr model produce autoantibodies which are specific for the disease, in this case rheumatoid factor and anti-DNA antibodies. Is the production due to nonspecific polyclonal B cell activation or specific autoantigen-driven B cell activation? The anti-DNA antibodies of the MRL/l mice bear a high frequency of a public idiotypic marker. Up to 50% of the serum anti-DNA antibodies share an idiotype termed H130, and its serum levels rise progressively during the course of the disease. Although this idiotype identifies a group of pathogenic antibodies, 75% of the serum immunoglobulins that carry this idiotype do not bind DNA (Rauch *et al.*, 1982). The V_H segment of MRL/l monoclonal anti-DNA antibody H130 was found to be identical in sequence to a BALB/c germ-line gene—indicating that anti-DNA V regions may be encoded by germ-line unmutated genes that are present in both normal and lupus-prone mice. Analyses of V gene sequences of additional anti-DNA antibodies derived from the MRL/l mice indicate that they are encoded by a large number of V_H and V_L genes—and that there is no single "anti-DNA" gene in these mice.

Several data point to the fact that at least the late phase of autoantibody production in the MRL mouse is an antigen-driven process. Klinman *et al.* (1990) analyzed the B cell repertoires of lpr mice over an 8-month period. The repertoire of mice under 12 weeks of age was dominated by IgM-secreting B cells that showed no bias toward production of specific autoantibodies. From 12 to 38 weeks, an increasing proportion of animals developed repertoires skewed toward reactivity against one or very few autoantigens. Bellon *et al.* (1987) found that autoantibodies produced from MRL-lpr/lpr mice demonstrate increased expression of V_H7183. This 3' bias suggested that the 3' V_H gene repertoire encoded germ-line, self-reactive autoantibodies, and that early expression of these autoantibodies may be important in autoantibody regulation later in life. Conversely, Kastner and colleagues (1989) found no evidence for 3' overrepresentation, while Komisar (1989) found that old lpr mice with severe autoimmune disease had overrepresentation of the J558 V_H family (5' skewing). Therefore, the hypothesis that autoimmune lpr mice have increased autoantibody production due to an inability to switch from 3' to 5' is still speculative.

Shlomchik *et al.* (1987) found that RF production in lpr mice resulted from oligoclonal expansion and somatic mutations of the RF autoantibodies. Similarly, analysis of the V regions of 31 monoclonal anti-DNA antibodies from MRL/l mice has revealed expression of somatic mutations defining specificity for DNA. Arginine residues were found to play an important role in defining this specificity. This led the authors to argue that the anti-DNA antibodies in the MRL/l mouse arise as a result of specific antigen-driven stimulation (Shlomchik et al., 1990).

The most outstanding example of the role of abnormal T-cell function in the pathogenesis of lupus is the MRL/l mouse. Immunoglobulin overproduction, secretion of autoantibodies, and immune hyperresponsiveness, together with the massive lymph node infiltration with helper phenotype T cells suggest that increased helper T-cell activity is instrumental in the immunopathogenesis of MRL/l lupus. Theofilopolous et al. (1980) found that addition of T-cell-enriched populations from old autoimmune MRL mice to syngeneic B cells provided significantly more help than controls. Naparstek et al. (1988) have shown that autoreactive T-cell clones derived from MRL/l mice induced B-cell proliferation and production of anti-DNA antibodies in vitro. Further support for T-cell-derived help is that without a neonatal thymus, lymphadenopathy does not occur, and production of anti-DNA antibodies, onset of immune nephritis, and mortality are significantly delayed (Steinberg et al., 1980). When a thymus graft is transplanted, autoimmune features develop (Theofilopoulos and Dixon, 1981). The factor by which T-help is mediated was found to be an antigen-nonspecific, B-cell differentiating factor (Prudhomme et al., 1983).

Insertion of the xid gene into the MRL/l model has also been studied. In contrast to the BW discussed above, hyperactivity and autoantibody production are not completely inhibited, and disease manifestations are only retarded, but not totally prevented (Cohen and Eisenberg, 1991).

One of the most interesting features of the lpr mouse model is the unusual phenotype and disordered function of the dominant T-cell infiltrating lymphoid tissue, namely CD4$^-$ CD8$^-$ Thy 1$^+$ cells (double negative, DN). Although the fraction of phenotypically normal cells bearing either marker (CD4$^+$ or CD8$^+$) decreases, the absolute number of these cells increases owing to the massive lymphoproliferation.

Double negative T cells bear Thy 1, CD3, and low levels of CD5, but also express certain B-cell surface markers, including B220. Several markers not usually appearing on normal, resting T cells are also present, which may serve to mark functional subsets (Kakkanaiah et al., 1990). Double negative T cells predominate also in the developing thymus, and are found in much smaller numbers also in the normal adult. Differences in functional behavior and differentiation, however, suggest only a superficial resemblance to the double negative lpr T cells (Budd et al., 1987; Igarashi et al., 1988).

The T-cell functions of the lpr double negative cells are markedly decreased on in vitro testing. Proliferation, interleukin-2 production, and acquisition of interleukin-2 receptors are profoundly deficient, and can only be partially resolved by phorbol ester and calcium ionophore. This poor function may be related to the lack of CD2 expression, which is involved in T-cell adhesion (Shirai *et al.*, 1990).

The V_β gene T-cell receptor (TCR) expression of the double negative T cells is diverse, and reflects appropriate intrathymic negative selection by Mls and I-E molecules (Kotzin *et al.*, 1988; Mountz *et al.*, 1990). Such selection requires expression of the CD4 by the T cell, suggesting that the precursor cells of the double negative T cells in the lpr once had CD4 present. Further support for this view is found in the study in which *in vivo* treatment of lpr mice with anti-CD4 antibody inhibited the accumulation of the abnormal CD4$^-$,8$^-$ TCR α/β^+ T cells (Santoro *et al.*, 1988). By similar reasoning, CD8 was also once present due to its role in class I restricted clonal deletion. A prior double positive marker status for the double negative T cell also explains another interesting finding, namely, the coexistence of immature (CD4$^-$,8$^-$), and mature (TCR α/β^+) markers on the cell surface. It seems that thymocytes destined to give rise to lpr cells passed at one stage of their development through a double positive stage in which tolerance-related clonal deletion occurred, giving rise to secondary double negative, but TCR α/β^+ T cells (Theofilopoulos *et al.*, 1989).

What is the mechanism for the loss of the accessory molecules from the lpr T cells? Several mechanisms have been proposed by Singer *et al.* and Singer and Theofilopoulos (1989, 1990). The "escape and backup tolerance" model suggests that highly autoreactive TCR-bearing cells are deleted from the repertoire, while those only moderately autoreactive escape deletion. However, as a backup form of tolerance, the lpr cells undergo downregulation of their accessory markers. The basis for autoimmunity in the lpr model, according to this hypothesis, is the moderate autoreactivity of lpr, which can induce clinically significant autoimmunity despite downregulation through reacquiring accessory molecules, or by production of B-cell differentiating factors. According to the second model of "failed positive selection," lpr cells express TCRs that are not self-reactive, and subsequently are not positively selected. Normally, these cells would be short lived, but lack of the normal intrathymic apoptosis due to the *lpr* mutation (see later discussion) allows them to accumulate. Autoimmunity is induced in this model by the activity of normal CD4$^+$ T cells stimulated by the large number of lpr cells.

Further insight into the molecular basis of the *lpr* mutation has been made possible by recent advances in techniques of molecular biology. The *lpr* gene is a single autosomal gene that is mainly recessive, with *lpr/lpr* homozygotes demonstrating the full clinical expression of autoimmune disease and lymphoproliferation. Nevertheless, heterozygotes (*lpr/+*) have some degree of autoimmunity, with increased autoantibody production (Jachez *et al.*, 1988) and mortality from lymphoid neoplasia. Phenotypic expression of *lpr* is strongly influenced by background genes, as shown by variation in lymphad-enopathy and autoantibodies in different inbred strains homozygous for *lpr* (Izui *et al.*, 1984). The *lpr* gene is greatly potentiated in the presence of *Yaa*, the Y chromosome gene responsible for autoimmunity in the BXSB mouse strain (Pisetsky *et al.*, 1985), and reduced in mice expressing *xid* (Cohen and Eisenberg, 1991). C57Bl/6 mice homozygous for *lpr* and the *nu* (nude) muta-tion do not develop lymphadenopathy, and exhibit only very low levels of autoantibodies (Mosbach-Ozmen *et al.*, 1985).

Another recently described mutation leading to an lpr-like disease with lymphoproliferation and autoimmunity is the *gld* (generalized lymphoproli-ferative disorder) (Roths *et al.*, 1984). The *gld* gene is also autosomal and recessive; however, *lpr* and *gld* are not allelic, and double heterozygotes are normal. The *gld* mutation maps to the long arm of chromosome 1 (Seldin *et al.*, 1988). Another more recently described lupus-inducing mutation is the *lpr*^{cg} gene, which is allelic to *lpr*. However, in contrast to *lpr*, *lpr*^{cg} complements the *gld* gene, so that *lpr*^{cg}/+, *gld*/+ mice have a lymphoproliferative disorder (Matsuzawa *et al.*, 1990).

Recent work by Wantanabe-Fukunaga and associates (1992) regarding the relation between the *lpr* gene and the Fas antigen has greatly advanced the understanding of the *lpr* gene and related mutations, and their relation to the lymphoproliferative and autoimmune phenotypes. Fas antigen is a cell-surface protein expressed in various tissues, including the thymus, which is important in the mediation of apoptosis. Almost no Fas mRNA was observed in homozygous *lpr* mice, owing to rearrangement of the structural gene for the Fas antigen. On the other hand, in *lpr*^{cg} Fas antigen, mRNA expression was normal, but a point mutation resulted in inability to transduce the apop-totic signal into cells. This defect may result in defective negative selection of self-reactive T cells in the thymus, excessive numbers of autoreactive T cells released to the periphery, and autoimmune disease.

These results can also elegantly explain the genetic basis for the pheno-type of double heterozygotes discussed earlier. Results of bone marrow trans-plantation suggest that *gld* and *lpr* affect an interacting pair of molecules (Allen *et al.*, 1990), leading Wantanabe-Fukunaga *et al.* (1992) to propose that the structural gene for *gld* may encode for the Fas antigen ligand. In *lpr* mice, Fas is not expressed and so cannot bind ligand. In *lpr*^{cg} mice, although the receptor is nonfunctional, it can still presumably bind ligand. Therefore, *lpr* cannot complement *gld* in double heterozygotes. However, in *lpr*^{cg}/+, *gld*/+, the nonfunctional receptor can compete for ligands, which decreases the effective concentration of ligands below normal to produce the lymphoproli-ferative phenotype.

Several cytokines have recently been implicated in the pathogenesis of lupus in the MRL strain. Interleukin-2 produced by T cells is believed to serve in a universal role for proliferation of activated T cells. Altman *et al.*

(1981) found reduced ConA-induced mitogenic response and interleukin production in several lupus strains, but the production defect was most severe in MRL/l. The defect appeared at 3–6 weeks of age and continued to progress thereafter. It was hypothesized that the uncontrolled proliferation of helper T cells seen in MRL/l lupus mice may be due to the lack of interleukin-2-dependent, T-cell differentiation (Dauphinee et al., 1981). Interestingly, in neonataly thymectomized CBA/H mice, high levels of human interleukin-2 introduced intraperitoneally induced conversion of double negative T cells to CD4$^+$ CD8$^-$ or CD4$^-$ CD8$^+$ single positive cells (Andreu-Sánchez et al., 1991). This may suggest a possible role for interleukin-2 deficiency in maintaining the double negative phenotype in the MRL lupus model. The T-cell abnormality can be reproduced on normal backgrounds by the insertion of the *lpr* gene into normal mouse strains. The mice then produce increased levels of autoantibodies, but the clinical expression is less severe than in the MRL.

Interleukin-3 regulates hematopoietic stem cell development and promotes early T- and B-cell differentiation. Spontaneous release of interleukin-3 activity was detected in supernatants from spleen cells of 6-week-old MRL/l mice, and titers increased with age (Palacios, 1984), although these findings could not be confirmed (Davignon et al., 1988). Peak interleukin-1 activity was markedly decreased in peritoneal cells from MRL/l mice, relative to MRL/n (Steinberg, 1984). On the other hand, interleukin-1 expression was found to be increased in renal tissue from this strain (Boswell et al., 1988b), and interleukin-1 administration enhanced the unique polyarthritis of the MRL (Hom et al., 1990).

Interferon acts upon resting macrophages to enhance Ia positivity, and thus stimulate T-cell release of colony-stimulating factor (Steinberg, 1984). Manolios et al. (1989) found enhanced interferon production in lymph node T cells from MRL/l and MRL/n mice, which supported the speculation that interferon may play a role in Ia hyperresponsiveness and consequent autoreactivity of the MRL strain (Rosenberg et al., 1986). Finally, attention has recently focused also upon tumor necrosing factor (TNF), with increased TNF-α expression in MRL/l Kupffer cells (Magilavy and Rothstein, 1988), and expression of TNF-β mRNA in MRL/l nephritic kidneys (Boswell et al., 1988a).

2. Viruses

Viruses are not thought to be involved in the primary pathogenesis of SLE in the MRL model. However, as in the BW, viruses may induce aberrant immune responses and subsequent autoimmune manifestations. Several mechanisms for this presumed effect have been proposed, including polyclonal B-cell activation, cytolysis, selective tropism for certain subsets of regulatory lymphocytes, and possible modification of autoantigens (Theofilo-poulos and Dixon, 1985).

Neonatal lymphocytic choriomeningitis virus was found to change the 50% mortality point in the MRL/n mice from 18 to 12 months. However, neonatal injection of the same virus into normal mice strains without a genetic predisposition to lupus did not cause an SLE-like disease over the 2 years of observation (Tonietti *et al.*, 1970). Interestingly, prostaglandin E_1 (PGE_1) was found to prevent development of fatal glomerulonephritis and massive lymphoproliferation in MRL/l mice (Izui *et al.*, 1980; Kelly *et al.*, 1981). Although the amount or type of anti-DNA antibodies did not change, the deposition of immune complexes containing anti-DNA was reduced (Kelly *et al.*, 1981). One suggested mechanism for the beneficial effect was PGE-mediated suppression in the MRL of the formation of circulating endogenous retroviral glycoprotein gp 70/anti-gp 70 immune complexes.

3. Sex Hormones

The influence of sex hormones on the development of murine lupus varies by strain. As we mentioned earlier, castration and hormonal modulation are most influential in modifying the disease course of the BW model. Sex is not a significant factor in determination of survival in the MRL model; 90% of female mice are dead by 7.3 months, while in males this point is reached in 8.6 months. However, some effects can be seen also in the MRL strain. Dihydrotestosterone and testosterone caused a significant reduction in anti-DNA, proteinuria, and mortality in male and female MRL mice, although lymphadenopathy developed in most (Steinberg *et al.*, 1980). Additional factors besides the *lpr* gene are instrumental in the mediation of susceptibility to sex hormones; background genes also play an important role. C57Bl/6-lpr female mice show significantly higher autoantibody levels than males of this strain, while in the C3H-lpr, no such difference exists (Warren *et al.*, 1984).

E. Summary

The MRL-lpr/lpr mouse is an important model in the study of lupus, and serves as a unique prototype for research concerning T-cell dysfunction and autoimmune disease. The link between a single gene abnormality and the autoimmune phenotype also increases the value of this particular strain. Important features include lymphoproliferation and infiltration of lymphoid tissues by T cells of the double negative phenotype. Clinically, major manifestations are immune glomerulonephritis similar to that of the BW, and massive enlargement of the lymph nodes and spleen. Another attractive clinical characteristic of the MRL strain, although not universally present, is rheumatoid arthritis-like manifestations, with production of rheumatoid factor. Parallels to human disease include lymphadenopathy and kidney disease, and specific anti-Sm and anti-ribosomal P antibody production, together with the anti-DNA response.

IV. Quantitation

Precise quantitation of the disease process in the various murine lupus strains serves several functions. Its primary importance of course is to enable the researcher to statistically compare groups of animals in assessing the benefits of any particular mode of experimental therapy. Other uses may be for the development of new strains (when cross breeding two known strains), for accurate follow-up of disease progression, and for a precise indication as to the clinicopathological stage of the sick mouse at any given time. Indeed, several attempts have been made in recent years to also quantitate human disease through the use of various scoring systems (Austin *et al.*, 1983; Petri *et al.*, 1992).

We are not aware of any one system composed of all the possible serological, chemical, clinical, and pathological parameters able to provide a global score for the activity of murine lupus. Rather, researchers usually have used scoring systems for single organ systems in which pathology is characteristic (e.g., kidney) or in which the focus of interest resided in that particular study. The grading is mostly semiquantitative, ranging from 0 to 1+ (absent to mild pathology) to 3+ to 4+ (severe involvement). For purposes of simplicity, we discuss the representative scoring systems used, according to organ pathology. The general features commonly reported include animal survival in days or weeks, cumulative survival until a certain date, median survival, and weight.

A. Grading Systems in Murine SLE

1. Laboratory Assessment

The serological, biochemical, hematological, and immunological disturbances present in murine lupus are protean, as is the case in the human counterpart. Actually, most of the unique features discussed earlier in the description of the disease have been used to follow its appearance and progression. They are summarized here.

    a. Autoantibodies.   Anti-ssDNA, anti-dsDNA, poly I, poly (dT) anti-Sm, anti-RNP, anti-SS-A (Ro), anti SS-B (La), anticardiolipin (Mendlovic *et al.*, 1988), IgM rheumatoid factor (Berden *et al.*, 1983), and positivity on Coombs test (Hahn *et al.*, 1973).

b. Hematological. Anemia, leukopenia, thrombocytopenia, increased sedimentation rate (Mendlovic *et al.*, 1988; Berden *et al.*, 1983).

c. Immunological. IgA, IgM, IgG 1, IgG 2a, IgG 2b, gp 70, percent immunoglobulin-bound gp 70, circulating immune complexes, serum complement hemolytic activity (CH_{50}), T-cell count, reverse passive Arthus reaction positivity with age (Wofsy *et al.*, 1985; Berden *et al.*, 1983).

2. Kidney

The organ most clearly and severely affected in the various models of murine SLE is the kidney. Grading in this organ is also relatively simple, and can be done by clinical, histological, or laboratory parameters. Therefore, there is a relative abundance of scoring systems to choose from in evaluating lupus nephritis in the mouse. Serum and urine values of importance are urine and plasma albumin, urine and plasma creatinine, and the creatinine clearance test (Bruijn *et al.*, 1988). Proteinuria can be directly measured, or colorimetrically estimated by the following dipstick system (Wofsy *et al.*, 1985): trace, 10 mg/dl; 1+ proteinuria, 30 mg/dl; 2+, 100 mg/dl; 3+, 300 mg/dl; and 4+, 1000 mg/dl. Similarly, the number of animals dying from renal disease can be stated (defined by death with a blood urea nitrogen above 20 mg/100 ml, or those with significant proteinuria, >+2).

The following pathological grading systems for kidney involvement have been used in murine lupus studies over the years:

a. Prickett et al. (1983). 0, normal; 1+, focal glomerular proliferation; 2+, diffuse glomerular proliferation; 3+, focal necrosis within the glomeruli, and 4 I, totally hyalinized glomeruli.

b. Berden et al. (1983). 0, normal; 1+, minimal thickening of the mesangium; 2+, noticeable thickening of the mesangium and glomerular swelling; 3+, as above, with superimposed inflammatory exudates and capsular adhesions; and 4+, obliteration of glomerular architecture of >70%, with extensive tubular cast formation.

c. Naparslek et al. (1990). 1+, mild glomerulonephritis, slight hypercellularity; 2+, moderate glomerulonephritis—glomeruli are hypercellular with focal changes, with foci of necrosis or crescents; 3+, diffuse changes with crescents and necrosis, some glomeruli completely destroyed or fibrotic.

d. Hurd et al. (1981). Separate scores of 0 to 4+ are given for each category of (1) glomerular cellularity, (2) amount of mesangial matrix, (3) size of epithelial crescents, (4) amount of interstitial infiltrate, and (5) fibrinoid and wire loops. These scores are added to give a composite score. The percentage of glomerular hyalinization is also given.

e. Hahn et al. (1973). 0, no abnormalities; 1+, most glomeruli normal, some abnormal with mesangial thickening, focal hypercellularity, and occasional wire loop changes, tubules are normal; 2+, majority of glomeruli abnormal, early tubular damage present; 3+, all glomeruli abnormal, some virtually replaced by fibrinoid material; marked tubular damage present, with chronic parenchymal inflammatory cell infiltration.

The intensity of fluorescent glomerular staining has also been graded on a 0 to 3+ scale, according to the immunoglobulin present (IgG or IgM) (Wofsy *et al.*, 1985).

3. Vascular Lesions

The two main types of vascular disease observed in murine lupus strains are degenerative vascular disease (*DVD) (including myocardial infarction) and necrotizing polyarteritis (*NPA). Berden *et al.* (1983) suggested the following system for both types of lesions:

a. DVD. Based upon the histological examination of four consecutive heart sections: 0, normal; 1+, minimal PAS-positive deposits along and within one coronary vessel wall; 2+, PAS-positive deposits causing narrowing in two or three coronary vessels; and 3+, deposits in three or more vessels.

b. NPA. A 0–3 system, corresponding to the number of affected small- to medium-sized muscular arteries and number of parenchymal organs involved (includes only vessels with necrotizing or exudative lesions of the intima and media): 0+, normal; 1+, one organ; 2+, three vessels in two organs; 3+, vascular involvement of more than three organs.

Berden *et al.* (1983) also classified the myocardial infarctions on a 1–3 scale, depending on the total depth of myocardial necrosis: grade 1, 1–2 mm; grade 2, 2–3 mm; and grade 3, >3 mm, often transmural. Another classification system for myocardial involvement was used by Yoshida *et al.* (1987), who tabulated: (1) number of animals with myocardial infarctions, (2) ratio of infarct area to total tissue area in different heart regions (e.g., right ventricular free wall, ventricular septum, etc.), (3) coronary arteries: percentage of significant stenoses, and (4) the histological stage (acute, chronic) of the lesions.

Immunofluoroscence in the coronary arteries can also be assessed on a 0 to 3+ system, grading IgA, IgM, IgG1, IgG2, IgG3, and gp 70 fluorescence (Berden *et al.*, 1983).

4. Lymphadenopathy

Lymph node hyperplasia is an important feature of certain lupus strains, particularly in the MRL model discussed above. Lymph node size, according to Wofsy *et al.* (1985), is ranked by: 0, no detectable lymphadenopathy; 1+, mild submandibular lymphadenopathy only; 2+, moderate submandibular lymphadenopathy; 3+, submandibular and one other palpable lymph node; and 4+, diffuse lymphadenopathy. This method is applicable even during life. After the animals are sacrificed, spleen, inguinal, and axillary lymph node weight and dimensions can be recorded (Moscovitch *et al.*, 1983).

5. Arthritis

MRL mice can be affected by a disease very similar to human rheumatoid arthritis. However, the disease might be hard to assess clinically and may only be evident on histological examination. The small size of the mouse joint may also contribute to difficulty in evaluation. A possible clinical scoring system can be applied from the mouse collagen arthritis model. Criteria of swelling, erythema, and deformities were recorded for the ankle and knee joints (Kamiya *et al.*, 1993). In this system, the grading is: 0, absence of arthritis; 1, swelling and erythema in a single joint; 2, swelling and erythema in more than one joint; and 3, severe swelling of the entire foot, or ankylosis. The sum of all four paws was calculated as an arthritis index, with a maximum possible score of 12/mouse. A score of 6–8 represents severe arthritis. A simpler clinical scoring system was proposed by Tarkowski *et al.* (1986). Here, only hind joint arthropathy is graded, with 0, normal; 1–3, slight to pronounced synovial proliferation and hyperplasia with occasional pannus formation and bone destruction.

Radiographic evaluation of the joints can be carried out after the animals are sacrificed (Nakamura *et al.*, 1991). According to a similar method of Nakagawa *et al.* (1993), osteoarthritic changes in the ankle joints and tarsal bones were graded from 0 to 2+. The grading was 0, no detectable osteoarthritic change; 1+, moderate changes such as joint erosion or narrowing of joint spaces; and 2+, severe osteoarthritic change such as ankylosis. Ossification of extraarticular regions was also scored on a 0 to 2+ scale.

6. Sjögren Syndrome

Sjögren syndrome appears in several different strains of autoimmune lupic mice, and is manifested by different grades of conjunctival inflammation, with cellular infiltration in lacrimal and salivary glands. Hoffman *et al.* (1984) proposed the following classification for Sjögren-like manifestations: Conjunctival inflammation on serial sections of ocular tissue was graded on a scale of 0–3: 0, normal; 1, minimal inflammation; 2, intermediate inflammation; and 3, diffuse infiltration of tissue with inflammatory cells. Lacrimal and salivary gland inflammation was given the same scoring system according to: 0, normal; 1, focal infiltration with mononuclear cells; 2, one-fourth of the gland replaced by mononuclear cells; 3, one-third of the gland replaced by mononuclear cells; 4, more than half of the gland replaced by mononuclear cells. A different system for grading the degree of sialadenitis has been suggested by Jonsson *et al.* (1988). This procedure involves enumerating the number of foci of inflammatory cell infiltrates consisting of at least 50 mononuclear cells per square millimeter of sections from salivary gland tissue. In addition to this scoring, the diameter of a random sample of focal infiltrates was measured. An inflammation index was then constructed, based on the area of infiltration by mononuclear cells related to total glandular area.

V. Conclusions

There is a striking similarity between human SLE and the murine models of the disease discussed here. Both MRL/l and the BW mice develop a chronic spontaneous autoimmune disease involving multiple systems, together with the appearance of hyperglobulinemia and anti-DNA antibodies—all features typical of the human disease.

Some properties of human SLE, such as its preponderance in females, are better represented in the BW model. On the other hand, other characteristics (polyarthritis, anti-SM antibodies) are unique, and are found only in the lpr model. In that aspect, neither animal strain seems distinctly superior as the "best" model for human disease. Moreover, although the clinical and pathological findings in the MRL/l and BW disease models are similar and have a lot in common with their human counterpart, the etiology and pathogenesis of the disease in the two strains of mice are clearly different. This indicates that distinct and differing mechanisms may lead to the common clinical syndrome of SLE in mice.

Human SLE is characterized by a wide variety of clinical manifestations and serological findings. Whether human SLE is a single disease entity or a syndrome representing the end result of different pathogenic mechanisms remains to be clarified. Thus, although murine models of SLE are invaluable in studying narrowly defined segments of the illness, the exact contribution of any of these models to the full understanding of the etiology and pathogenesis of human disease is as yet unclear.

Acknowledgment

Yaakov Naparstek is the incumbent of the Leifferman Chair in Rheumatology. This work was supported in part by the Gablinger Fund for Research in Autoimmunity, and the U.J.A., Canada branch.

References

Abdelmoula, M., Spertini, F., Shibata, T., et al. (1989). J. Immunol. 143, 526–532.
Accinni, L., and Dixon, F. J. (1979). Am. J. Pathol. 96, 477–486.

Akizuki, M., Reeves, J. P., Steinberg, A. D., *et al.* (1978). *Clin. Immunol. Immunopathol.* **10**, 247–250.

Allen, R. D., Marshall, J. D., Roths, J. B., *et al.* (1990). *J. Exp. Med.* **172**, 1367–1375.

Altman, A., Theofilopoulos, A. N., Weiner, R., *et al.* (1981). *J. Exp. Med.* **154**, 791–808.

Andreu-Sánchez, J. L., Moreno de Alboran, I. M., Marcos, M. A., Sanchez-Movilla, A., Martinez, A.-C., and Kroemer, G. (1991). Interleukin 2 abrogates the non-responsive state of T cells expressing a forbidden T cell repertoire and induces autoimmune disease in neonatally thymectomized mice. *J. Exp. Med.* **173**, 1323–1329.

Andrews, B. S., Eisenberg, R. S., Theofilopoulos, A. N., *et al.* (1978). *J. Exp. Med.* **148**, 1198–1215.

Austin, H. A., Muenz, L. R., Joyce, K. M., *et al.* (1983). *Am. J. Med.* **75**, 382–391.

Bach, J. F., Dardenne, M., and Salomon, J. C. (1973). *Clin. Exp. Immunol.* **14**, 247–256.

Behar, S. M., and Scharff, M. D. (1988). *Proc. Natl. Acad. Sci. USA* **85**, 3970–3974.

Bellon, B., Manheimer-Lory, A., Monestier, M., *et al.* (1987). *J. Clin. Invest.* **79**, 1044–1053.

Berden, J. H. M., Hang, L. M., McConahey, P. J., *et al.* (1983). *J. Immunol.* **130**, 1699–1705.

Bielschowsky, M., and Goodall, C. M. (1970). *Cancer Res.* **30**, 834–835.

Bonfa, E., Marshak-Rothstein, A., Weissbach, H., *et al.* (1988). *J. Immunol.* **140**, 3434–3437.

Boswell, J. M., Yui, M. A., Burt, D. W., *et al.* (1988a). *J. Immunol.* **141**, 3050–3054.

Boswell, J. M., Yui, M. A., Endres, S., *et al.* (1988b). *J. Immunol.* **141**, 118–124.

Bruijn, J. A., Van Elven, E. H., Hogendoorn, P. C. W., *et al.* (1988). *Am. J. Pathol.* **130**, 639–641.

Budd, R. C., Schreyer, M., Miescher, G. C., *et al.* (1987). *J. Immunol.* **139**, 2200–2210.

Carteron, N. L., Wofsy, D., Schimenti, C., and Ermak, T. H. (1990). F(ab')2 anti-CD4 and intact anti-CD4 monoclonal antibodies inhibit the accumulation of CD4$^+$ T cells, CD8$^+$ T cells, and B cells in the kidneys of lupus-prone NZB/NZW mice. *Clin. Immunol. Immunopathol.* **56**, 373–383.

Cohen, P. L., and Eisenberg, R. A. (1991). *Ann. Rev. Immunol.* **9**, 243–269.

Crieghton, W. D., Katz, D. H., and Dixon, F. J. (1979). *J. Immunol.* **123**, 2627–2636.

Dang, H., and Herbeck, R. J. (1984). *Clin. Immunol. Immunopathol.* **30**, 265–278.

Dauphinee, M. S., Kipper, S. B., and Wofsy, D. (1981). *J. Immunol.* **127**, 2483–2487.

Davidson, A., Shefner, R., Livneh, A., *et al.* (1987). *Ann. Rev. Immunol.* **5**, 85–108.

Davignon, J. L., Kimoto, M., Kindler, V., *et al.* (1988). *Eur. J. Immunol.* **18**, 1367–1372.

Diamond, B., and Scharff, M. D. (1984). *Proc. Natl. Acad. Sci. USA* **81**, 5841–5844.

Dixon, F. J. (1981). *Immunol. Today* **2**, 145–146.

Ebling, F. M., and Hahn, B. H. (1980). *Arthr. Rheum.* **23**, 392–403.

Eilat, D. (1990). *Mol. Immunol.* **27**, 203–210.

Eilat, D., Schecter, A. N., and Steinberg, A. D. (1976). *Nature* **259**, 141–143.

Eilat, D., Ben Sasson, S. A., and Laskov, R. (1980). *Eur. J. Immunol.* **10**, 841–845.

Eilat, D., Webster, D. M., and Rees, A. R. (1988). *J. Immunol.* **141**, 1745–1753.

Eisenberg, R. A., Tan, E. M., and Dixon, F. J. (1978). *J. Exp. Med.* **147**, 582–587.

Elkon, K. B., Bonfa, E., Llovet, R., *et al.* (1989). *J. Immunol.* **143**, 1549–1554.

Gioud, M., Kotzin, B. L., Rubin, R. L., *et al.* (1983). *J. Immunol.* **131**, 269–274.

Gregory, C. D., Dive, C., Henderson, S., *et al.* (1990). *Nature* **349**, 612–614.

Hahn, B. H. (1987). *In* "Dubois' Lupus Erythematosus" (D. J. Wallace and E. L. Dubios, Eds.), 3rd edition, pp. 130–157. Lea & Febiger, Philadelphia.

Hahn, B. H., and Ebling, F. M. (1987). *J. Immunol.* **138**, 2110–2117.

Hahn, B. H., Bagby, M. K., Hamilton, T. R., *et al.* (1973). *Arthr. Rheum.* **16**, 163–170.

Hahn, B. H., Knotts, L., Mary, N. G., *et al.* (1975). *Arthr. Rheum.* **18**, 145–148.

Hang, L. M., Theofilopoulos, A. N., and Dixon, F. J. (1982). *J. Exp. Med.* **155**, 1690–1701.

Hardin, J., and Thomas, J. O. (1983). *Proc. Natl. Acad. Sci. USA* **80**, 7410–7414.

Heyler, B. J., and Howie, J. B. (1963). *Nature* **197**, 197.

Hoffman, R. W., Yang, H. K., Waggie, K. S., *et al.* (1983). *Arthr. Rheum.* **26**, 645–652.

Hoffman, R. W., Alspaugh, M. A., Waggie, K. S., *et al.* (1984). *Arthr. Rheum.* **27**, 157–165.

Hom, J. T., Cole, H., and Bendele, A. M. (1990). *Clin. Immunol. Immunopathol.* **55**, 109–119.
Howie, J. B., and Heyler, B. J. (1968). *Adv. Immunol.* **9**, 215–266.
Hurd, E. R., Johnston, J. M., Okita, J. R., *et al.* (1981). *J. Clin. Invest.* **67**, 476–485.
Igarashi, S., Takiguchi, M., Kariyone, A., *et al.* (1988). *Int. Arch. Allergy Appl. Immunol.* **86**, 249–255.
Izui, S., Kelly, V. E., McConahey, P. J., *et al.* (1980). *J. Exp. Med.* **152**, 1645–1658.
Izui, S., Kelly, V. E., Masuda, K., *et al.* (1984). *J. Immunol.* **133**, 227–233.
Jachez, B., Montecino-Rodriguez, E., Fonteneau, P., *et al.* (1988). *Immunology* **64**, 31–36.
Jacob, C. O. and McDevitt, H. O. (1988). Tumoui necrosis factor-alpha in murine autoimmune lupus nephritis. *Nature* **331**, 356–358.
Jonsson, R., Tarkowski, A., and Backman, K. (1988). *Agents Actions* **25**, 368–374.
Kakkanaiah, V. N., Nagarkatti, M., and Nagarkatti, P. S. (1990). *Cell. Immunol.* **127**, 442–457.
Kamiya, M., Sohen, S., Yamane, T., *et al.* (1993). *J. Rheumatol.* **20**, 225–230.
Kastner, D. L., McIntyre, T. M., Mallett, C. P., *et al.* (1989). *J. Immunol.* **143**, 2761–2767.
Kelly, V. E., Winkelstein, A., Izui, S., *et al.* (1981). *Clin. Immunol. Immunopathol.* **21**, 190–203.
Kincade, P. W., Jyonouchi, H., Landreth, K. S., *et al.* (1982). *Immunol. Rev.* **64**, 81–98.
Klinman, D. M., Ishigatsubo, Y., and Steinberg, A. D. (1988). *J. Immunol.* **141**, 801–806.
Klinman, D. M., Eisenberg, R. A., and Steinberg, A. D. (1990). *J. Immunol.* **144**, 506–511.
Komisar, J. L., Leung, K. Y., Crawley, R. R., *et al.* (1989). *J. Immunol.* **143**, 340–347.
Kotzin, B. L., Babcock, S. K., and Heron, L. R. (1988). *J. Exp. Med.* **168**, 2221–2229.
Krakauer, R. S., Waldman, T. A., and Storber, W. (1976). *J. Exp. Med.* **144**, 662–673.
Krakauer, R. S., Strober, W., Rippeon, D. L., *et al.* (1977). *Science* **196**, 56–59.
Krieg, A. M. (1991). *In* Steinberg, A. D., moderator: Systemic lupus erythematosus. *Ann. Intern. Med.* **115**, 548–559.
Krieg, A. M., and Steinberg, A. D. (1990a). *J. Autoimmun.* **3**, 137–166.
Krieg, A. M., and Steinberg, A. D. (1990b). *J. Clin. Invest.* **86**, 806–816.
Krieg, A. M., Gause, W. C., Gourley, M. F., *et al.* (1989). *J. Immunol.* **143**, 2448–2451.
Lambert, P. H., and Dixon, F. J. (1968). *J. Exp. Med.* **127**, 507–521.
Levy, J. A. (1973). *Science* **182**, 1151–1153.
Levy, J. A., and Pincus, T. (1970). *Science* **170**, 326–327.
Magilavy, D. B., and Rothstein, J. L. (1988). *J. Exp. Med.* **168**, 789–794.
Manolios, N., and Schrieber, L. (1986). *Aus. N.Z. J. Med.* **16**, 729–743.
Manolios, N., Schrieber, L., Nelson, M., *et al.* (1989). *Clin. Exp. Immunol.* **76**, 301–306.
Matsuzawa, A., Moriyama, T., Kaneko, T., *et al.* (1990). *J. Exp. Med.* **171**, 519–531.
Mellors, R. C., and Huang, C. Y. (1967). *J. Exp. Med.* **126**, 53–62.
Mellors, R. C., Aoki, T., and Heubner, R. J. (1969). *J. Exp. Med.* **129**, 1045–1062.
Mendlovic, S., Brocke, S., Shoenfeld, Y., *et al.* (1988). *Proc. Natl. Acad. Sci. USA* **85**, 2260–2264.
Milich, D. R., and Gershwin, M. E. (1980). *Semin. Arthritis Rheum.* **10**, 111–147.
Mosbach-Ozmen, L., Fonteneau, P., and Loor, F. (1985). *Thymus* **7**, 233–245.
Moscovitch, M., Rosenmann, E., Neeman, Z., *et al.* (1983). *Exp. Mol. Pathol.* **38**, 33–47.
Mountz, J. D., Smith, T. M., and Toth, K. S. (1990). *J. Immunol.* **144**, 2159–2166.
Murphy, E. D., and Roths, J. B. (1977). *In* "Topics in Hematology: Proceedings of the 16th International Congress in Hematology" (S. Seno, F. Takaku, and S. Irino, Eds.), pp. 69–72. Excerpta Medica, Amsterdam, Holland.
Nakamura, K., Kashiwazaki, S., Takagishi, K., *et al.* (1991). *Arthr. Rheum.* **34**, 171–177.
Nakagawa, T., Nagata, N., Hosaka, N., *et al.* (1993). *Arthr. Rheum.* **36**, 263–268.
Naparstek, Y., Andre-Schartz, J., Manser, T., *et al.* (1986). *J. Exp. Med.* **164**, 614–626.
Naparstek, Y., Baur, K., Reis, M. D., *et al.* (1988). *J. Mol. Cell. Immunol.* **4**, 35–43.
Naparstek, Y., Ben-Yehuda, A., Madaio, M. P., *et al.* (1990). *Arthr. Rheum.* **33**, 1554–1559.
Norton, J. I., Siegel, B. V., and Moore, R. D. (1975). *Transplantation* **19**, 464–469.

Palacios, R. (1984). *Eur. J. Immunol.* **14**, 599–605.
Pansky, B., and Freimer, E. H. (1974). *Arthr. Rheum.* **17**, 403–408.
Petri, M., Hellman, D., and Hochberg, M. (1992). *J. Rheumatol.* **19**, 53–59.
Pisetsky, D. S., McCarty, G. A., and Peters, D. V. (1980). *J. Exp. Med.* **152**, 1302–1310.
Pisetsky, D. S., Klatt, C., Dawson, D., *et al.* (1985). *Clin. Immunol. Immunopathol.* **37**, 369–376.
Prickett, J. D., Robinson, D. R., and Steinberg, A. D. (1983). *Arthr. Rheum.* **26**, 133–139.
Prudhomme, G. J., Park, C. L., Fieser, T. M., *et al.* (1983). *J. Exp. Med.* **157**, 730–742.
Rauch, J., Murphy, E., Roths, J. B., *et al.* (1982). *J. Immunol.* **129**, 236–241.
Raveche, E. S., Steinberg, A. D., DeFranco, A. L., *et al.* (1982). *J. Immunol.* **129**, 1219–1226.
Rosenberg, Y. J., Goldsmith, P. K., Ohara, J., *et al.* (1986). *Ann. N.Y. Acad. Sci.* **475**, 251–266.
Roths, J. B., Murphy, E. D., Eichler, E. M., *et al.* (1984). *J. Exp. Med.* **159**, 1–20.
Roubinian, J. R., Talal, N., Greenspan, J. S., *et al.* (1978). *J. Exp. Med.* **147**, 1568–1583.
Roubinian, J., Talal, N., Siiteri, P. K., *et al.* (1979). *Arthr. Rheum.* **22**, 1162–1169.
Santoro, T. J., Portanova, J. P., and Kotzin, B. L. (1988). *J. Exp. Med.* **167**, 1713–1718.
Scher, I. (1982). *Immunol. Rev.* **64**, 117–136.
Seldin, M. F., Morse, H. C., III, Reeves, J. P., *et al.* (1988). *J. Exp. Med.* **167**, 688–693.
Shirai, T., and Mellors, R. C. (1972). *Clin. Exp. Immunol.* **12**, 133–152.
Shirai, T., Abe, M., Yagita, H., *et al.* (1990). *J. Immunol.* **144**, 3756–3761.
Shlomchik, M. J., Marshak-Rothstein, A., Wolfowicz, C. B., *et al.* (1987). *Nature* **328**, 805–811.
Shlomchik, M., Mascelli, M., Shan, H., *et al.* (1990). *J. Exp. Med.* **171**, 265–297.
Singer, P. A., and Theofilopoulos, A. N. (1990). *Immunol. Rev.* **118**, 103–127.
Singer, P. A., Balderas, R. S., McEvilly, R. J., *et al.* (1989). *J. Exp. Med.* **170**, 1869–1877.
Slack, J. H., Hang, L. M., Barkley, J., *et al.* (1984). *J. Immunol.* **132**, 1271–1275.
Smith, H. R., and Steinberg, A. D. (1983). *Ann. Rev. Immunol.* **1**, 175–210.
Steinberg, A. D. (1984). *Ann. Intern. Med.* **100**, 714–727.
Steinberg, A. D., Law, L. W., and Talal, N. (1970). *Arthr. Rheum.* **13**, 369–377.
Steinberg, A. D., Roths, J. B., Murphy, E. D., *et al.* (1980). *J. Immunol.* **125**, 871–875.
Steinberg, B. J., Smather, P. A., Fredrikson, K., *et al.* (1982). *J. Clin. Invest.* **70**, 587–597.
Steinberg, A. D. (1992). *Clin. Immunol. Immunopathol.* **63**, 19–22.
Steward, M. W., and Hay, F. C. (1976). *Clin. Exp. Immunol.* **26**, 363–370.
Tarkowski, A., Gunnarsson, L. A., Nilsson, L. A., *et al.* (1986). *Arthr. Rheum.* **29**, 1405–1409.
Theofilopoulos, A. N., and Dixon, F. J. (1981). *Immunol. Rev.* **55**, 179–216.
Theofilopoulos, A. N., and Dixon, F. J. (1985). *Adv. Immunol.* **37**, 269–390.
Theofilopoulos, A. N., Shawler, D. J., Eisenberg, R. A., *et al.* (1980). *J. Exp. Med.* **151**, 446–466.
Theofilopoulos, A. N., Balderos, R. S., Hang, L. M., *et al.* (1983). *J. Exp. Med.* **158**, 901–919.
Theofilopoulos, A. N., Kofler, R., Singer, P. A., *et al.* (1989a). *Adv. Immunol.* **46**, 61–109.
Theofilopoulos, A. N., Singer, P. A., Kofler, R., *et al.* (1989b). *Springer Semin. Immunopathol.* **11**, 335–368.
Tonietti, G., Oldstone, M. B. A., and Dixon, F. J. (1970). *J. Exp. Med.* **132**, 89–109.
Wantanabe-Fukunaga, F., Brannan, C. I., Copeland, N. D., *et al.* (1992). *Nature* **356**, 314–317.
Warren, R. W., Caster, S. A., Roths, J. B., *et al.* (1984). *Clin. Immunol. Immunopathol.* **31**, 65–77.
Wofsy, D., Ledbetter, J. A., Hendler, P. L., *et al.* (1985). *J. Immunol.* **134**, 852–857.
Woods, J. I., Jr., and Zvaifler, N. J. (1989). *In* "Textbook of Rheumatology" (E. N. Kelly, Ed.), pp. 1077–1100. WB Saunders, Philadelphia.
Yoshida, H., Fujiwara, H., Fujiwara, T., *et al.* (1987). *Am. J. Pathol.* **129**, 477–485.

Chapter 15

Experimental Systemic Lupus Erythematosus: Role of the Idiotypic Network

Edna Mozes[1] and Yehuda Shoenfeld[2]

[1]Department of Chemical Immunology, The Weizmann Institute of Science, Rehovot 76100 Israel

[2]Research Unit of Autoimmune Diseases, Department of Medicine 'B', Sheba Medical Center, Sackler Faculty of Medicine, Tel-Aviv University, Tel-Hashomer 52621, Israel

I. History of the Model

Systemic lupus erythematosus (SLE) is a multisystem disease involving among other organs, the kidneys, brain, synovial membrane, skin, and joints. The serological markers of the disease are the anti-DNA antibodies, but it is characterized by more than 50 other autoantibodies (Isenberg *et al.*, 1984b). So far, SLE has been reported only in mouse strains prone to this disease (Shoenfeld, 1989). The characteristics of these spontaneously developing mouse strains are summarized in Table I.

Table I

Selected Features of Systemic Lupus Erythematosus-Prone Mouse Strains[a]

Strain	Haplotype	Mean life span (months)	Major clinical features	Autoantibodies	Other immunological abnormalities
NZB	$H-2^d$	15–18	Hemolytic anemia, glomerulonephritis, lymphomas, pulmonary infiltrates	Anti-DNA, cryoglobulins, rheumatoid factor	Thymic atrophy, IgM and IgG overproduction
(NZB/NZW)F$_1^b$	$H-d^{d/z}$	7–9	Severe glomerulonephritis, pulmonary infiltrates	Anti-DNA, rheumatoid factor	Thymic atrophy, IgM and IgG overproduction
MRL-lpr/lpr^b	$H-2^k$	3–5	Glomerulonephritis, vasculitis, arthritis, myocardial infracts	Anti-DNA, anti-Sm, rheumatoid factor (high titer), cryoglobulins	Thymic atrophy, IgM and IgG overproduction lymphoid hyperplasia
BXSB^c	$H-2^b$	4–6	Glomerulonephritis, myocardial infracts, hemolytic anemia	Anti-DNA, antierythrocyte	Thymic atrophy, IgM and IgG overproduction lymphoid hyperplasia
Motheaten	$H-2^b$	1	Pulmonary infiltrate, hair loss, mild glomerulonephritis	Anti-DNA, antierythrocyte, rheumatoid factor	Thymic atrophy, IgM and IgG overproduction, general immunosuppression leading to infections
Palmerston-North	$H-2^q$	10–12	Polyarteritis nodosa, glomerulonephritis	Anti-DNA	IgM and IgG overproduction
Swan	$H-2^k$	18	Mild glomerulonephritis	Anti-DNA	Early thymic atrophy

[a] From Shoenfeld and Isenberg (1988). The Mosaic of Autoimmunity, Elsevier, The Netherlands, 1989; with permission.
[b] Female.
[c] Male.

Until 1988 the only induced SLE model was graft-versus-host (GVH)-induced SLE. SLE-GVH disease is not associated with exacerbations or remissions, and there are no sex predilections (Portanova *et al.*, 1988; Bruijn *et al.*, 1988).

A. Induction by the 16/6 Idiotype of Anti-DNA Antibodies

The human monoclonal immunoglobulin M (IgM) anti-DNA antibody 16/6 was generated by the hybridoma technique from a patient with cold agglutinin disease who also had anti-DNA antibodies (Shoenfeld *et al.*, 1982; Shoenfeld *et al.*, 1983). The 16/6 idiotype (Id) was found to be a cross-reactive Id of anti-DNA antibodies (Shoenfeld *et al.*, 1983a) and to appear in many diseases, including infectious ones (Shoenfeld *et al.*, 1992; Konikoff *et al.*, 1987; El-Roeiy *et al.*, 1987; Sela *et al.*, 1987). However, the titers of the 16/6 Id in the serum of SLE patients was found to correlate with disease activity (Isenberg *et al.*, 1984a) and the Id could be detected in affected organs of patients with SLE, for example, skin, kidneys, and brain (Isenberg *et al.*, 1985a,b).

Since the idiotypic network was shown to play a role in regulating immune responses (Jerne, 1974) it has been suggested that idiotypic-anti-idiotypic antibodies may be involved in the induction and progression of autoimmunity (Bona, 1981). Based on the above, the 16/6 Id appeared to be a good candidate for attempts to induce experimental SLE.

In 1988 Mendlovic *et al.* immunized C3H.SW mice in the hind footpads with 1 μg of 16/6 Id emulsified in Freund's adjuvant and 3 weeks later boosted the mice with the same amount of the Id in phosphate-buffered saline (PBS). During the next 5 months of follow-up, the mice became sick, generating high titers of anti-DNA antibodies and 16/6 Id. The disease that evolved was subsequently characterized as experimental SLE (Mozes *et al.*, 1990; Shoenfeld *et al.*, 1990).

II. Animals and Housing

The disease can be induced in mice; however, experiments were not carried out to see whether it can be induced in other species too. The original mouse in which it was induced is the C3H.SW strain (Mendlovic *et al.*, 1988). Subsequently, it was found that the disease could be induced in other mouse strains, such as BALB/c, AKR, C3H/eB, DBA/2 and SJL. The following strains were found to be relatively resistant to SLE induction: C57BL/6, C3H/HeJ, and (BALB/c $\times$ C57BL/6)F_1 (Mendlovic *et al.*, 1990). When NZB/W F_1 mice (which are spontaneously prone to develop SLE) were immunized with the 16/6 Id, the regular parameters of their SLE appeared earlier and they died sooner than non-16/6 Id-immunized NZB/W F_1 mice (Mendlovic *et al.*, 1990). Recently a similar phenomenon was reported in rabbits (Rombach *et al.*, 1992).

A. Sex

The disease has a female predilection (Mendlovic *et al.*, 1988, 1990; Mozes *et al.*, 1990; Shoenfeld and Mozes, 1990). Sex hormones may significantly affect induction. The disease appears earlier (3 months) in females and orchiectomized males treated with estrogens (Blank *et al.*, 1990a). Testosterone-treated BALB/c females and orchiectomized males developed a classic response to the human anti-DNA antibody (16/6 Id^+), but failed to develop fulminant SLE-like disease (Blank *et al.*, 1990a).

This result was supported by treatment of mice in which experimental SLE induced with the estrogen antagonist tamoxifen had a beneficial effect on the clinical manifestations of the murine experimental SLE. This tamoxifen treatment prevented the hematological disturbances as well as the kidney damage that is typical for experimental SLE (Mozes *et al.*, 1992).

B. Age

Usually we have used 2- to 3-month-old mice (Mendlovic *et al.*, 1988, 1990; Blank *et al.*, 1990a,b). We have demonstrated that when experimental SLE was induced in aging mice (12–24 months old), the antibody responses were significantly lower and disease manifestations were milder than in the young mice (Tomer *et al.*, 1991; Segal *et al.*, 1992).

C. Conditions

The mice were housed in regular facilities and fed a normal mouse diet. No special preparations are required.

III. Genetic Background

In one study (Mendlovic *et al.*, 1990), we analyzed seven strains of mice (C3H.SW, C57BL/6, BALB/c, AKR, C3H/eB, C3H/He, and SJL). Two out of the seven strains failed to develop the disease (C57BL/6 and C3H/He). These two strains did not produce antibodies specific to the 16/6 Id, while the other five strains produced high titers of anti-16/6 Id antibodies. The anti-16/6 Id antibody response, followed by the induction of the disease, was found not to be linked to major histocompatibility complex (MHC) or an Ig heavy chain allotype (Mendlovic *et al.*, 1990). F_1 hybrids between a resistant strain and two of the susceptible mouse strains (BALB/c and SJL) were shown to be resistant. Thus, susceptibility is inherited as a recessive trait (Mendlovic *et al.*, 1990).

In an attempt to map the gene(s) responsible for the susceptibility to experimental SLE induction, we have followed 20 of the recombinant inbred B × D strains for autoantibody production and disease manifestations following immunization with the 16/6 Id. The parental strains of the latter are DBA/2 susceptible, and C57BL/6 resistant to the induction of experimental SLE. The recombinant inbred strains could be clearly separated into susceptible and resistant strains. Analysis of the results suggested that at least two genes mapping to chromosomes 7 and 14, respectively, control susceptibility to disease induction and development.

IV. Disease Induction

Classical induction involves immunization with 1 μg of anti-DNA antibody carrying the 16/6 Id (Mendlovic *et al.*, 1988). In the first injection, the antibody is emulsified with Freund's adjuvant (Difco, Detroit, Michigan). The boost given 3 weeks later has the same amount of antibody in PBS. Both injections should be carried out intradermally in the hind footpads.

The disease was also induced with the following agents:

1. Other anti-DNA antibodies carrying the 16/6 idiotype, for example:

SA-1—a human monoclonal anti-DNA antibody generated from a patient with polymyositis (Blank *et al.*, 1991a), carrying the 16/6 Id (Blank *et al.*, 1990c).

TB-68—a mouse monoclonal antituberculous glycolipid antibody having anti-DNA properties (Blank *et al.*, 1988) and carrying the 16/6 Id (Blank *et al.*, 1990c).

4B4—a human anti-Sm antibody, carrying the 16/6 Id (Blank *et al.*, 1990c).

Polylconal IgG anti-DNA—an antibody derived from a patient with active SLE and carrying the 16/6 Id (Tincani *et al.*, 1993).

Murine monoclonal 5G12-4—an anti-anti-16/6 Id (Ab3) monoclonal antibody found to bind to DNA and to harbor the 16/6 Id. The latter antibody could induce an experimental disease similar to that induced by the human monoclonal 16/6 Id (Mozes *et al.*, 1992; Waisman *et al.*, 1993).

2. A monoclonal murine anti-16/6 Id antibody, termed 1A3-2, was derived from C3H.SW mice immunized with the 16/6 Id. The murine monoclonal anti-16/6 Id was found to be more effective than the human monoclonal 16/6

Id in inducing experimental SLE, and caused an earlier onset of proteinuria and renal damage (Mendlovic *et al.*, 1989).

3. A monoclonal anti-La antibody (2D/2) was derived by the hybridoma technique from a mouse in which experimental SLE was induced by the 1A3-2 murine monoclonal anti-16/6 Id (Offen *et al.*, 1990). This monoclonal antibody was found to induce experimental SLE similar to the disease obtained by using the human or murine 16/6 Id monoclonal antibodies (Fricke *et al.*, 1989).

4. A monoclonal anticardiolipin antibody that binds to DNA as well (2C4C2) (16/6 Id negative) was derived from mice afflicted with experimental SLE following immunization with the murine monoclonal 1A3-3 anti-16/6 Id. Immunization with the monoclonal 2C4C2 anticardiolipin antibody led to an early onset of experimental SLE with antiphospholipid syndrome (Sthoeger *et al.*, 1993). (See Chapter).

5. A single transfusion of 5×10^6, 16/6 Id-specific, T-helper cell lines in PBS into the tail vein of the mouse led to the induction of experimental SLE with all the typical manifestations (Fricke *et al.*, 1991). The injection of a smaller number of cells led to delayed onset and reduced severity of symptoms of the disease. However, even injection of 10^4 cells per animal led to elevated titers of anti-16/6 Id, 16/6 Id, and anti-DNA antibodies (Fricke *et al.*, 1991).

6. A single transfusion of 1×10^7 T-helper cell lines specific against SA-1 (anti-DNA, 16/6 Id-positive human IgM) and tuberculin (TB)-68 (anti-DNA, 16/6 Id positive, antituberculous glycolipid, mouse IgG) (Blank *et al.*, 1991a) was used.

7. Immunization with MIV-7 (a human IgM monoclonal anti-DNA and anti-gp 52 of the mouse mammary tumor (MMT virus) (Blank *et al.*, 1991a) led to the induction of SLE with a secondary antiphospholipid syndrome (see Chapter) (Blank *et al.*, 1992b).

V. Course of the Disease

The disease usually appears after 4–5 months from the time of boost injections, although the serological markers (anti-16/6 Id antibodies, 16/6 Id, anti-DNA antibodies, etc.) are detected earlier (starting 1 week following the boost). It is characterized by three parameters:

A. Serology

Most mice will develop high titers of anti-16/6 Id antibodies, 16/6 Id, anti-single-stranded DNA, anti-Sm, anti-ribonucleoprotein (RNP), antihistones, anti-Ro, and anti-La, and anticardiolipin antibodies.

B. Clinical and Other Laboratory Findings

One can find an increased sedimentation rate (determined by diluting the heparinized blood in PBS at a ratio of 1:1. The diluted blood is then passed to a micro sampling pipet, and the sedimentation is measured 6 hr later). The mice develop various degrees of leukopenia (2000–4000 cells/mm^3) and thrombocytopenia (<600,000 platelets/mm^3). After 4–5 months the mice may develop proteinuria (measured by a semiquantitative method using a Combistix kit from Ames Co., Elkhart, Indiana). Some of the mice (about 5%) may develop paralysis after a long period (10–12 months) as an indication of central nervous system (CNS) involvement. The female mice suffer from low fecundity and may develop a secondary antiphospholipid syndrome. Some of the mice may develop alopecia (Tincani et al., 1993). (See Chapter).

Experimental SLE was found to be associated with dysregulation of cytokine secretion. Thus a significant increase is found in the levels of the inflammatory-related cytokines interleukin-1 (IL-1) and tumor necrosing factor (TNF) in the SLE-afflicted mice, and a decrease in the levels of IL-2 and IL-4 secreted (Mozes et al., 1990).

The neonatal lupus erythematosus (NLE) syndrome can be diagnosed in a high percentage of the offspring of SLE-afflicted BALB/c mothers. Electrocardiograms recorded from groups of neonates indicated defects in the conduction system, including first-, second-, and third-degree heart block, significant bradycardia, and a wide QRS complex compared with normal patterns observed in the offspring of healthy mothers (Kalush et al., 1992).

C. Histopathology

The 16/6 Id carrying immunoglobulin can be shown to be deposited in the mesangial cells in the kidneys (Mendlovic et al., 1988, 1989, 1990; Blank et al., 1990c, 1991a,b; Tomer et al., 1991; Bona, 1981; Segal et al., 1992; Sthoeger et al., 1993; Tincani et al., 1993; Fricke et al., 1989, 1991) by immunofluorescent and immunoperoxidase staining. Electron-dense deposits could also be shown (Mendlovic et al., 1988; Fricke et al., 1991; Blank et al., 1991a,b, 1992). Some of the glomeruli may develop sclerosis and atrophy (Mendlovic et al., 1988, 1990). Deposition of Ig was also detected in the epidermal–dermal junction of the skin (Tincani et al., 1993). The disease seems to be chronic without the classic relapses noted in human SLE.

VI. Resistance to the Disease

Susceptibility to disease induction is strain dependent but not MHC or Ig allotype linked (Mendlovic et al., 1990). Therefore, one should use the proper strain. Although environmental factors were claimed to be important in induction, the authors of the article (Isenberg *et al.*, 1991) did not strictly follow the protocol for induction, namely, employing a pathogenic antibody, using the proper concentration of antibody (1 μg/mouse), following the time schedule (boost 3 weeks after first immunization), and intradermal injection into the hind footpads. Indeed, in an experiment in which the mice were not immunized according to previous studies (Mendlovic *et al.*, 1988, 1990; Mozes *et al.*, 1990; Blank *et al.*, 1988, 1990a,b,c, 1991a,b, 1992; Tomer *et al.*, 1991; Shoenfeld *et al.*, 1986; Tincani *et al.*, 1993; Fricke *et al.*, 1989, 1991), the mice developed adjuvant arthritis (Isenberg *et al.*, 1992). Other laboratories have reported results similar to ours (Tincani *et al.*, 1993).

C3H/Hej mice were found to be resistant to disease induction by the human monoclonal 16/6 Id (Mendlovic *et al.*, 1990). However, the disease could be induced in these mice when the A3-2 murine monoclonal anti-16/6 Id (Ab 2) was utilized (Mendlovic *et al.*, 1989).

Furthermore, C57BL/6 mice are resistant to SLE induction by either the human 16/6 Id or the murine anti-16/6 Id. Nevertheless, the disease can be induced in these mice by administration of 5×10^6 cells of the C3H.SW (*H-2* matched), 16/6 Id-specific, T-cell line (Fricke *et al.*, 1991).

VII. Manipulation of the Disease

The disease was found to be affected by sex hormones (e.g., estrogen accelerated and androgen abrogated the induction of the disease; Blank *et al.*, 1990a) and drugs affecting estrogen and androgen (e.g., tamoxifen had a beneficial effect on the clinical manifestations of the disease; Mozes *et al.*, 1992; Sthoeger *et al.*, 1993). AS-101, a drug known to increase interleukin-2 production, when given to mice did not seem to affect either the induction of experimental SLE or the course of the disease (Blank *et al.*, 1990b).

T-suppressor (Ts) cells and clones specific for the 16/6 Id-carrying antibody, when infused into mice after 16/6 Id immunization, could abrogate the disease (Blank *et al.*, 1991b). Cyclosporin-A, a drug known to affect T-helper (Th) cell activity, when given early after disease induction, was able to completely inhibit the emergence of serological and clinical manifestations. However, given when the disease was already fully manifested, the drug was of no avail (Blank *et al.*, 1992a).

Treatment of mice with monoclonal anti-CD4 antibodies starting 1 week before immunization through a period of 18 weeks significantly reduced the autoantibody titers and prevented the development of clinical manifestations (Sthoeger *et al.*, 1993).

Infusion of mouse anti-16/6 Id antibody could also inhibit induction of disease. The binding of a cytotoxic agent showed an effect additive to the use of anti-16/6 antibody alone (Blank *et al.*, 1991).

VIII. Lessons

The new experimental SLE model is very similar to human SLE, yet it differs in several respects. It lacks the remission and exacerbation pattern of many patients with the disease. At the same time, the mice have all the types of autoantibodies found in different patients with SLE. Not all clinical manifestations of human SLE have been identified in the induced disease in the mouse (e.g., arthritis, pleuritis).

The model shows that (1) SLE can be induced by external immunization, and most mouse strains are susceptible without an MHC restriction; (2) Idiotypes of anti-DNA and other autoantibodies may be instrumental in SLE initiation; (3) Immunization with an antibody (or Id) in special conditions (intradermal, long follow-up) may lead to the production of the same antibody (Id) as the immunizing agent; (4) Both T-helper and T-suppressor cells play an important role in the pathogenesis of SLE; (5) Some treatments for SLE (e.g., cyclosporin A) should be employed at an early stage of disease induction, rather than when the immunological damage is already done; and (6) Susceptibility to disease induction and development is controlled by at least two genes, mapped to chromosomes 7 and 11, respectively.

Acknowledgment

We thank Ms. Shira Lancry for her excellent secretarial assistance.

References

Avinoach, I., Amital-Teplizki, H., Kuperman, O., Isenberg, D. A., and Shoenfeld, Y. (1990). *Isr. J. Med. Sci.* **26**, 367–373.

Blank, M., Mendlovic, S., Mozes, E., and Shoenfeld, Y. (1988).*J. Autoimmun.* **1**, 683–691.

Blank, M., Mendlovic, S., Fricke, H., Mozes, E., Talal, N., and Shoenfeld, Y. (1990a).*J. Rheumatol.* **17**, 311–317.

Blank, M., Sredni, B., Albeck, M., Mozes, E., and Shoenfeld, Y. (1990b). *Clin. Exp. Immunol.* **79**, 443–447.

Blank, M., Krup, M., Mendlovic, S., Fricke, H., Mozes, E., Talal, N., Coates, A. R. M., and Shoenfeld, Y. (1990c). *Scand.J. Immunol.* **31**, 45–52.

Blank, M., Mendlovic, S., Mozes, E., Coates, A. R. M., and Shoenfeld, Y. (1991a). *Clin. Immunol. Immunopathol.* **60**, 471–483.

Blank, M., Ben-Bassat, M., and Shoenfeld, Y. (1991b). *Cell. Immunol.* **137**, 474–486.

Blank, M., Monsoagi,J., and Shoenfeld, Y. (1994). *Clin. Exp. Immunol.* (in press).

Blank, M., Smorodinsky, N. I., Keydar, I., Chaitchik, S., and Shoenfeld, Y. (1991c). *Immunol. Lett.* **28**, 65–72.

Blank, M., Ben-Bassat, M., and Shoenfeld, Y. (1992a). *Arthr. Rheum.* **35**, 1350–1354.

Blank, M., Krause, I., Ben-Bassat, M., and Shoenfeld, Y. (1992b). *J. Autoimmun.* **5**, 495–509.

Bona, C. A. (1981). *In* (C. A. Bona, Ed.), pp. 156–182. Academic Press, New York.

Bruijn, J. A., Van Ellen, E. H., Hogendoom, P. C. W., Corver, W. E., Hoedemarker, P. J., and Fleuren, G. J. (1988). *Am. J. Pathol.* **130**, 639–645.

El-Roeiy, A., Sela, O., Isenberg, D. A., Kennedy, R. L., and Shoenfeld, Y. (1987). *Clin. Exp. Immunol.* **67**, 507–515.

Fricke, H., Offen, D., Mendlovic, S., Shoenfeld, Y., Bakimer, R., Sperling, J., and Mozes, E. (1989). *Int. Immunol.* **2**, 225–230.

Fricke, H., Mendlovic, S., Blank, M., Shoenfeld, Y., Ben-Bassat, M., and Mozes, E. (1991). *Immunology* **73**, 421–427.

Isenberg, D. A., and Collins, C. (1985). *J. Clin. Invest.* **76**, 287–294.

Isenberg, D. A., Shoenfeld, Y., Madaio, M., Reichlin, M., Stollar, B. D., and Schwartz, R. S. (1984a). *Lancet* **2**, 418–422.

Isenberg, D. A., Shoenfeld, Y., and Schwartz, R. S. (1984b). *Arthr. Rheum.* **27**, 132–138.

Isenberg, D. A., Dundeney, D., Wojnsruska, F., Bhogal, B. S., Rauch, J., Schattner, A., Naparstek, Y., and Duggan, D. (1985). *J. Immunol.* **135**, 261–263.

Isenberg, D. A., Katz, D., le Page, S., Knight, D., Tucker, L., Maddison, P., Hutchings, F., Watts, R., Andae-Schwartz, J., Schwartz, R. S., and Cooke, A. (1991). *J. Immunol.* **147**, 4139–4177.

Jerne, N. K. (1974). *Ann. Immunol. (Paris)* **125c**, 373–389.

Kalush, K., Rimon, E., and Mozes, E. (1992). *Am. J. Rep. Immunol.* **28**, 264–268.

Knight, B., Katz, D. R., Isenberg, D. A., Ibrahim, M. A., Le Page, S., Hutchings, P., Schwartz, R. S., and Cooke, A. (1992). *Clin. Exp. Immunol.* **90**, 459–465.

Konikoff, F., Isenberg, D., Kennedy, R. C., Kuperman, O., and Shoenfeld, Y. (1987). *Clin. Immunol. Immunopathol.* **43**, 265–270.

Mendlovic, S., Brocke, S., Shoenfeld, Y., Ben-Bassat, M., Meshorer, A., Bakimer, R., and Mozes, E. (1988). *Proc. Natl. Acad. Sci. USA* **85**, 2260–2264.

Mendlovic, S., Fricke, H., Shoenfeld, Y., and Mozes, E. (1989). *Eur. J. Immunol.* **19**, 729–734.

Mendlovic, S., Brocke, S., Fricke, H., Shoenfeld, Y., Bakimer, R., and Mozes, E. (1990). *Immunology* **69**, 228–236.

Mozes, E., Kalush, F., and Tartakovsky, B. (1990a). *In* "Progress in Leukocyte Biology Vol. 10B. The Physiological and Pathological Effects of Cytokines" (Dinarello, Kluger, Powanda and Oppenheim, Eds.). Wiley-Liss, Inc. pp. 111–116.

Mozes, E., Mendlovic, S., Kalush, F., Waisman, A., Shoenfeld, Y., and Fricke, H. (1990b). *Isr. J. Med. Sci.* **26**, 688–691.

Mozes, E., Waisman, A., Levite, M., Zinger, H., Reismer, Y., and Sthoeger, Z. (1992). *Isr. J. Med. Sci.* **28**, 136–138.

Offen, D., Mendlovic, S., Fricke, H., Sperling, R., Sperling, J., and Mozes, E. (1990). *J. Autoimmun.* **3**, 701–713.

Portanova, J. P., Arndt, R. E., and Kutzin, B. L. (1988). *J. Immunol.* **140**, 755–759.

Rombach, E., Stetler, D. A., and Brown, J. C. (1992). *Autoimmunity* **13**, 291–302.

Ruiz, P., and Mozes, E., submitted for publication.

Segal, R., Globerson, A., Zinger, H., and Mozes, E. (1992). *J. Clin. Immunol.* **12**, 341–346.

Sela, O., El-Roeiy, A., Isenberg, D. A., Kennedy, R. C., Colaco, C. B., Pinkhas, J., and Shoenfeld, Y. (1987). *Arthr. Rheum.* **30**, 50–55.

Shoenfeld, Y. (1989). *Curr. Opinion Rheumatol.* **1**, (3): 360–368.

Shoenfeld, Y., and Mozes, E. (1990). *FASEB J* **4**, 2646–2651.

Shoenfeld, Y., Hsu-Lin, S. C., Gabriel, J. E., Silberstein, L. E., Furie, B. C., Furie, B., Stollar, B. D., and Schwartz, R. S. (1982). *J. Clin. Invest.* **70**, 205–208.

Shoenfeld, Y., Rauch, J., Massicotte, H., Datta, S. K., Schwartz, J. A., Stollar, B. D., and Schwartz, R. S. (1983a). *New Engl. J. Med.* **308**, 414–420.

Shoenfeld, Y., Isenberg, D. A., Rauch, J., Madaio, M. P., Stollar, B. D., and Schwartz, R. S. (1983b). *J. Exp. Med.* **158**, 718–730.

Shoenfeld, Y., Wilner, Y., Coates, A. R., Rauch, J., Lavie, G., and Pinkhas, J. (1986). *J. Clin. Exp. Immunol.* **66**, 255–261.

Shoenfeld, Y., Slor, H., Shafrir, S., Krause, I., Granados, J., Villarreal, G. M., and Alarcon-Segovia, D. (1992). *Ann. Rheum. Dis.* **51**(5), 611–618.

Sthoeger, Z., Tartakovsky, B., Bentwich, Z., and Mozes, E. *J. Clin. Immunol.*, in press.

Sthoeger, Z., Zinger, H., and Mozes, E. (1994). *J. Clin. Immunol.* **13**, 127–138.

Tincani, A., Balesterieri, G., Allegri, F., Cattaneo, R., Formasieri, A., Lim, Sinico, A., and D'Amico, G. (1993). *Clin. Exp. Rheumatol.* **17**, 129–136.

Tomer, Y., Mendlovic, S., Kukulansky, T., Mozes, E., Shoenfeld, Y., and Globerson, A. (1991). *Mech. Ageing Develop.* **58**, 233–244.

Waisman, A., Mendlovic, S., Ruiz, P. J., Zinger, H., Meshorer, A., and Mozes, E., (1993). *Int. J. Immunol.* **5**, 1293–1300.

Chapter 16

Autoimmune Vasculitis

Michael N. Hart and Zsuzsanna Fabry

Department of Pathology, Division of Neuropathology,
University of Iowa, College of Medicine, Iowa City, Iowa 52242

I. Introduction and History of the Model

This autoimmune vasculitis model was developed by Hart and collaborators in the 1980s using endothelial (En) cells in an allogeneic system (Hart *et al.*, 1983). It was later shown that BALB/c splenocytes would become activated in coculture with brain-derived, BALB/c microvessel smooth muscle/pericytes (SM/Ps) and that passive transfer of the activated spleen cells resulted in vasculitis in host syngeneic mice (Hart *et al.*, 1985). The model establishes that SM/Ps are capable of an immunologic role as antigen-presenters and presumably as targets for immunocompetent cells.

II. Animals

Brain microvessel SM/P cell cultures are derived from 1- to 3-month-old BALB/c female mice by an established technique (Moore *et al.*, 1984). Spleen cells are harvested from the BALB/c mice at any age under sterile conditions for coculture with the SM/Ps. Host mice (recipients of passively transferred, activated lymphocytes) are of BALB/c origin, usually between 3 and 6 months of age. No special preparation is necessary, although the number of vasculitic lesions in the recipient mice can be increased if the mice donating the splenocytes are treated with cyclophosphamide (25 mg/kg) 2–3 days before spleen cells are removed for coculture, and if the recipients are treated with 200 mg/kg of cyclophosphamide just before passive transfer of activated splenocytes.

III. Genetic Background

The genetic background has not been worked out. In addition to the BALB/c syngeneic system, the only other system that has been attempted was an SJL/ j syngeneic. Vasculitic lesions were seen in the SJL/j recipient mice, but to a lesser degree than in the BALB/c.

IV. Disease Induction

Culture of BALB/c microvessel SM/Ps is difficult but can be accomplished with diligence (Moore *et al.*, 1984). Mouse brain emulsions are strained through a 153-micron mesh nylon filter which traps small muscular vessels. The microvessels are then plated onto plastic dishes and covered with Dulbecco's modified Eagle's medium (DMEM) (GIBCO, Grand Island, New York) with 20% fetal calf serum and treated for 2 min with 1 mg/ml of collagenase. Cells migrate from these vessels and proliferate sufficiently to be passed in 2–3 weeks. On many occasions SM/P cells do not grow from these vessels, whereas endothelial (En) cells do. If a particular isolate shows a majority of smooth muscle cells, attempts are made to ablate the contaminating En cells individually. By three to four passages, a sufficient number of cells has usually accumulated to sort by flow cytometry for contaminating En cells. En cells are labeled with the lectin *Griffonia* (Bandieraea) *simplicifolia* agglutinin (GSA) which is specific for En in the mouse brain (Sigma Chemical Co., St. Louis, Missouri) and negatively sorted. Aliquots of SM/P are identified with an anti-SM/P-specific α-actin by microfluorometry, and subsequent passages of SM/P cells are generally 95–99% pure. Astrocytes are not a contamination problem because they do not grow well in DMEM and, after three to four passages, the number of contaminating hematopoietic cells is probably less than 0.5%.

The irradiated (2000 rads) SM/P are cocultured for 5–7 days with syngeneic spleen cells that are removed aseptically from mice. The viable spleen cells are separated by centrifugation (2500 rpm for 10 min) through lympholyte M solution (Cedar Lane Laboratories, Hornsby, Ontario) to obtain the cell suspension. Cells are then washed three times in Hank's balanced salt solution (HBSS) before being added to the coculture. At the time of coculture, the SM/Ps in a T-75 flask are switched to RPMI 1640 medium with

5% fetal calf serum (KC Biological Co., Lenexus, Kansas); the usual ratio is 10 splenocytes per SM/P. One hundred U/ml penicillin, 100 μg/ml streptomycin, 0.2 mM glutamine, and 5 × 10^{-5} M2-ME are added. (Successful cocultures have been carried out without any foreign antigens, using only 0.5% BALB/c mouse serum.) After the coculture period, the splenic cells are removed from the SM/P by gentle agitation, washed, and concentrated by centrifugation. Three × 10^6 cells are passively transferred to BALB/c recipients by tail vein injection. The mice can usually tolerate 0.1 ml injections. Larger injections will often result in death from congestive heart failure.

Studies in our laboratory have shown that up to 35% of the SM/P express class II antigen, which can be increased to 80% or more by incubating SM/P for 3–4 days with interferon-γ (IFNγ) (Hart et al., 1987; Fabry et al., 1990). Other studies have shown that, after 1 week of syngeneic coculture of SM/P with splenocytes, the only cells that increase in number from the original splenocyte mixture are CD4$^+$ [T helper (Th) cells]. The SM/P can activate CD4$^+$ lymphocytes in an antigen-specific manner and the activation is inhibited with anti-major histocompatibility complex (anti-MHC) class II monoclonal antibody (Fabry et al., 1990a, 1990b). CD8$^+$ cells, monocytes and macrophages, and B cells are not in evidence following 1 week of coculture. It has been subsequently shown that the SM/P preferentially activate a Th1 subset. This is in contrast to brain-derived, microvessel endothelium, which in a similar system will preferentially activate a Th2 subset (Fabry et al., 1993). The Th1 subset of T-cells activated by SM/P also demonstrate restricted T-cell receptor (TCR) usage. Thirty-seven percent show Vβ8.2, 18% show Vβ8.3, and 16% show Vβ14 TCR (unpublished studies).

V. Lesion and Course of the Disease

Following passive transfer of activated lymphocytes, the recipient mice usually do not become obviously ill. Sacrifice of the recipient mice between 4 and 8 days following passive transfer will reveal vasculitic lesions in lungs and liver primarily, with other organs sometimes being affected. The vasculitic lesions are never seen in the brain or the skeletal muscle, in spite of the fact that the presumptive antigen to which they are being activated is present on brain SM/P. Lesions are found predominantly in medium-sized arterioles and venules, and consist of cellular infiltrates in the media of vessels, often with lymphocytes adherent to the endothelium (Figure 1). Occasionally the lesions are destructive, with disruption of the elastica in the more muscular vessels. The cells found in the lesions are predominantly mononuclear, with large activated lymphocytes and monocyte-appearing cells apparent. Granulocytes can also be found, however. Mice autopsied at 2–3 weeks show little

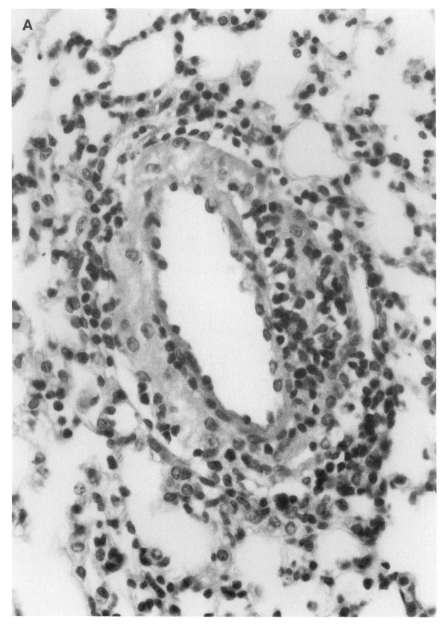

Figure 1. (A) Early lesion in a small vessel with a polymorphic inflammatory cell infiltrate and mural edema. Hematoxylin and eosin stain (H-E). ×100. (B) Lymphocytic cuffing and mural invasion. H-E. ×100. (C) Granulomatous-like vasculitis in large pulmonary vessel. This type of vasculitis is seen exclusively in the smooth muscle model. H-E. ×50.

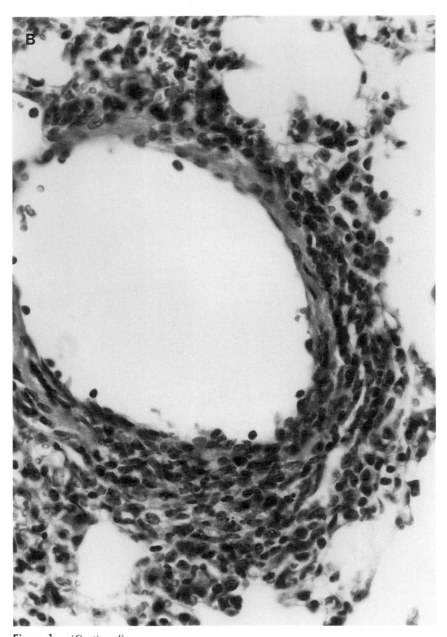

Figure 1. *(Continued)*

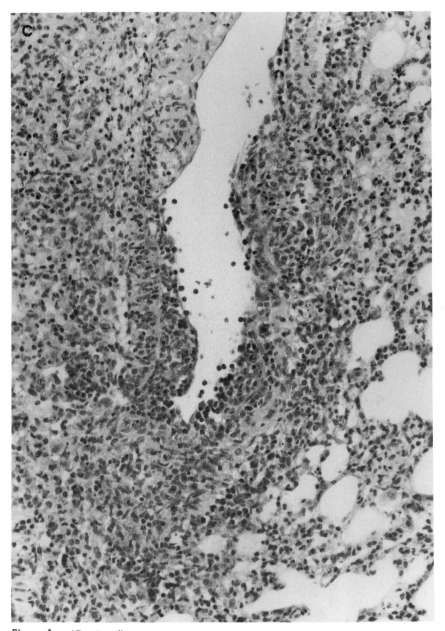

Figure 1. (*Continued*)

inflammation and occasional scarred vessels, indicating that there is a self-healing process and that the disease is self-limited. Attempts to reproduce the disease in these healed mice have not been done. The active disease can be prolonged if activated lymphocytes are passively transferred weekly for 3–4 weeks. This does not appear to increase the severity of the disease. The number of mice developing active vasculitic lesions can be increased with the use of cyclophosphamide, as mentioned earlier.

The affected mice all develop an IγG2a (complement-fixing) antibody that reacts with mouse SM/P from both BALB/c and SJL/j but to a lesser degree with En. It does not appear to react with fibroblasts or astrocytes. Rat hybridomas have been developed that produce IgM anti-SM/P. Unfortunately, these antibodies cross-react with endothelial cells. Further characterization of the antigen by Western blotting and immunoprecipitation is now being performed.

The severity of the lesions is quantified using a subjective scale of 1–4 on which 1 represents evidence of infiltration into the vessel wall by mononuclear cells with evidence of some deleterious effect to the vessel, such as edema. A 4+ reaction represents severe destruction of the vessel wall with fragmentation of elastica and/or obliteration of the lumen with inflammatory cells. Perivascular inflammatory infiltrates are not considered as vasculitis and are not counted. It was found following a complete autopsy that approximately 30–35% of injected animals had developed vasculitis.

The factors that contribute to disease resistance in two-thirds of the animals are not known. It is also not known why the lesions are never seen in the brain or the skeletal muscle, but it is speculated that the En barrier to inflammatory cells is different in these two organs. Conversely, it is assumed that lesions are most often seen in the lungs and the liver because these are the drainage sites following tail-vein injection, and the En shows sufficient fenestrations in the microvessels of these organs to allow the injected lymphocytes to more or less immediately come in contact with smooth muscle. In fact, studies in our laboratory have shown that chromium-labeled lymphocytes injected by tail vein into mice can be seen at autopsy 2 hr later in the lungs and liver, beneath the En, and occasionally in the other organs. In these studies, lymphocytes were also never found in the brain or in the skeletal muscle.

The vasculitic lesions in the mouse resemble a small spectrum of human vasculitides. On the one hand, some mouse vessels are infiltrated only by lymphocytes and quite closely resemble the mononuclear vasculitides seen in small vessels of many organs in association with human collagen vascular diseases, such as lupus erythematosis and rheumatoid arthritis. On the other hand, the severe involvement of some vessels, particularly the larger and more muscular vessels in the lungs, with destruction of elastica and a granulomatous-appearing infiltrate, resemble human vasculitides, such as Churg-Strauss syndrome or a Wegner's picture. It will be important in future studies to determine exactly what the triggering antigen is on the SM/P and also to determine whether this antigen is ever expressed *in vivo*.

VI. Autoimmune Myositis

A separate model from the vasculitis model is one that we have developed coculturing splenocytes with skeletal muscle isolates (Hart *et al.*, 1987). This model has not been well characterized but may be important as a model for human autoimmune myositis (inflammatory myopathy) because it can be produced in 80% of the animals of one strain (SJL/j) but not at all in another strain of mouse (BALB/c). The difficulties in working with this model include foremost the problem of producing pure cultures of myocytes. Myocytes are cultured from newborn mice but even at that age are contaminated by fibroblasts, making it difficult to determine the relative role of skeletal muscle versus that of fibroblasts in activating lymphocytes. Nevertheless, when splenocytes from SJL/j mice are cocultured for 7 days with syngeneic cultures of myocytes that have reached the stage where they display striations and actively contract in culture, and then are passively transferred to syngeneic hosts, a myositis develops in the skeletal muscle of the host. Vasculitis does not develop and there are no lesions in other organs. The lesions usually consist of perivascular accumulations of lymphocytes, with focal destruction of myofibers. In the SJL/j mouse, there are normally numerous muscle fibers that appear to be in a regenerative state, and one has to be careful in the interpretation of these fibers and not count them as inflammatory lesions.

The myositic lesions very closely resemble those seen in humans in a wide variety of nonspecific inflammatory myopathies, including those considered secondary to collagen-vascular disease states of autoimmunity. When BALB/c splenocytes are cocultured with BALB/c skeletal muscle, the lymphocytes appear to become activated to the same degree as they do in the SJL/j system, but myositis is never seen upon passive transfer to hosts.

References

Fabry, Z., Waldschmidt, M. M., Moore, S. A., and Hart, M. N. (1990a). *J. Neuroimmunol.* **28**, 63–71.

Fabry, Z., Waldschmidt, M. M., Van Dyk, L., Moore, S. A., and Hart, M. N. (1990b). *J. Immunol.* **145**, 1099–1104.

Fabry, Z., Sandor, M., Gajewski, T. F., Herlein, J. A., Waldschmidt, M. M., Lynch, R. G., and Hart, M. N. (1993). *J. Immunol.* **151**, 38–47.

Hart, M. N., Sadewasser, K. L., Cancilla, P. A., and DeBault, L. (1983). *Lab. Invest.* **48**, 419–428.

Hart, M. N., Tassell, S. K., Sadewasser, K. L., Schelper, R. L., and Moore, S. A. (1985). *Am. J. Pathol.* **119**, 448–455.

Hart, M. N., Linthicum, D. S., Waldschmidt, M. M., Tassell, S. K., and Schelper, R. L. (1987). *J. Neuropathol. Exp. Neurol.* **46**, 511–521.

Hart, M. N., Waldschmidt, M. M., Hyde, J. M., Moore, S. A., and Kemp, J. (1987). *J. Immunol.* **138**, 2960–2963.

Moore, S. A., Straunch, A. R., Yoder, E. J., Rubenstein, P. A., and Hart, M. N. (1984). *In Vitro* **20**, 512–520.

Chapter 17

Testicular and Ovarian Autoimmune Diseases

Kenneth S. K. Tung,[1] Osamu Taguchi,[2] and Cory Teuscher[3]

[1]Department of Pathology, University of Virginia, Charlottesville, Virginia 22906
[2]Aichi Cancer Center Research Institute, Nagoya 464, Japan
[3]Department of Microbiology, Brigham Young University, Provo, Utah, 84602

I. Introduction

Experimental autoimmune diseases of the testis (autoimmune orchitis) and ovary (autoimmune oophoritis) develop in mice following immunization with the corresponding organ-specific antigen in adjuvant. The orchitogenic antigen has not been identified, whereas an oophoritogenic peptide has been characterized. Studies based on these autoimmune models have yielded new information on the genetic control of organ-specific autoimmune disease and on the mechanism of antigen mimicry at the level of T-cell receptor.

Gonadal autoimmune diseases also occur in common normal laboratory mice following manipulations of their immune system, without the requirement of antigen challenge or use of complex adjuvants. These extremely novel autoimmune models provide opportunities for research on the pathogenic self-reactive T cells and on their regulation in a relatively physiological setting.

Autoimmune diseases of the testis and the ovary are known causes of spontaneous infertility in domestic animals and are likely causes of human infertility (Tung and Lu, 1991). In testes of infertile men, granulomatous orchitis and testicular immune complexes are found that resemble changes in experimental autoimmune orchitis. Evidence for human ovarian autoimmune disease rests on firmer ground; both ovarian autoantibodies and idiopathic oophoritis have been documented in women with premature ovarian failure (Tung and Lu, 1991). Most important, orchitis and especially oophoritis are well-established components of the human polyendocrine autoimmunity syndromes (LaBerbera *et al.*, 1988).

This chapter describes murine autoimmune orchitis and oophoritis elicited by immunization with organ-specific antigens in adjuvant, followed by a description of models of autoimmune oophoritis that involve manipulating the normal immune system, including (1) neonatal thymectomy, (2) transfer of normal T-cell populations to athymic *nu/nu* mice, and (3) engraftment of fetal rat thymuses in the *nu/nu* mice.

II. Experimental Autoimmune Orchitis

A. Historical Aspects

Experimental autoimmune orchitis (EAO) is one of the classic tissue/adjuvant autoimmune disease models, first reported in the guinea pig by Voisin *et al.* (1951). A more detailed description of the disease by Freund *et al.* (1953, 1955) and Waksman (1959) soon followed. Kohno *et al.* (1983) described a reproducible model of murine EAO.

B. Animals

The (C57BL/6 × A/J)F$_1$ (B6AF$_1$) mice from the Jackson Laboratory (Bar Harbor, Maine) or the National Cancer Institute (Frederick, Maryland) are highly susceptible to EAO. B6AF$_1$ mice kept in an environment positive or negative for mouse hepatitis virus develop EAO.

C. Genetic Control of EAO Susceptibility and Resistance

A study based on a large number of independent inbred mouse strains indicates that EAO is under polygenic control involving H-2-linked and non-H-2-linked genes (Teuscher *et al.*, 1985, 1987b; Teuscher, 1985).

Mice with the H-2^s haplotype develop mainly testicular inflammation (orchitis), whereas mice of the H-2^k haplotype develop pathology mainly in the epididymis (epididymitis) and the vas deferens (vasitis) (Tung *et al.*, 1984, 1985). This difference in response is also demonstrated by studies using the BXH series of recombinant inbred lines derived from the EAO-susceptible C57BL/6J and the EAO-resistant C3H/HeJ strains (Person *et al.*, 1992). Orchitis tends to segregate with the *D17Tu20* or *D17Tu52* loci on chromosome 17, whereas autoimmune epididymovasitis has maximal concordance with *MARK-1* (Watson and Paigen, 1990), an androgen-regulated locus on chromosome 7. Further genetic studies on EAO have uncovered three additional orchitis-susceptible genes: *Orch-1*, *Orch-2*, and *Orch-3*.

Orch-1 is an orchitis-susceptibility gene mapping within the H-2^s/H-2^D interval (Teuscher *et al.*, 1985, 1990a), between the *Ir* gene controlling antibody responsiveness to trinitrophenyl-Ficoll (*TNP-Ficoll*) and the locus encoding tumor necrosing factor-α (TNF-α) (Teuscher *et al.*, 1990a). Recently, *Orch-1* has been mapped to a 50–60-kb segment from *Hsp 70.1* to a region proximal to *G7* (Person *et al.*, 1992; Snoek *et al.*, 1993) that encompasses the *Hsp 70.1*, *Hsp70.3*, *Hsc70t*, *G7b*, and *G7a/Bat6* genes.

Genes outside the MHC strongly influence EAO susceptibility. DBA/2J (H-2^d) mice are resistant to EAO (Teuscher *et al.*, 1985; Teuscher, 1985), and BALB/cByJ (H-2^d) mice are susceptible to EAO, whereas (BALB/cByJ × DBA/2J)F$_1$ (CD2F$_1$) mice are resistant. Among the CD2F$_1$ × BALB/cByJ BC1 population ($n = 172$), 54% of the animals can be classified as resistant (average PI = 0.2) while 46% are susceptible (average PI = 3.9). Thus dominant resistance appears to be controlled by a single gene, *Orch-2* (Teuscher *et al.*, 1985). Further study on radiation-chimeric mice suggests that the physiological compartment conferring EAO resistance in DBA/2J mice is marrow derived and probably not a function of the nonmarrow-derived component of the testis.

Significant differences in susceptibility to EAO exist among sublines of BALB/c mice (Teuscher *et al.*, 1987a,b). BALB/cByJ is a responder, whereas less than 20% of BALB/cJ mice develop very mild orchitis. Disease resistance, inherited as a recessive trait, has been shown by segregation analysis to be associated with a single genotypic difference, *Orch-3* (Person *et al.*, 1992). *Orch-3* is not related to elevated levels of serum alpha-fetoprotein in adult BALB/cJ animals (Olsson *et al.*, 1977; Teuscher *et al.*, 1987b), or to the *Bphs* locus that governs hypersensitivity response to the *Bordetella pertussis* toxin

(Teuscher *et al.*, 1987b). Rather, the mutation appears to define a unique immunoregulatory locus required for full expression of EAO susceptibility in wild-type BALB/c substrains. The role of immunoregulatory cells in EAO resistance in BALB/cJ mice has been demonstrated as follows: (1) BALB/cJ mice pretreated with low-dose cyclophosphamide and low-dose whole-body irradiation 2 days prior to inoculation showed enhanced disease severity; and (2) BALB/cJ mice immunized with testis antigen in adjuvant generated Thy1+ CD4+ cells in the spleen, which, when transferred to naive BALB/cByJ recipients, suppressed EAO induction in the recipients (Teuscher *et al.*, 1990b; Mahi-Brown and Tung, 1990).

D. Disease Induction

1. Active Immunization

Severe EAO occurs only in mice immunized with homologous testis antigens, whereas testis antigens from other species are ineffective. Both testis homogenate (TH) and mouse epididymal spermatozoa are active; TH prepared from sexually mature B6AF$_1$ mice kept in a clean environment is pathogenic. When lyophilized and kept in a desiccator at 4°C, TH remains active for 2–3 years. A high incidence of EAO is accomplished by a single injection of 10 mg of TH emulsified in complete Freund's adjuvant (CFA) that contains a final concentration of 4.5 mg/ml of *Mycobacterium tuberculosis* (H37Ra from Difco, Detroit, Michigan). A simultaneous i.p. injection of *B. pertussis* toxin is required for maximum EAO induction. To prepare TH/CFA homogenate, preweighed TH powder is carefully scraped into an empty plastic syringe barrel, and the plunger carefully inserted to firmly compress the dry TH. A second syringe containing an equal volume of distilled water is connected to the TH syringe via a double "female" leurlock syringe connector (Rainin Inst. Co., Woburn, Massachusetts). An even suspension of TH, created by passing the mixture 10 times between the two syringes, is delivered into one syringe. The empty syringe is replaced by a syringe containing an equal volume of CFA with 9 mg/ml of well-suspended *Mycobacterium tuberculosis* powder. The CFA and the TH are mixed by passing the contents between the two syringes to attain a thick emulsion that forms indispersable droplets in water. Under general anesthesia, mice are injected with TH in CFA through a 23-gauge needle, 0.1 ml per mouse, distributed in both hind footpads and two bilateral subcutaneous sites. This is followed by an i.p. injection of *B. pertussis* extract or toxin.

A great deal of variation in toxicity and adjuvanticity exists among *B. pertussis* preparations, and mouse strain variation in susceptibility to *B. pertussis* toxicity is documented (Teuscher, 1985). The two reliable *B. pertussis* preparations are (1) *B. pertussis* extract prepared according to Munoz and Arai (1982), at a dose of 5 μg (for B6AF$_1$ mice) in 0.5 ml of a 0.025 M Tris buffer containing 0.5 M NaCl and 0.017% Triton X-100 (pH 7.6); and (2) purified pertussigen, about 100 ng, i.v. (List Lab. Biol., Campbell, California).

A method for EAO induction in the C3H mice by injecting testicular cells without adjuvants has been described recently (Sakamoto *et al.*, 1985; Itoh *et al.*, 1991).

2. Adoptive Transfer

Adoptive transfer of EAO to untreated normal syngeneic recipients by testis antigen-specific lymph node T cells, T cell lines, and T cell clones (Mahi-Brown *et al.*, 1987, 1988; Yule and Tung, 1993) is detailed here. Adoptive transfer of EAO and generation of T cell clones with crude testis antigen depend on successful *in vitro* induction of proliferative response of testis antigen-specific lymphocytes. To assay for lymphocyte proliferative response (LPR) against testicular cell and spermatozoa antigens, lymphoid cells are obtained from regional lymph nodes and/or the spleen 10 to 14 days after immunization. T cells enriched by passage through a nylon wool column are stimulated by irradiated syngeneic testicular cells or epididymal spermatozoa, with irradiated syngeneic normal spleen cells as antigen-presenting cells. Four days later, cell proliferation is determined by uptake of tritiated thymidine. For optimal LPR, 3×10^6/ml lymphocytes are incubated with 6×10^6/ml irradiated spleen cells and 4×10^6/ml testicular cells in RPMI 1640 (GIBCO Labs, Santa Clara, California) supplemented with 10% fetal calf serum (FCS), 1 mM sodium pyruvate, 2 mM L-glutamine, 0.1 mM nonessential amino acids, 100 U/ml penicillin, 100 μg/ml streptomycin, and 5×10^{-5} M 2-mercaptoethanol (complete medium). Carefully pretested FCS and fresh 2-mercaptoethanol are critical ingredients for low background T-cell proliferation and high antigen-specific responses.

Single testicular cells are obtained as antigens in the LPR by shaking decapsulated testes from normal syngeneic mice at room temperature in collagenase (1 mg/ml; Type II, Sigma Chemical Co., St. Louis, Missouri) for 15 min in Hanks balanced salt solution (HBSS) without FCS, washed three times in HBSS, followed by trypsin (type III-S, Sigma) at 2.5 mg/ml and DNase (type I, Sigma) at 100 μg/ml for 10 min. For stimulation of bulk T-cell culture, decapsulated testes are frozen in liquid nitrogen, thawed, and homogenized in a tissue grinder. The insoluble particulate material is washed twice in HBSS and resuspended in complete medium. The same number of testes is used as would yield 4×10^6 testicular cells/ml. Epididymal spermatozoa are recovered from bisected cauda epididymides of mature B6AF$_1$ mice.

Adoptive transfer of EAO is highly reproducible in the B6AF$_1$ mice and is less consistent among BALB/cBy mice. The major requirements are that the donors be immunized with a testis or sperm antigen in appropriate adjuvants (CFA and *B. pertussis* toxin, or incomplete CFA and *B. pertussis* toxin) and that the lymphocytes be stimulated *in vitro* before transfer. The recipients are not treated in any way except for the i.p. or i.v. injection of the lymphocytes in serum-free HBSS. Disease transfer can be effected with as few as 5×10^6 cells, and signs of disease appear as early as day 5 after transfer. CD4+ T cells are required during *in vitro* stimulation, and their removal even after *in vitro* stimulation greatly reduces the severity of EAO in recipients.

Despite the use of crude TH for immunization and for *in vitro* selection, 100% of the sixteen T-cell clones (or oligoclonal T-cell lines) derived from B6AF$_1$ mice are orchitogenic (Yule and Tung, 1993). These CD4+ T cells produce interleukin-2 (IL-2) and interferon-γ (IFNγ) but not IL-4 upon stimulation, and disease transfer is attenuated if recipient mice also receive neutralizing monoclonal antibody to TNF but not antibody to IFNγ.

Transfer of antibodies results in immunoglobulin G (IgG) binding to germ cells, presumably preleptene spermatocytes, outside the blood–testis barrier (Yule *et al.*, 1988). This finding documents the existence of autoantigenic target cells outside the blood–testis barrier. However, antibody binding to germ cells per se does not lead to EAO.

E. Immunopathology and Pathology Index

While many mice with EAO become infertile, clinical assessment of the infertility is cumbersome, and the demonstration of EAO occurrence relies on histopathological findings. The whole gonad, including the testis, the epididymis, and the vas deferens, is fixed in Bouin's fixative for 24 to 48 hr, and embedded *en bloc* in paraffin. The tissue block is trimmed on the microtome until the testis, the epididymis, and the vas deferens are bisected, whereupon serial 5-micron sections are obtained and stained with hematoxylin/eosin stain.

Actively induced EAO and EAO elicited by passive transfer of orchitogenic T cells consist of orchitis, epididymitis, and/or vasitis (Figure 1). However, distribution of orchitis differs between active EAO and passive EAO (Tung *et al.*, 1987a). The inflammatory foci in active EAO occur at random, with accumulations of lymphoid cells around blood vessels in the interstitium, outside the seminiferous tubules. Lymphocytes, macrophages, polymorphonuclear neutrophils, and eosinophils invade the seminiferous tubules through disrupted Sertoli cell tight junctions. Desquamation of spermatocytes and spermatids occurs adjacent to inflammatory foci (aspermatogenesis). However, aspermatogenesis also occurs independently of orchitis, and the formation of giant spermatids is observed in these tubules. In testes with severe orchitis, complete aspermatogenesis and necrosis are found. The severity of

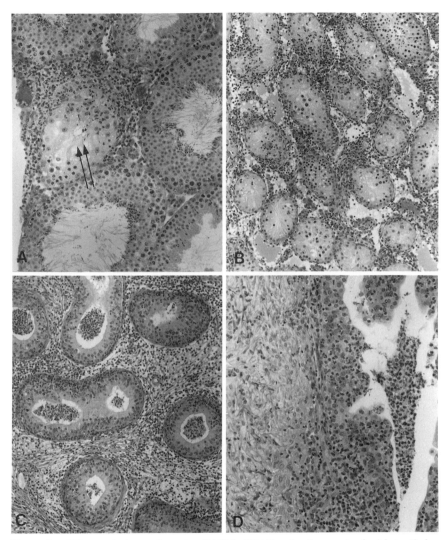

Figure 1. Histopathology of murine EAO in B6AF₁ mice immunized with testis homogenate in CFA and *B. pertussis* extract. Orchitis ranges from focal (A, ×400) to diffuse in distribution and is often associated with aspermatogenic seminiferous tubules (B, ×100). Inflammation also affects the epididymis (C, ×100) and the vas deferens (D, ×100). Arrows in (A) point to the only inflamed tubule found in this testis.

orchitis is semiquantified from grades 1 to 10. A single inflammatory focus is noted in grade 1. About 50% of the testis is involved in grade 5. Grades 2 to 4 denote increasing inflammation between grades 1 and 5. Grades 9 and 10 EAO are those with complete aspermatogenesis and/or necrosis. Grades 6 to 8 denote increasing histopathology between grades 5 and 9. All slides are read as unknown, coded specimens.

In passive EAO, the predominant testicular pathology occurs around the straight tubules, the rete testis, and the ductus efferentes. This blocks the passage of tubular spermatozoa and fluids, leading to the dilation of seminiferous tubules. Severe orchitis spreads centripetally to involve peripheral seminiferous tubules, and ultimately it causes testicular atrophy and necrosis. Vasitis also develops. The pathology of passive EAO is graded as 1–5: grade 1, mild lymphocytic infiltration only in the region of the straight tubules; grade 2, early infiltration of the rete testis; grade 3, presence of either severe inflammation of the rete testis or extension of inflammation to adjacent seminiferous tubules; grade 4, extensive orchitis; grade 5, extensive necrosis.

In the normal mouse testis, MHC II-positive macrophages are sparse, but form a cuff around the straight tubules, where orchitogenic T cells probably encounter germ-cell peptides to initiate passive EAO. After immunization with adjuvant, the number, size, and MHC class II staining intensity of macrophages increase dramatically in interstitial spaces throughout the testis. This change occurs 5–6 days after immunization, 7 days before onset of orchitis (Tung et al., 1987a). Simultaneously, IgG antibody is detected bound to preleptotene spermatocytes outside the blood–testis barrier (Yule et al., 1988).

Epididymitis occurs in the caput, corpus, and/or the cauda epididymides and consists of infiltration of lymphoid cells between and within epididymal ducts, with disappearance of spermatozoa from the lumen. Vasitis is characterized initially by small clusters of inflammatory infiltrates in the submucosal site (Fig. 1). The cells then spread into the muscularis mucosae, invade the vas lumen, and, in severe cases, form large abscesses.

F. Course of the Disease

The inflammation is biphasic. Thus, after 20 to 30 days, most inflammation has receded. The amount of residual normal testicular tissue is inversely related to the extent of orchitis. Spermatogenesis may not resume in aspermatogenic tubules.

G. Recent Studies Based on EAO

Recent studies have clearly refuted the long-held dogma that testis autoantigens are completely sequestered behind the blood–testis barrier. Antigenic peptides recognized by CD4+ T cells are accessible in unique regions of the mouse testis. Moreover, preleptotene spermatocytes, located outside the blood–testis barrier, possess self-surface antigens that are immunogenic. In addition, considerable advances in our understanding of the genetic control of susceptibility and resistance to EAO have been made. The mapping of genes inside and outside the MHC that regulate autoimmune disease susceptibility will clarify not only EAO but other organ-specific autoimmune diseases.

III. Experimental Autoimmune Oophoritis

A. Historical Aspects

Delayed-type hypersensitivity skin reactions to ovarian antigens and autoimmune oophoritis were reported by Jankovic et al. (1973) in rats immunized with bovine ovarian homogenate; a similar pathology was later reported in rats immunized with rat ovarian antigens (Vajnstangl et al., 1979). In 1992, Rhim et al. (1992) induced murine autoimmune oophoritis by a well-defined synthetic peptide from murine ZP3. ZP3, a glycoprotein with sperm receptor activity, is localized in the zona pellucida that surrounds the developing and mature oocytes (Dean, 1992).

B. Animals

B6AF$_1$ female mice from the National Cancer Institute or the Jackson Laboratory are highly susceptible to autoimmune oophoritis. Outbred Swiss mice and occasional A/J and BALB/cBy mice also develop disease, and C57BL/6 is a nonresponder.

C. Disease Induction

1. Active Induction

Ovarian autoimmune disease is induced by a single injection of the ZP3 peptide in CFA. The most active ZP3 peptide is a 13-mer peptide that corresponds to the sequence 330–342 of murine ZP3 (NSSSSQFQIHGPR) (Table I). The carboxyl 7-mer sequence (FQIHGPR) is a B-cell epitope recognized by a monoclonal antibody raised against murine ZP3 (Millar et al., 1989). However, the B epitope is not required for induction of T-cell response or oophoritis, and the shortest oophoritogenic peptide is an 8-mer peptide (NSSSSQFQ) (Rhim et al., 1992). Because an overlapping peptide (SSSQFQIHGPR) also induces oophoritis, there are at least two overlapping

Table I

Immune Response of B6AF$_1$ Mice to ZP3 328-342 and Truncated Derivatives[a]

Position in ZP3	Amino acid sequence	Oophoritis—incidence and graded severity					Antibody titer to ZP3$^{328\text{-}342}$[b]	T-Cell Response		
		Incidence (No. of mice)	1	2	3	4	ELISA (SE)	LPR: Mean (SE)[c]	Line ZP3A[d]	Line ZP3B[d]
328–342	CSNSSSSQFQIHGPR	86% (56)	20	14	11	3	133.4 (19.9)	25,442 (5958)	135,020	59,336
328–340	CSNSSSSQFQIHG	55% (20)	5	4	1	1	1.5 (0.3)	14,504 (3265)	45,797	5,474
328–338	CSNSSSSQFQI	43% (28)	3	7	2	0	2.1 (0.8)	−345 (358)	38,046	31,640
328–336	CSNSSSSQF	0% (9)	—	—	—	—	1.1 (0.3)	−29 (108)	323	313
330–342	NSSSSQFQIHGPR	97% (20)	4	8	10	6	31.0 (7.7)	29,438 (5087)	108,593	53,760
332–342	SSSQFQIHGPR	14% (14)	2	0	0	0	0.8 (0.1)	7,242 (2297)	10,280	3,597
330–340	NSSSSQFQIHG	92% (13)	3	6	0	3	3.9 (1.8)	6,784 (1936)	106,043	60,776
330–339	NSSSSQFQIH	77% (13)	1	3	4	2	2.1 (0.8)	3,589 (246)	31,877	34,973
330–338	NSSSSQFQI	56% (16)	2	3	3	1	1.3 (0.3)	−649 (361)	15,977	1,096
330–337	NSSSSQFQ	57% (21)	4	5	3	0	0.9 (0.1)	508 (230)	300	280
331–339	SSSSQFQIHG	72% (18)	0	6	5	2	1.1 (0.1)	2,104 (340)	37,007	19,127
331–340	SSSSQFQIH	0% (18)	—	—	—	—	1.2 (.2)	954 (561)	223	330

[a] Reproduced from Rhim *et al.* (1992) with permission of the *Journal of Clinical Investigation* by copyright permission of the American Society for Clinical Investigation.

[b] Antibody titer detected by ELISA to ZP3$^{328\text{-}342}$ expressed as mean percent binding of standard antiserum to ZP3$^{328\text{-}342}$.

[c] dpm of [^{3}H]thymidine incorporation in lymphocyte proliferation assay (LPR) in mice immunized with ZP3 peptides.

[d] Mean dcpm of three determinations of [^{3}H]thymidine (dpm) incorporated in the T-cell line (ZP3A and ZP3B) after stimulation with 30–100 μm peptide.

oophoritogenic epitopes within the ZP3 330–342 peptide (Rhim *et al.*, 1992). Whether the whole murine ZP3 protein induces autoimmune oophoritis and whether ZP3 330–342 is a T cell epitope in the context of the ZP3 protein have not been determined.

To induce oophoritis, 0.1 ml of the peptide/adjuvant is distributed in both hind pads, or between one hind pad and bilateral subcutaneous sites in the back. With a single injection of 5 nM of ZP3 330–342 in CFA, over 90% of B6AF$_1$ mice develop oophoritis 12–15 days later. Adjuvant preparation and immunization follow the same procedures as described in EAO induction. However, oophoritis differs from murine EAO and experimental autoimmune encephalomyelitis in that equally severe oophoritis occurs in mice immunized with the ZP3 peptide in incomplete Freund's adjuvant, and *B. pertussis* toxin is *not* required for maximum disease.

The peptides for this study are synthesized by solid-phase synthesis using the RAMPS synthesizer (Dupont Inst., Boston, Massachusetts) and purified by high-pressure liquid chromatography on a C18 reverse-phase column. The peptide composition is verified by amino-acid analysis, and the sequence and purity of selected peptides are determined by mass spectroscopy (Hunt *et al.*, 1992).

2. Adoptive Transfer by ZP3 330–342 Specific T-cell Lines and T-cell Clones

As shown in Table I, only lymph node cells of B6AF$_1$ mice immunized with the longer ZP3 peptides proliferate in response to ZP3 330–342. However, the shorter peptides stimulate ZP3 330–342 specific T-cell lines or T-cell clones to proliferate *in vitro*.

After they have been activated *in vitro* by the ZP3 peptide, lymph node CD4+ T cells readily transfer severe oophoritis to untreated syngeneic recipients (Rhim *et al.*, 1992). Oophoritogenic T-cell lines and T-cell clones against ZP3 330–342 are uniformly CD4+, and produce IL-2, TNF, and IFNγ upon stimulation. Severe ovarian pathology develops within 48 hr in cell recipients, and <1 × 10^6 cells per recipient are sufficient for disease (Luo *et al.*, 1993). As in EAO, coinjection of neutralizing antibodies in TNF also blocks transfer of oophoritis. While the ZP3 peptide-specific CD4+ T cells are clearly sufficient for induction of oophoritis, the role of antibodies in this disease has not been determined.

D. Immunopathology and Pathology Index

Murine oophoritis is characterized by ovarian inflammation, followed, in severe cases, by loss of ovarian follicles and ovarian atrophy (Figure 2). Inflam-

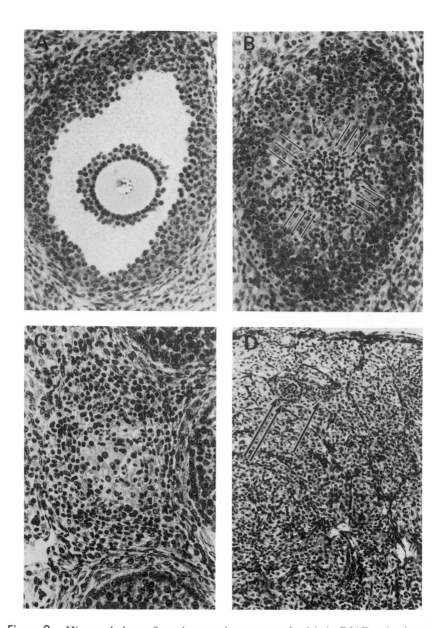

Figure 2. Histopathology of murine autoimmune oophoritis in B6AF$_1$ mice immunized with ZP3 peptide in CFA. (A) Normal ovarian graafian antral follicle with oocyte (×200). (B) Oophoritis with invasion of lymphoid cells inside graafian follicle in mice 10 days after immunization with 50 nmol of ZP3 328-342 (×200). Note accumulation of neutrophils and macrophages in the region of the oocyte (arrows). (C) Granuloma in interfollicular area of B6AF$_1$ mouse ovary after immunization with ZP3 328-342 (×400). (D) 21 days after immunization with ZP3 328-342 (×100). Note loss of oocytes in small ovarian follicles (arrows). (Reproduced from Rhim *et al.*, 1992, with permission of the *Journal of Clinical Investigation* by copyright permission of the American Society for Clinical Investigation.)

matory infiltrates are noted in atretic ovarian follicles within interstitial tissue; others are found inside the Graafian follicles. Among the lymphocytes, there are more CD4+ than CD8+ T cells, and only rare B cells. T-cell infiltrates are colocated with numerous class II MHC-positive, activated macrophages. Granulomatous inflammation with multinucleated giant cells is a frequent finding. In pathologic Graafian follicles, numerous T cells infiltrate the granulosa cell layer, and the oocyte is replaced by macrophages or neutrophils. Oophoritis is graded from 1 to 4. Grades 1, 2, and 3 denote inflammation of focal, intermediate, and diffuse severity, respectively. In grade 4 disease, inflammation has receded and only occasional follicles remain in the atrophic ovary. Oophoritis, first detected on day 6 after immunization, reaches plateau severity by days 12–15. The disease is biphasic, and in severe cases (about 10% of immunized mice), ovarian atrophy with loss of oocytes is apparent by days 25–30.

Oophoritis is almost invariably associated with deposits of IgG antibody in the zona pellucida of the normal Graafian follicles and within atretic follicles. Among individual mice, the intensity of antibody staining closely parallels the severity of oophoritis ($p = 10^{-5}, n = 145$).

E. Recent Studies on Murine Autoimmune Oophoritis

Recent studies on the new autoimmune oophoritis model have yielded several interesting findings. Four randomly positioned amino acids in a nanomer ZP3 330–338 peptide are critical for induction of ovarian disease and T-cell response. Nonovarian peptides that share three of these critical residues are sufficient to stimulate a ZP3 330–338-specific T-cell clone, and the responses are restricted by the same MHC II molecule. Moreover, such nonovarian peptides elicit autoimmune oophoritis (Luo *et al.*, 1993). Further, polyalanine peptide inserted with the critical residues of the ZP3 peptide is fully oophoritogenic. Thus antigen mimicry at the level of T-cell receptor has clearly been demonstrated in a study based on the ZP3 peptide. The finding also predicts induction of autoimmune disease as a potential problem of peptide vaccines.

When B6AF$_1$ female mice are immunized with the ZP3 330–342 peptide from which the B-cell epitope (336–342) has been partially deleted, they still develop oophoritis but do not produce antibodies against the ZP3 336–342 domain. However, these mice produce antibodies against the native ZP3 protein, which are detectable in serum and bound to the ovarian zona pellucida (Lou and Tung, 1993). Endogenous ovarian antigens are required for this unexpected amplified antibody response, since mice that have been ovariectomized do not produce the antibody. Thus immunization with a self-peptide, a pure T-cell epitope, is sufficient to trigger immunologic events beyond T-cell response and autoimmune disease. Interestingly, mice immunized with the nonovarian peptides that mimic the ZP3 peptide also produce amplified autoantibodies against the zona pellucida.

IV. Autoimmune Oophoritis Following Manipulation of the Normal Murine Immune System

Manipulations that elicit autoimmune oophoritis include: (1) neonatal thymectomy, (2) infusion of T cells from normal mice to athymic *nu/nu* mice, and (3) engraftment of fetal rat thymus into athymic *nu/nu* mice. In addition to autoimmune oophoritis, these maneuvers result in autoimmune disease in testis, thyroid, stomach, prostate, adrenal gland, pancreatic islet, salivary and lacrimal glands, and the eye (Table II). Although the immune defects created in these models may differ, the resultant immunopathologies share common characteristics, and as a group they offer insight into tolerance mechanisms against self-antigens.

A. Model 1: Thymectomy Days 1–4 after Birth

1. Historical Aspects

Nishizuka and Sakakura (1969) observed that chemical carcinogen-induced mammary carcinoma did not occur in neonatally thymectomized mice. Subsequently, neonatal thymectomy was found to result in autoimmune oophoritis, and without ovarian steroid hormones, the mammary glands (targets of the carcinogen) failed to develop.

2. Animals

B6AF$_1$ mice from breeding colonies housed in both conventional and pathogen-free rooms, subjected to thymectomy 3 days after birth (D3TX), develop severe oophoritis and ovarian atrophy without additional treatment.

3. Genetics of Disease Susceptibility

A limited number of *H-2* congenic strains, as well as the CXB series of recombinant inbred lines, have been used to attempt to identify the genes controlling disease susceptibility (Kojima and Prehn, 1981). The results suggest that multiple genes are involved and that, for the most part, *H-2*-linked genes had minimal effect in determining disease outcome. In these studies, severe penetrance problems in most mouse strains studied have made meaningful genetic analysis difficult at best. However, autoimmune oophoritis is inherited as a dominant trait with complete penetrance in B6AF$_1$ mice (Tung *et al.*, 1987b). Ninety-five percent of B6AF$_1$ mice developed disease, whereas

Table II

Induction of Autoimmune Diseases by Manipulation of the Normal Immune System[a]

Manipulation of normal immune system	Mouse strain	Disease	Incidence (%)	Autoantibody specificity	References
Day 3 thymectomy	AJ, (C3H × 129)F₁	Thyroiditis	25	Epithelium, colloid	1
	AJ, B6AF₁	Oophoritis	90	Oocyte, ZP, others	2
	BALB/c	Gastritis	40	Parietal cells, ATPAse	3
	SWR, A/J, SWRAF₁	Orchitis	35	Sperm	4
	AJ, (C3H × 129)F₁	Prostatitis	70	Epithelium, secretions	5
Neonatal female spleen cells	Into BALB/c nu/nu	Oophoritis	73	Oocytes, ZP	6
Adult CD5-depleted female spleen T cells	Into BALB/c nu/nu	Gastritis	53	Parietal cells, ATPase	6
	Gastritis	Oophoritis	74	Oocytes, ZP	7
Adult female thymocytes	Into BALB/c nu/nu	Oophoritis	32	Parietal cells, ATPase	7
		Gastritis	73	Oocytes, ZP	8
Adult male spleen cells	Into BALE/c nu/nu	Oophoritis	50	Parietal cells, ATPase	9
		Prostatitis	0	Not specific	10
Adult female spleen cells	Into BALB/c nu/nu	Oophoritis	0	Not specific	11
		Prostatitis	90		12
Fetal rat thymic graft	Into BALB/c nu/nu	Thyroiditis	60	Epithelium, colloid	13
		Gastritis	80	Parietal cells, mucous cells, chief cells	14
		Sialoadenitis	80	Epithelium	15
		Lacrimalitis	90	Epithelium	16
		Uveoretinitis	70	Retina, cornea	17
		Adrenalitis	20	Cortical cells	18
		Oophoritis	90	Oocytes, ZP	18
		Orchitis	20	Spermatozoa	18
		Prostatitis	40	Epithelium, secretions	18

[a] References: (1) Nishizuka et al. (1973); Kojima et al. (1976); Kojima and Prehn (1981). (2) Nishizuka and Sakakura (1969); Nishizuka and Sakakura (1971); Sakakura and Nishizuka (1972); Kojima et al. (1973); Kojima et al. (1977); Taguchi et al. (1980); Taguchi and Nishizuka (1980); Tung et al. (1987b,c); Sakaguchi et al. (1982); Nyake et al. (1988); Smith et al. (1991). (3) Kojima et al. (1980); Suzuki et al. (1981); Kubota et al. (1986); Taguchi and Nishizuka (1987); Tung et al. (1987b,c); Fukuma et al. (1988); Kontani et al. (1992). (4) Taguchi and Nishizuka (1981); Kojima and Spencer (1983); Tung et al. (1987b,c). (5) Taguchi et al. (1985); Taguchi and Nishizuka (1987). (6) Smith et al. (1992). (7) Sakaguchi et al. (1985); Smith et al. (1992). (8) Kojima et al. (1982); Smith et al. (1992). (9) Kojima et al. (1980); Kojima et al. (1982); Smith et al. (1992). (10) Kojima et al. (1977); Kojima et al. (1982). (11) Taguchi and Nishizuka (1987). (12) Kojima et al. (1982); Smith et al. (1992). (13) Taguchi et al. (1986); Taguchi and Nishizuka (1987); Taguchi et al. (1986); Iwasaki et al. (1990). (15) Taguchi, unpublished data. (16) Ichikawa et al. (1991a,b). (17) Taguchi et al. (1986, 1987).

8% of C57BL/6 mice had disease after D3TX. Among 85 (C57BL/6J × A/J)F$_1$ × C57BL/6J backcross (BC1) mice studied after D3TX, 37 mice exhibited disease equivalent in severity to that of the B6AF$_1$ hybrids, whereas 48 others were resistant.

4. Disease Induction and Prevention

The mouse's age at thymectomy is absolutely critical and must fall within the narrow time window of 1 to 4 days after birth in all the strains of mice studied. The incidence and severity of tissue damage are greatly reduced when mice are thymectomized at day 0 or day 5.

Mice are anesthetized with ether inhalation or by cooling in a container immersed in ice. Their legs, arms, and the upper jaw are held down on a cork board by four crisscrossed rubber bands, and under the dissecting microscope, with the head toward the operator, a 3–4 mm longitudinal incision is made below the sternal notch to expose the superior mediastinum. By retracting the overlying muscle, the thymic lobes are visualized and removed by one of two approaches. After the thymus is picked up at its inferior pole with a fine cotton applicator, it can be removed by a rolling motion. Alternatively, the thymus is aspirated by mechanical suction through a fire-polished glass pipet. The chest wound is closed with a continuous 7-0 silk suture. Ophthalmological instruments, including needle holders, fine-toothed forceps, and fine iris scissors are used in the thymectomy procedure. Before being returned to the mother, the thymectomized mice are kept for 2 to 4 hr under a warm (approximately 30°C) lamp. With experience, mortality from surgery is less than 5%. However, residual thymic tissue is left even by experienced operators, and its presence must be assessed histologically.

Autoimmune oophoritis is passively transferred by T cells from D3TX mice to normal B6AF$_1$ mice. The transfer of spleen cells obtained from D3TX mice at 6 to 8 weeks of age to syngeneic mice that are less than 10 days old or to adult syngeneic athymic nude mice (5 to 20 × 10^6 per mouse) results in oophoritis (Taguchi and Nishizuka, 1980; Kojima *et al.*, 1980; Sakaguchi *et al.*, 1982, 1991). Severe oophoritis is detected in almost 100% of cell recipients 10 to 14 days later. The disease is not transferable to recipients older than 15 days unless the cells have been activated *in vitro* by concanavalin A, and CD4+ and not CD8+ T cells are required for disease transfer (Smith *et al.*, 1991).

D3TX-induced autoimmune oophoritis is also prevented by introducing syngeneic T cells from normal mice, either by thymic graft or by a single i.p. injection of spleen or lymph node cells from normal adult female mice. For effective disease suppression, cells must be transferred within 10 days after thymectomy of the cell recipients (Nishizuka and Sakakura, 1969; Sakakura and Nishizuka, 1972; Kojima *et al.*, 1976; Sakaguchi *et al.*, 1982; Smith *et al.*, 1991). Moreover, disease suppression depends on the transfer to normal

CD4+ T cells that express intermediate to high levels of CD5 (Smith *et al.*, 1991).

5. Immunopathology and Pathology Index

Oophoritis first appears 3 weeks after D3TX and is characterized by heavy infiltrates of lymphoid cells in the hilar region of the ovary, within ovarian interstitium, and inside Graafian follicles (Tung *et al.*, 1987b). About equal numbers of CD4+ and CD8+ T cells are detected, though their tissue distributions are somewhat different. B cells form rare, isolated clusters in the ovarian interstitial space. The inflammatory process is biphasic and lasts for 6 to 8 weeks. By 2 months, the ovaries are atrophic, most oocytes having disappeared, and the ovary interstitium is filled with luteinized cells of unknown origin. The severity of oophoritis is graded as 1 when inflammation is confined to the ovarian hilum, as 2 when inflammation is more diffuse, and as 3 when there is ovarian atrophy. Depositions of immunoglobulin and complement around the basement membrane have been detected in diseased ovaries (Taguchi and Nishizuka, 1981).

Following the onset of oophoritis, serum autoantibodies against oocytes, the zona pellucida, and steroid-producing cells are detected by indirect immunofluorescence. Antibody frequency and titer correlate well with the histopathologic grade and clinicopathological course of the disease (Taguchi *et al.*, 1980; Taguchi and Nishizuka, 1981; Taguchi *et al.*, 1985; Tung *et al.*, 1987c).

6. Clinical Findings

The onset of the first estrus in normal mice occurs at the age of 32–40 days. In D3TX mice, estrous cycles spontaneously cease at 40–60 days after a period of a few or several weeks of irregular estrous cycles (Miyake *et al.*, 1988), and mice with severe oophoritis become sterile (Kojima *et al.*, 1973). The time course of the disease and its clinicopathological features are comparable to those in patients with premature ovarian failure in whom increased serum gonadotropin and failure of estrogen secretion are documented. In D3TX mice, higher levels of plasma LH, FSH, and prolactin are demonstrated by radioimmunoassay (Michael *et al.*, 1980, 1981). Furthermore, there is abnormal production of androgenic hormones by luteinized interstitial cells (Nishizuka *et al.*, 1973).

B. Model 2: Transfer of T Cells from Normal Syngeneic Mice to BALB/c *nu/nu* Mice

1. Historical Aspects

Since 1977, investigators have elicited autoimmune oophoritis in normal BALB/c *nu/nu* mice by transfer of lymphoid cells from normal *nu/+*

littermates (Table II). More recently, this experimental approach has been used to investigate the pathogenetic basis of autoimmune diseases that follow D3TX. Following is a summary of pathogenic T cells that have been identified in normal mice and a description of the experimental method.

2. Self-Reactive T Cells in Normal Mice Can Elicit and Prevent Autoimmune Oophoritis in BALB/c *nu/nu* Mice

The transfer of thymocytes (10^6 to 4×10^7) from syngeneic neonatal or adult *nu*/+ female mice to BALB/c *nu/nu* recipients results in autoimmune oophoritis in 75% of the recipients (Table II) (Kojima *et al.*, 1982; Smith *et al.*, 1992). Analysis of adult thymocyte subpopulations has shown that the mature CD4+CD8-thymocytes are responsible for disease induction (Smith *et al.*, 1992).

Spleen cells from untreated adult female mice do not elicit autoimmune oophoritis in *nu/nu* recipients. However, T cells from normal female mice will transfer oophoritis under two experimental conditions. First, spleen cells (10 to 20×10^6) from untreated 3-day-old female mice elicit oophoritis in 75% of recipients, and CD4+ (not CD8+) T cells are responsible for disease induction (Smith *et al.*, 1992). Second, the same number of normal adult female spleen cells that have been treated with Lyt1 (CD5) antibody and complement also transfer severe oophoritis to 75% of BALB/c *nu/nu* recipients (Sakaguchi *et al.*, 1985; Smith *et al.*, 1992). T cells are responsible, since disease induction is abrogated by further treatment of the cells with Thy1 antibody and complement (Sakaguchi *et al.*, 1985). Two-color, flow cytometric analysis with CD5 and CD4 antibodies demonstrates a wide range of CD5 expression on CD4+ T cells from normal murine lymph nodes and spleens. Treatment with CD5 antibody and complement eliminates 95% of the CD4+ T cells that express intermediate and high levels of CD5; the residual T cells express low levels of CD5. Thus autoimmune oophoritis appears to be elicited by adult female T cells expressing a low level of CD5 (Smith *et al.*, 1992).

Autoimmune oophoritis is also induced in athymic nude mice by a single injection of small numbers (10^5 to 4×10^6) of spleen or lymph node lymphocytes from syngeneic normal male mice, or adult female mice that have been ovariectomized at birth (Kojima *et al.*, 1977, 1982; Taguchi and Nishizuka, 1987).

Finally, although neonatal spleen T cells elicit autoimmune oophoritis when transferred to *nu/nu* mice, cotransfer of these cells with spleen cells from adult female spleens completely abrogates disease transfer (Smith *et al.*, 1992).

3. Experimental Method

Spleen cell donors are BALB/c *nu/+* mice and recipients are the BALB/c *nu/nu* littermates. Adult mice used in these studies are 6 to 8 weeks old, and the ages of neonates range from 3 to 10 days. BALB/c *nu/nu* mice from the National Cancer Institute consistently develop oophoritis, gastritis, and corresponding serum autoantibodies. Spleen cells from normal BALB/cAnn mice (from which the BALB/c *nu/nu* mice were derived) also transfer oophoritis to BALB/c *nu/nu* mice, but they should not be used, since the cell recipients also develop varying degrees of graft-versus-host disease. All animals are kept in a pathogen-free environment, housed in sterile boxes in a laminar flow hood, handled with sterile gloves, and fed sterile food pellets and water.

Suspensions of spleen cells or thymocytes, released by mincing with scissors in HBSS and 5% newborn calf serum, are obtained either by pressing tissue segments between the frosted ends of two microscope slides or by grinding them with the blunt end of a sterile syringe plunger on a petri dish and filtering them through a nylon mesh. Erythrocytes are lysed by 0.1% ammonium chloride, and viable cells counted in a hemocytometer. A cell suspension in a 0.1-ml volume is injected i.v. or i.p. into a recipient mouse. Pathology and serum antibodies are detectable as early as 30 days, but maximum incidence is noted at 2 months.

C. Model 3: Engraftment of Fetal Rat Thymus in BALB/c *nu/nu* Mice

1. Historical Aspects

To investigate murine thymic function, rat thymuses from 15-day-old embryos were transplanted to 4-week-old BALB/c *nu/nu* mice. The thymuses had normal morphology and were populated with rat epithelial cells and mouse thymic lymphocytes, macrophages, and dendritic cells. Skin grafts from syngeneic mice and thymic donor rat strains were accepted as self. Unexpectedly, these mice developed autoimmune diseases with features similar to, and of greater severity, organ distributions, and incidence than those observed in D3TX mice (Table II) (Taguchi *et al.*, 1986; Taguchi and Nishizuka, 1987).

2. Animals

Fetal thymuses, obtained from rats of the F344 or ACI strain, are grafted in 4-week-old BALB/c *nu/nu* recipients. All mice are housed in a pathogen-free environment.

3. Disease Induction and Prevention

Fifteen days after mating (dated by the vaginal plug), rat embryos are removed under the dissecting microscope. A wide triangle of the anterior chest wall, including the adherent thymus and the heart, is excised. The thymic lobes that measure 300 to 500 μm in diameter are located slightly to the side in front of the heart. Under transmitted light, the thymic lobes are removed by very fine dissecting scissors and placed in phosphate-buffered saline (PBS) with 2% FCS on ice. The fetal rat thymuses are transplanted under the renal capsule of anesthetized 3- to 5-week-old BALB/c *nu/nu* mice. The recipient's kidney is exposed through a loin incision. Under the dissecting microscope, a small incision is made in the kidney capsule, and one or two thymic lobes are inserted under the capsule. The abdominal wall is closed with 5-0 silk.

Autoimmune oophoritis develops in 90% of mice by 3 months of age, and the disease is transferable by their CD4+ T cells to normal BALB/c *nu/nu* recipients. Serum autoantibodies similar to those found in D3TX mice are also detected. Autoimmune oophoritis is completely prevented by transfer of CD4+ T spleen T cells from normal syngeneic adult mice.

D. Elucidation of Self-Tolerance Mechanisms Based on These Autoimmune Models

Two hypothetical mechanisms have been proposed to explain the requirement of a narrow time window for thymectomy-induced oophoritis. First, the neonatal T cell repertoire may be enriched with self-reactive T cells; thymectomy would fix the T-cell repertoire, which in turn would endow the D3TX mice with the propensity for autoimmune diseases, including oophoritis. Second, population(s) of suppressor or regulatory T cells may develop later than self-reactive pathogenic T cells, and D3TX would preempt their development. These hypotheses are not mutually exclusive.

The first hypothesis is initially supported by a study based on mice that express the endogenous, superantigen, mouse mammary, retroviral peptide and the MHC class II IE molecule (Smith *et al.*, 1989). Expression of this superantigen in the adult thymus prevents the development of Vβ11+ T cells. However, because of the late ontogeny of this superantigen, thymic deletion of Vβ11+ T cells does not occur in the first 10 days of life (Schneider *et al.*, 1989; Smith *et al.*, 1989; Jones *et al.*, 1990; Signorelli *et al.*, 1992). Moreover, lymph nodes of adult D3TX mice are found to contain excessive Vβ11+ T cells (Smith *et al.*, 1989; Jones *et al.*, 1990). However, the enriched Vβ11+ T cells in D3TX mice appear anergic, unresponsive to stimulation by Vβ11+ antibody *in vitro* (Jones *et al.*, 1990); moreover, Vβ11+ T cells are not required for the transfer of oophoritis from D3TX mice to neonates (Smith *et al.*, 1992). Since oophoritis is elicited in the BALB/c *nu/nu* mice by CD4+CD8- adult thymocytes, the pathogenic T cells are not deleted in the adult thymus.

Therefore, compared with adults, the neonatal T cell repertoire appears to be enriched for self-reactive T cells, but the difference is not accounted for by major differences in the ontogeny of negative thymic selection of oophoritogenic T cells.

There is also compelling evidence for the importance of the immunoregulatory or suppressor T cells that normally regulate the pathogenic T cells. For example, oophoritis induced by all three methods of manipulating the immune system is effectively prevented by normal CD4+ T cells. In a similar rat autoimmune model, T cells that express high levels of the CD45 isoform with the C exon are found to transfer autoimmune disease to athymic rats, and the disease is abrogated by the cotransfer of T cells expressing low levels of the CD45 isoform (Fowell et al., 1991). At present, the nature of the regulatory or suppressor T cells is unknown. The finding of autoimmune oophoritis in BALB/c nu/nu mice engrafted with fetal rat thymus suggests that perhaps the development of suppressor T cells normally requires interaction between developing thymocytes with syngeneic thymic epithelial cells. If a low level of CD45 with the C exon indeed marks rat T cells that produce IL-4 and not IL-2, then the suppressor cell may belong to the T helper (Th2) T-cell subset. This finding would be consistent with the known cross-regulation of Th1 and Th2 T cells by cytokines from the CD4+ T-cell subsets.

V. Summary and Conclusions

Several new, interesting, but not yet well-known models of autoimmune disease of the testis and the ovary are in existence. Autoimmune oophoritis is a highly reproducible experimental ovarian disease induced by a well-characterized self-peptide. Studies on this model have permitted structure and functional analysis of T-cell peptides and the reassessment of molecular mimicry as an autoimmune disease mechanism. In addition, a novel mechanism of autoantibody induction has been uncovered. Recent studies on autoimmune orchitis have mapped new genes outside the class I or class II MHC that strongly influence disease susceptibility and resistance, and the functions of these genes are beginning to be defined.

A group of highly reproducible autoimmune models that includes a high prevalence of autoimmune oophoritis can be elicited in common laboratory mice following perturbation of their normal immune function. Recent studies on these novel disease models indicate that they are likely to be powerful tools for testing the reality of self-tolerance mechanisms.

Research on gonadal autoimmunity has been underrepresented. Indeed, its description is often omitted from standard immunology textbooks. This is unfortunate inasmuch as these diseases cause infertility in humans and animals, which, though they do not cause death, preempt life. Moreover, gonadal antigens are likely to attract more attention because they are candidate molecules in the current efforts to develop animal and human contraceptive vaccines.

Acknowledgments

We are extremely grateful to the following colleagues who participated in many studies described in this chapter. They include Adeyemi O. Adekunle, Stephen Estes, John Griffith, M. Izawa, Kevin Livingstone, Ya-Huan Lou, An-Ming Luo, Cherri Mahi-Brown, Nathan Meeker, Pamela Person, Hedy Smith, Jayce Sudweeks, Zheng Yi, Terecita Yule, and Zhao-Zong Zhou. Our work was supported in part by the Special Coordination Fund from the Science and Technology Agency, Japan and grants-in-aid for scientific research and cancer research from the Ministry of Education and Culture, Japan (O.T.) and National Institutes of Health grants HD21926 and HD27275 (C.T.) and HD14504 and HD29099 (K.T.).

References

Dean, J. (1992). *J. Clin. Invest.* **89**, 1055–1059.

Fowell, D., McKnight, A. J., Powrie, F., Dyke, R., and Mason, D. (1991). *Immunol. Rev.* **123**, 37.

Freund, J., Lipton, M. M., and Thompson, G. E. (1953). *J. Exp. Med.* **97**, 711–725.

Freund, J., Thompson, G. E., and Lipton, M. M. (1955). *J. Exp. Med.* **101**, 591–603.

Hunt, D. F., Henderson, R. A., Shabanowitz, J., Sakaguchi, K., Michel, H., Sevilir, N., Cox, A. L., Appella, E., and Engelhard, V. H. (1992). *Science* **255**, 1261–1263.

Ichikawa, T., Taguchi, O., Takahashi, T., Ikeda, H., Takeuchi, M., Tanaka, T., Usui, M., and Nishizuka, Y. (1991a). *Clin. Exp. Immunol.* **85**, 112–117.

Ichikawa, T., Tanaka, T., Sakai, J., Usui, M., Taguchi, O., Ikeda, H., Takahashi, T., and Nishizuka, Y. (1991b). *In* "Ocular Immunology Today" (M. Usui, S. Ohno, and K. Aoki, Eds.), pp. 183–186. Excerpta Medica, Amsterdam.

Ikeda, H., Taguchi, O., Takahashi, T., Itoh, G., and Nishizuka, Y. (1988). *J. Exp. Med.* **168**, 2397–2402.

Itoh, M., Hiramine, C., and Hojo, K. (1991). *Clin. Exp. Immunol.* **83**, 137–142.

Iwasaki, A., Yoshikai, Y., Sakamoto, M., Himeno, K., Yuuki, H., Kumamoto, M., Sueishi, K., and Nomoto, K. (1990). *J. Immunol.* **145**, 28–35.

Jankovic, B. D., Markovic, B. M., Petrovic, S., and Isakovic, K. (1973). *Eur. J. Immunol.* **3**, 375–377.

Jones, L. A., Chin, T., Merriam, G. R., Nelson, L. M., and Kruisbeck, A. M. (1990). *J. Exp. Med.* **139**, 1277–1285.

Jukuma, K., Sakaguchi, S., Kuribayashi, K., Chen, W.-L., Morishita, R., Sekita, K., Uchino, H., and Masuda, T. (1988). *Gastroenterology* **94**, 274–285.

Kohno, S., Munoz, J. A., Williams, T. M., Teuscher, C., Bernard, C. C. A., and Tung, K. S. K. (1983). *J. Immunol.* **130**, 2675–2582.

Kojima, A., and Prehn, R. T. (1981). *Immunogenetics* **14**, 15–27.

Kojima, A., and Spencer, C. A. (1983). *Biol. Reprod.* **29**, 195–205.

Kojima, A., Sakakura, T., Tanaka, Y., and Nishizuka, Y. (1973). *Biol. Reprod.* **8**, 358–361.

Kojima, A., Tanaka-Kojima, Y., Sakakura, T., and Nishizuka, Y. (1976). *Lab. Invest.* **34**, 550–557.

Kojima, A., Tanaka-Kojima, T., and Nishizuka, Y. (1977). *In* "Proceedings of the Second International Workshop on Nude Mice" (T. Nomura, P. E. Bigazzi, and N. L. Warner, Eds.), pp. 127–137. University of Tokyo Press, Tokyo.

Kojima, A., Taguchi, O., and Nishizuka, Y. (1980). *Lab. Invest.* **482**, 387–395.
Kojima, A., Taguchi, O., and Nishizuka, Y. (1982). *In* "Proceedings on the Third International Workshop on Nude Mice" (N. Reed, Ed.), pp. 245–254. Gustav Fischer, New York.
Kontani, K., Taguchi, O., and Takahashi, T. (1992). *Clin. Exp. Immunol.* **89**, 63–67.
Kubota, H., Taguchi, O., Suzuki, Y., Matsuyama, M., and Nishizuka, Y. (1986). *Jpn. Soc. Gastroenterol.* **21**, 122–128.
LaBerbera, A. R., Miller, M. M., Ober, C., and Rebar, R. W. (1988). *Am. J. Reprod. Immunol.* **16**, 115–122.
Lou, Y. H., and Tung, K. S. K. (1993). *J. Immunol.* **151**, 5790–5799.
Luo, A. M., Garza, K. M., Hunt, D., and Tung, K. S. K. (1993). *J. Clin. Invest.* 92, 2117–2123.
Mahi-Brown, C. A., and Tung, K. S. K. (1990). *J. Reprod. Immunol.* **18**, 247–257.
Mahi-Brown, C. A., Yule, T. D., and Tung, K. S. K. (1987). *Cell. Immunol.* **106**, 408–419.
Mahi-Brown, C. A., Yule, T. D., and Tung, K. S. K. (1988). *Am. J. Reprod. Microbiol. Immunol.* **16**, 165–170.
Michael, S. D., Taguchi, O., and Nishizuka, Y. (1980). *Biol. Reprod.* **22**, 343–350.
Michael, S. D., Taguchi, O., and Nishizuka, Y. (1981). *Endocrinology* **108**, 2375–2380.
Millar, S. E., Chamow, S. M., Baur, A. W., Oliver, C., Robey, F., and Dean, J. (1989). *Science* **246**, 935–938.
Miyake, T., Taguchi, O., Ikeda, H., Sato, Y., Takeuchi, S., and Nishizuka, Y. (1988). *Am. J. Obstet. Gynecol.* **158**, 186–192.
Munoz, J. J., and Arai, H. (1982). *In* "Seminar in Infectious Diseases" (J. B. Robbins, J. C. Hill, and J. C. Sadoff, Eds.), p. 396. Thieme-Stratton, Inc., New York.
Nishizuka, Y., and Sakakura, T. (1969). *Science* **166**, 753–755.
Nishizuka, Y., and Sakakura, T. (1971). *Endocrinology* **89**, 888–893.
Nishizuka, Y., Tanaka, Y., Sakakura, T., and Kojima, A. (1973). *Experientia* **29**, 1396–1398.
Niyake, T., Taguchi, O., Ikeda, H., Sato, Y., Takeuchi, S., and Nishizuka, Y. (1988). *Am. J. Obstet. Gynecol.* **158**, 186–192.
Olsson, M., Lindahl, G., and Rouslahti, E. (1977). *J. Exp. Med.* **145**, 819–827.
Person, P. L., Snoek, M., Demant, P., Woodward, S. R., and Teuscher, C. (1992). *Reg. Immunol.* **4**, 284–297.
Rhim, S. H., Millar, S. E., Robey, F., Dean, J., Allen, P., Tung, K. S. K., Luo, A. M., Lou, Y. H., and Yule, T. D. (1992). *J. Clin. Invest.* **89**, 28–35.
Sakaguchi, S., Takahashi, T., and Nishizuka, Y. (1982). *J. Exp. Med.* **156**, 1565–1576.
Sakaguchi, S., Fukuma, K., Kuribayashi, K., and Masuda, T. (1985). *J. Exp. Med.* **161**, 72–87.
Sakakura, T., and Nishizuka, Y. (1972). *Endocrinology* **90**, 431–437.
Sakamoto, Y., Himeno, K., Sanui, H., Yoshida, S., and Nomoto, K. (1985). *Clin. Immunol. Immunopathol.* **37**, 360–368.
Schneider, R., Lees, R. K., Pedrazzini, T., Zinkernagel, R. M., and Hengartner, H. (1989). *J. Exp. Med.* **169**, 2149.
Signorelli, K., Benoist, C., and Mathis, D. (1992). *Eur. J. Immunol.* **22**, 2487–2493.
Smith, H., Chen, I.-M., Kubo, R., and Tung, K. S. K. (1989). *Science* **245**, 749–752.
Smith, H., Sakamoto, Y., Kasai, K., and Tung, K. S. K. (1991). *J. Immunol.* **147**, 2928–2933.
Smith, H., Lou, Y.-H., Lacy, P., and Tung, K. S. K. (1992). *J. Immunol.* **149**, 2212–2218.
Snoek, M., Jansen, M., Olavessen, M. G., Campbell, D., Teuscher, C., and van Vugt, H. (1993). *Genomics* **15**, 350–356.
Suzuki, Y., Taguchi, O., Kojima, A., Matsuyama, M., and Nishizuka, Y. (1981). *Lab Invest.* **45**, 209–217.
Taguchi, O., and Nishizuka, Y. (1980). *Clin. Exp. Immunol.* **42**, 324.
Taguchi, O., and Nishizuka, Y. (1981). *Clin. Exp. Immunol.* **46**, 425–434.
Taguchi, O., and Nishizuka, Y. (1987). *J. Exp. Med.* **165**, 146–156.

Taguchi, O., Nishizuka, Y., Sakadura, T., and Kojima, A. (1980). *Clin. Exp. Immunol.* **40**, 540–553.

Taguchi, O., Kojima, A., and Nishizuka, Y. (1985). *Clin. Exp. Immunol.* **60**, 123–129.

Taguchi, O., Takahashi, T., Masao, S., Namikawa, R., Matsuyama, M., and Nishizuka, Y. (1986). *J. Exp. Med.* **164**, 60.

Teuscher, C. (1985). *Immunogenetics* **22**, 417–425.

Teuscher, C., Smith, S. M., Goldberg, E. H., Shearer, G. M., and Tung, K. S. K. (1985). *Immunogenetics* **22**, 323–333.

Teuscher, C., Blankenhorn, E. P., and Hickey, W. F. (1987a). *Cell. Immunol.* **110**, 294–304.

Teuscher, C., Smith, S. M., and Tung, K. S. K. (1987b). *J. Reprod. Immunol.* **10**, 219–230.

Teuscher, C., Gasser, D. L., Woodward, S. R., and Hickey, W. F. (1990a). *Immunogenetics* **32**, 337–344.

Teuscher, C., Hickey, W. F., and Korngold, R. (1990b). *Immunogenetics* **32**, 34–40.

Tung, K. S. K., Ellis, L. E., Childs, G. V., and Dufau, M. (1984). *Endocrinology* **114**, 922–929.

Tung, K. S. K., Yule, T. D., Mahi-Brown, C. A., and Listrom, M. B. (1987a). *J. Immunol.* **138**, 752–759.

Tung, K. S. K., Smith, S., Teuscher, C., Cook, C., and Anderson, R. E. (1987b). *Am. J. Pathol.* **126**, 293–302.

Tung, K. S. K., Smith, S., Matzner, P., Kasai, K., Oliver, J., Feuchter, F., and Anderson, R. E. (1987c). *Am. J. Pathol.* **126**, 303–314.

Tung, K. S. K., and Lu, C. Y. (1991). *In* "Pathology of Reproductive Failure," pp. 308–333. Williams and Wilkins, New York.

Vajnstangl, M., Petrovic, S., and Jankovic, B. D. (1979). *Periodicum Biologorum* **81**, 249–251.

Voisin, G. A., Delauney, A., and Barber, M. (1951). *Ann. Inst. Pasteur* **81**, 48–63.

Waksman, B. H. (1959). *J. Exp. Med.* **109**, 311–324.

Watson, G., and Paigen, K. (1990). *Mol. Cell. Endocrinol.* **68**, 67–74.

Yule, T. D., and Tung, K. S. K. (1993). *Endocrinology*, **133**, 1098–1107.

Yule, T. D., Montoya, G. D., Russell, L. D., Williams, T. M., and Tung, K. S. K. (1988). *J. Immunol.* **141**, 1161–1167.

Chapter 18

Allogeneic Diseases

Sandrine Florquin and Michel Goldman

Laboratoire Pluridisciplinaire de Recherche Experimentale Biomédicale et Service d'Immunologie, Hôpital Erasme, Université Libre de Bruxelles, B-1070 Brussels, Belgium

I. Chronic Graft-versus-Host Disease

A. History of the Model

The response of adult unirradiated F_1 hybrid mice to the injection of parental T cells depends upon differences in the donor and host major histocompatibility complex (MHC), and donor cell inoculum size and T-cell phenotype. The administration of donor cells that differ from the F_1 recipient at both class I and class II MHC loci leads to a rapidly fatal, acute graft-versus-host reaction (GVHR). When donor inoculum is depleted of $CD8^+$ cells, the course of the disease is changed to a chronic form of GVHR characterized by the development of autoimmune features reminiscent of systemic lupus erythematosus (SLE). This chronic GVHR also arises when recipient and donor animals differ only at class II MHC loci or when donor cells fail to mount an antirecipient cytotoxic T-lymphocyte response (Via and Shearer, 1988). The immunopathology associated with chronic graft-versus-host disease (GVHD) was first described by Lewis *et al.* (1968) in (BALB/c × A/J)F_1 mice injected with BALB/c spleen cells. In this strain combination, experimental animals develop an immune complex glomerulonephritis of the membranous type which is responsible for a severe nephrotic syndrome.

B. The Animals

A/J (H-$2^{k/k}$), BALB/c (H-$2^{d/d}$), C57BL/10 (H-$2^{b/b}$), DBA/2 (H-$2^{d/d}$) and F_1 hybrids can be purchased from several commercial animal breeders. Eight to 10-week-old female mice are suitable as recipient and donor animals. In the parent-into-F_1 combinations described below, recipients never display symptoms of acute GVHD ("runt disease"). Therefore, mice can be bred in the usual animal facilities on standard laboratory chow.

C. Genetic Background

A chronic GVHD with high serum levels of immunoglobulin G (IgG) antibodies to DNA and histones is generally obtained when cells of an H-2^d parent are injected into F_1 hybrids obtained by breeding H-2^d mice with other H-2 strains (Portanova et al., 1988). A single incompatibility between donor and F_1 recipients at the I-E locus, which is the murine analog of HLA-D/DR, is sufficient to trigger the production of autoantibodies (van Rappard-van der Veen et al., 1982). However, no correlation exists between the production of autoantibodies and the occurrence of progressive renal disease. Indeed, the susceptibility for renal involvement in murine chronic GVHD depends on several factors. Fatal glomerulonephritis was first thought to be restricted to F_1 mice bearing H-2^b class II MHC molecules (Portanova et al., 1988). However, using congenic strains created by combining the H-2 region of one strain (B.10S, H-$2^{s/s}$) with the non-MHC background of another strain (C57BL/10, H-$2^{b/b}$), it has been shown that non-H-2 factors also determine the difference in susceptibility to renal disease in murine chronic GVHD (Bruijn et al., 1989).

D. The Disease

1. Active Induction

Optimal induction of SLE-like GVHD in (C57BL/10 × DBA/2)F_1 hybrid recipient mice depends on the number and composition of the DBA/2 parental donor cells administered. Doses of 100×10^6 to 200×10^6 spleen and lymph node cells (two parts spleen cells for one part lymph node cells) appear the most appropriate to induce the autoimmune syndrome (van Rappard-van der Veen et al., 1983). Single-cell suspensions are prepared by mincing spleens and lymph nodes (mesenteric, cervical, inguinal) in phosphate-buffered saline, gently pressing the fragments through a nylon sieve, and passing the cells through a Pasteur pipet loosely packed with sterile cotton wool. The proportion of viable donor cells must be higher than 90%. The total amount of cells is given in two injections in the tail vein on day 0 and day 5. The presence of thymocytes in the donor inoculum allows one to reproducibly induce a long-lasting disease with a high incidence of immunoglobulin deposits in the skin and glomerulosclerosis. Typically, 120×10^6 splenocytes are administered together with 60×10^6 thymocytes and 30×10^6 lymph node cells given as four divided doses at intervals of 3 or 4 days (Bruijn et al., 1989).

2. Course of Disease

We first describe the disease occurring in the DBA/2 $\rightarrow$ (C57BL/10 $\times$ DBA/2)F_1 combination. The lack of acute GVHD in this particular model has been related to the relative inability of T cells from DBA/2 mice to mount anti-C57BL/10 cytotoxic responses. In contrast, DBA/2 CD4$^+$ T cells that recognize host MHC class II alloantigens are functional and persistently activate B cells of the host to produce immunoglobulins. The reaction of donor helper T cells against MHC class II disparate B cells of the host leads to a preferential secretion of IgG autoantibodies characteristic of SLE as well as to high serum levels of IgE (hyperIgE) (Goldman et al., 1991). Some of the cytokines involved in these interactions between T cells and B cells have been identified. Spleen cells from mice undergoing GVHR spontaneously produce interleukin-5 (IL-5) as well as B151TRF2, another B-cell tropic factor (Dobashi et al., 1987). Furthermore, the serum hyperIgE is prevented by the in vivo administration of anti-IL-4 antibody, suggesting that IL-4 is another mediator of B-cell activation in this model (Doutrelepont et al., 1991).

As far as autoimmunity is concerned, GVH mice produce antibodies to nuclear antigens, double-stranded DNA, thymocytes, erythrocytes, skin basement membrane, and glomerular basement membrane as well as to brush border of proximal renal tubuli (van Rappard-van der Veen et al., 1983; Bruijn et al., 1990). These autoantibodies appear in the serum 2 weeks after induction of the GVHR and the highest titers are generally found 14 to 16 weeks after the cell transfer. In contrast, organ-specific antibodies such as antibodies to smooth muscle, intracytoplasmic antigens of gastric parietal cells, mitochondrial antigens, or microsomal and colloid antigens of the thyroid gland are typically absent (Elson, 1982; Gleichmann et al., 1982).

At autopsy, most of the GVH F_1 mice show evidence of lymphoid stimulation with enlargement of spleen, lymph nodes, and lymphocyte infiltrations in several tissues such as the portal tracts of the liver, the bile duct epithelium, the salivary glands, the lungs, and the pancreas. Moreover, from weeks 1 to 7 all GVHF$_1$ mice show periarteritis in their kidneys. This lesion is occasionally seen in other organs, such as lungs and pancreas (Gleichmann *et al.*, 1982). About 80% of 12-week-old GVH mice display autoantibody deposits along the basement membrane of the skin in a linear fashion (van Elven *et al.*, 1981). During the course of the GVHR, the linear immunofluorescent staining of the basement membrane of the skin increases from an initially weak and discontinuous staining to a continuous and strongly positive one. The presence of cortisone-resistant thymocytes (mature T cells) in the donor inoculum is critical for triggering the appearance of linear IgG deposits in the skin.

The *in vivo* deposition of IgG antibodies at the dermo-epidermal junction correlates well with the development of a severe immune-complex glomerulonephritis. Indeed, the kidneys show glomerular mesangial, segmental, and diffuse proliferative lesions and occasionally membranous nephritis. In the most severe cases, global glomerulosclerosis in the form of accumulation of extracellular matrix components (Bergijk *et al.*, 1992) and extensive tubular atrophy is observed after 3 months. With immunofluorescence, deposits of immunoglobulins (IgM, IgG 1 and IgG 2a) and complement are observed 2 weeks after the first injection of parental lymphocytes. These deposits are located in the mesangium and along the glomerular capillary walls, where they are organized in a linear pattern until week 6. After 6 to 8 weeks, this distribution changes to a granular pattern. Electron microscopy reveals the presence of mesangial and subepithelial electron-dense deposits with various degrees of spike formation and incorporation of electron-dense material in the glomerular basement membrane. Kidneys of animals with proliferative changes have electron-dense deposits in subendothelial localization as well (Rolink *et al.*, 1983; Bruijn *et al.*, 1990). These glomerular lesions are responsible for a massive proteinuria starting after 4 weeks and culminating around week 10. At this time, GVH mice present hypoalbuminemia sometimes associated with edema of the feet. Furthermore, renal insufficiency develops together with variable degrees of anemia. This renal syndrome is responsible for an increased mortality in GVH mice. Indeed, the mean survival of GVH F_1 mice is about 16 weeks after the first injection of donor cells.

About one-third of mice with chronic GVHD also develop lymphocytic sialoadenitis, reminiscent of human Sjögren syndrome (Fujiwara *et al.*, 1991). The submandibular gland lesions are characterized by the infiltration of mononuclear cells around interlobular ducts, often complicated by parenchymal destruction. The submandibular gland lesions do not contain immunoglobulin deposits and are neither correlated with the degree of proteinuria nor with the presence of autoantibodies. The occurrence of sialoadenitis might indeed involve a cell-mediated immunopathogenesis.

In the BALB/c → (BALB/c × A/J)F_1 combination, the GVHR results in a chronic progressive polyarthritis. Twelve months after cell transfer, about

50% of F_1 recipients display arthritis in the interphalangeal joints of the feet characterized by lymphoid infiltration, synovial proliferation, and pannus formation. In severe cases, articular erosion and bone destruction also develop. This arthritis is associated with prominent juxtaarticular lesions, including perivascular infiltrates, peritendinitis, myositis, and inflammatory nodules. Moreover, 75% of the recipients develop skin lesions characterized by dermal fibrosis and loss of skin appendages, thereby resembling scleroderma (Pals *et al.*, 1985; Gelpi *et al.*, 1990). See Table I for more details on the various types of chronic GVHD.

E. Quantitation

GVHR is invariably associated with hypergammaglobulinemia, which can be easily determined by solid-phase enzyme-linked immunosorbent assay (ELISA). Elevated proteinuria is good evidence of severe glomerulonephritis and reflects the severity of the autoimmune syndrome. Renal morphological alterations can be classified according to the World Health Organization's (WHO) morphologic classification of lupus nephritis (Bruijn *et al.*, 1988). The development of linear IgG deposits at the dermo-epidermal junction appears to be a good indicator for the existence of autoantibodies and immune complex glomerulonephritis (van Elven *et al.*, 1981). Splenomegaly at the time of sacrifice is also good evidence for GVHD but does not predict the degree of severity of the disease.

F. Expert Experience

C57BL/10 and (C57BL/10 × DBA/2)F_1 mice can be replaced with C57BL/6 and (C57BL/6 × DBA/2)F_1 mice respectively, inasmuch as similar outcomes are observed. Males and females can be equally used. However, it is crucial to always use and breed mice from the same commercial source.

II. Host-versus-Graft Disease

A. History of the Model

Allogeneic interactions are involved in another murine model of systemic autoimmunity, namely, the host-versus-graft disease (HVGD) that develops in BALB/c mice injected at birth with spleen cells from either (C57BL/6 × BALB/c)F_1 or (A/J × BALB/c)F_1 hybrids. About 20 years ago, Hard and Kullgren (1970) described hematological disorders in C3H mice neonatally injected with 10^8 spleen cells from (C3H × T6)F_1 hybrids. The resulting

Table I

Various Types of Chronic GVH[a]

Donor	Recipient	Inoculum	AutoAb	Pathology	References
BALB/c $H-2^{d/d}$	(BALB/c × A/J) $H-2^{d/k}$	4 inj. 50×10^6 S	+[b]	Immune complex GN (100%)	Lewis et al. (1968)
BALB/c $H-2^{d/d}$	(BALB/c × A/J) $H-2^{d/k}$	4 inj. 25×10^6 S	+[b]	Arthritis (50%), sialoadenitis (80%) scleroderma (75%), ICGN (50%)	Pals et al. (1985)
BALB/c $H-2^{d/d}$	(BALB/c × A/J) $H-2^{d/k}$	Not given	+	Arthritis (50%), membranous GN (30%), purpura (55%)	Gelpi et al. (1990)
A/J $H-2^{d/k}$	(BALB/c × A/J) $H-2^{d/k}$	Not given	+	Membranous GN (50%), purpura (25%)	Gelpi et al. (1990)
DBA/2 $H-2^{d/d}$	$H-2^{d/d}$ $H-2^{d/k}$	2 inj. 50×10^6 S:LN	+	No GN	Portanova et al. (1988)
DBA/2 $H-2^{d/d}$	(C57Bl/ × DBA/2) $H-2^{b/d}$	4 inj. 50×10^6 S:LN:T	+	Proliferative GN (100%)	Bruijn et al. (1990)
DBA/2 $H-2^{d/d}$	(C57Bl/ × DBA/2) $H-2^{b/d}$	2 inj. $100 \times$ 10^6 S	+	Sialoadenitis (33%), proteinuria (100%)	Fujiwara et al. (1991)
DBA/2 $H-2^{d/d}$	[(B10 × B10.S) × DBA/2] $H-2^{b/d}$	4 inj. 50×10^6 S:LN:T	+	GN (80%)	Bruijn et al. (1989)
DBA/2 $H-2^{d/d}$	[(B10 × B10.S) × DBA/2] $H-2^{b/d}$	4 inj. 50×10^6 S:LN:T	+	GN (65%)	Bruijn et al. (1989)
B10.A(2R) $H-2^{k}$ (I-E^y)	[B10.A(2R) × B10.A(4R)] $H-2^{k}$ (I-E$^{t/b}$)	2 inj. 50×10^6 S:LN	−	ND	van Rappard-van der Veen et al. (1982)
B10.A(4R) $H-2^{k}$ (I-E^y)	[B10.A(2R) × B10.A(4R)] $H-2^{k}$ (I-E$^{t/b}$)	2 inj. 50×10^6 S:LN	+	ND	van Rappard-van der Veen et al. (1982)

[a] inj, injections; S, splenocytes; LN, lymph node cells; T, thymocytes; Ab, antibodies; GN, glomerulonephritis; ND, not done. [b] S. Pals, personal communication.

HVGD is characterized by lymphosplenomegaly, hemolytic anemia, thrombocytopenia, and fatal intestinal hemorrhage. Splenectomy at 14 days prevents hemorrhagic death, and about 50% of the surviving HVG mice develop full-blown nephrotic syndrome secondary to an immune complex glomerulonephritis (Hard et al., 1973). In other strain combinations, the neonatal injection of semiallogeneic spleen cells induces nonlife-threatening pathological changes, including lymphosplenomegaly (Simpson et al., 1974) and SLE-like syndrome (Goldman et al., 1983).

B. The Animals

C57Bl/6 (H-$2^{b/b}$), BALB/c (H-$2^{d/d}$), A/J (H-$2^{k/k}$), and F_1 hybrids can be purchased from several commercial animal breeders. Eight-to 12-week-old F_1 mice are used as donor animals. Donor and recipient mice can be kept under standard animal facility conditions.

C. Genetic Background

Semiallogeneic F_1 hybrid cells are used to induce neonatal tolerance because their inoculation does not lead to the fatal runt disease observed with fully allogeneic cells. Host-versus-graft reaction (HVGR) is best attained when cells of an H-$2^{d/k}$ donor are injected into an H-$2^{d/d}$ recipient. The combination H-$2^{b/d} \rightarrow H$-$2^{d/d}$ leads to the same results.

D. The Disease

1. Active Induction

HVG disease is induced by intraperitoneal inoculation of 1×10^8 (A/J × BALB/c)F_1 hybrid spleen cells in newborn BALB/c mice (less than 24 hr after birth). Spleen cell suspensions are prepared as described for GVHD induction. Cells are resuspended in buffered RPMI 1640 (pH 7.2–7.4) before injection.

2. Course of Disease

Neonatal injection of semiallogeneic cells [(BALB/c × C57Bl/6)F_1 or (BALB/c × A/J)] in BALB/c mice induces a state of tolerance toward donor alloantigens, as indicated by deletion and/or anergy of donor-specific cytolytic T cells and of donor-specific T helper (Th) cells secreting IL-2 and interferon-γ (IFNγ). As a consequence, donor cells are not rejected, so neonatally injected mice become chimeric. Allotolerance in this model is indeed incomplete, as indicated by the persistence of alloreactive CD4$^+$ T cells of the Th2 type (Goldman *et al.*, 1991). *In vivo* activation of donor B cells by these Th2 cells results in a preferential production of IgG 1 and IgE (Abramowicz *et al.*, 1988) and an increased expression of class II MHC antigens on B cells (Abramowicz *et al.*, 1990b), IL-4 being the predominant cytokine involved in this HVGR between host T cells and donor F_1 B cells (Abramowicz *et al.*, 1990a, Schurmans *et al.*, 1990).

As early as 2 weeks after injection of semiallogeneic cells, HVG mice display hypergammaglobulinemia, serum hyperIgE, circulating immune complexes, cryoglobulins, and various autoantibodies. These immunological disorders are at least detectable until week 24. Antinuclear antibodies are observed with a high incidence (80%) (Goldman *et al.*, 1983) and experiments with IgH-congenic BALB/c mice established that most of the anti-DNA antibodies are produced by F_1 donor B cells (Luzuy *et al.*, 1986). Other autoantibodies produced by HVG mice include anti-ssDNA, thymocytotoxic and rheumatoid factor-like antibodies, as well as antibodies to antigens of the glomerular basement membrane and of the renal tubular epithelium (Florquin *et al.*, 1991). In addition, thrombocytopenia and a positive direct Coomb's test are often present.

Serum C3 values are within the normal range while increased albuminuria is detected in about 70% of 4-week-old animals and persists at least until week 12 in 50% of HVG mice. At autopsy, chimeric animals show generalized lymphadenopathy and splenomegaly. Granular deposits of IgG are detected in the choroid plexus as early as 2 weeks after neonatal injection. IgG deposits are also observed at the dermo–epidermal junction of the skin with a linear pattern (Goldman *et al.*, 1983). In the kidneys, HVG mice also display linear deposits of IgG along the glomerular capillary walls from week 4 to week 6. Later on, the immunofluorescence pattern of IgG deposits changes from linear to granular. At this stage, light microscopy and electron microscopy reveal irregularities of the capillary walls with spike formation and electron-dense deposits in a subepithelial position, all features characteristic of membranous glomerulopathy. At week 12, this immune complex nephritis is complicated in one-half of the mice by focal and segmental glomerulosclerosis which involves about 60% of the glomeruli (Florquin *et al.*, 1991). The mean survival of HVG mice is about 14 weeks.

E. Quantitation

Chimerism can easily be demonstrated by the detection of immunoglobulins bearing allotypes of the donor strain. This can be done using either hemagglutination or ELISA. Evaluation of the immunopathological syndrome can be performed as described for the GVHD.

F. Expert Experience

It is crucial to inject newborn mice less than 24 hr after birth. Later, they are more immunocompetent and able to reject semiallogeneic inoculum, leading to a lower incidence of HVGR induction. All precautions must be taken in manipulating newborn animals (sterile and buffered cell suspensions, gloves, quiet environment).

III. Lessons

There are many similarities between murine allogeneic diseases and human SLE. From an immunopathological point of view, GVH or HVG mice display cutaneous and renal changes resembling those observed in SLE. In GVHD, the SLE-like syndrome may occur together with lesions characteristic of other inflammatory diseases, including rheumatoid arthritis, Sjögren syndrome, scleroderma, and sclerosing cholangitis (Gleichmann et al., 1982). The spectrum of autoantibodies produced by HVG or GVH mice is very similar to that encountered in human SLE. Furthermore, autoantibodies characteristic of scleroderma are secreted by GVH mice, among them anti-small ribonucleoprotein (snRNP) antibodies, including antifibrillarin antibodies. Incompatibility at the *I-E* locus alone provides the stimulus that leads to the massive formation of autoantibodies characteristic of SLE. Because *I-E* appears to be the murine analog of *HLA-D/DR*, this finding is in keeping with the increased frequency of certain *HLA-DR* alleles in SLE patients. Experimental allogeneic diseases differ, however, from human SLE in some aspects: mice do not display the sex-dependent predisposition and the exacerbations and remissions characteristic of the human disease.

GVHD and HVGD represent relevant models for analyzing the role of T cells in the induction of systemic autoimmune diseases. Indeed, in both models, $CD4^+$ T cells recognizing foreign class II MHC molecules on B cells are responsible for the induction of autoantibody production. The profile of cytokines produced by these T cells corresponds to the definition of Th2 cells because they produce high levels of IL-4 and IL-10 and low levels of IL-2 and IFNγ. Current studies aim at defining the factors leading to the preferential differentiation of alloreactive T cells into Th2-like cells in experimental allogeneic diseases.

In human SLE too, there is good evidence that T cells play a central role in the pathogenesis of the disease. A variety of T-cell changes have indeed been reported in SLE, the most relevant being the demonstration in peripheral blood of activated T cells eventually able to induce immunoglobulin hyperproduction by B cells (Volk *et al.*, 1986; Huang *et al.*, 1988). Therefore, murine allogeneic diseases represent excellent models for studying the pathogenesis of human SLE and related autoimmune syndromes and for designing new therapeutic approaches.

References

Abramowicz, D., Van Der Vorst, P., Bruyns, C., Lambert, P., and Goldman, M. (1988). *Nephrol. Dial. Transplant.* **3**, 399–405.

Abramowicz, D., Vandervorst, P., Bruyns, C., Doutrelepont, J., Vandenabeele, P., and Goldman, M. (1990a). *Eur. J. Immunol.* **20**, 1647–1653.

Abramowicz, D., Doutrelepont, J., Lambert, P., Van Der Vorst, P., Bruyns, C., and Goldman, M. (1990b). *Eur. J. Immunol.* **20**, 469–476.

Bergijk, E., Munaut, C., Baelde, J., Prins, F., Foidart, J., Hoedemaeker, P., and Bruijn, J. (1992). *Am. J. Pathol.* **140**, 1147–1156.

Bruijn, J., van Elven, E., Hogendoorn, P., Corver, W., Hoedemaeker, P., and Fleuren, G. (1988). *Am. J. Pathol.* **130**, 639–641.

Bruijn, J., van Elven, E., Corver, W., Oudshoorn-Snoek, M., and Fleuren, G. (1989). *Clin. Exp. Immunol.* **76**, 284–289.

Bruijn, J., Hogendoorn, P., Corver, W., van den Broek, L., Hoedemaeker, P., and Fleuren, G. (1990). *Clin. Exp. Immunol.* **79**, 115–128.

Dobashi, K., Ono, S., Murakami, S., Takahama, Y., Katoh, Y., and Hamaoka, T. (1987). *J. Immunol.* **138**, 780–787.

Doutrelepont, J., Moser, M., Leo, O., Abramowicz, D., Vanderhaegen, M., Urbain, J., and Goldman, M. (1991). *Clin. Exp. Immunol.* **83**, 133–136.

Elson, C. (1982). *Immunol. Today* **3**, 181–182.

Florquin, S., Abramowicz, D., de Heer, E., Bruijn, J., Doutrelepont, J., Goldman, M., and Hoedemaeker, P. (1991). *Kidney Int.* **40**, 852–861.

Fujiwara, K., Sakaguchi, N., and Watanabe, T. (1991). *Lab. Invest.* **65**, 710–718.

Gelpi, C., Martinez, A., Vidal, S., Algueró, A., Juarez, C., Hardin, J., and Rodriguez-Sanchez, J. (1990). *Clin. Immunol. Immunopathol.* **56**, 298–310.

Gleichmann, E., van Elven, E., and van der Veen, J. (1982). *Eur. J. Immunol.* **12**, 152–159.

Goldman, M., Feng, H., Engers, H., Hochman, A., Louis, J., and Lambert, P. (1983). *J. Immunol.* **131**, 251–258.

Goldman, M., Druet, P., and Gleichmann, E. (1991). *Immunol. Today* **12**, 223–227.

Hard, R., and Kullgren, B. (1970). *Am. J. Pathol.* **59**, 203–224.

Hard, R., Moncure, C., and Still, W. (1973). *Lab. Invest.* **28**, 468–476.

Huang, Y., Perrin, L., Miescher, P., and Zubler, R. (1988). *J. Immunol.* **141**, 827–833.

Lewis, R., Armstrong, M., André-Schwartz, J., Muftuoglu, A., Beldotti, L., and Schwartz, R. (1968). *J. Exp. Med.* **128**, 653–667.

Luzuy, S., Merino, J., Engers, H., Izui, S., and Lambert, P. (1986). *J. Immunol.* **136**, 4420–4426.

Pals, S., Radaszkiewicz, T., Roozendaal, T., and Gleichmann, E. (1985). *J. Immunol.* **134**, 1475–1482.

Portanova, J., Ebling, F., Hammond, W., Hahn, B., and Kotzin, B. (1988). *J. Immunol.* **141**, 3370–3376.

Rolink, A., Gleichmann, H., and Gleichmann, E. (1983). *J. Immunol.* **130**, 209–215.

Schurmans, S., Heusser, C., Qin, H.-Y., Merino, J., Brighouse, G., and Lambert, P. (1990). *J. Immunol.* **145**, 2465–2473.

Simpson, E., O'Hopp, S., Harrison, M., Mosier, D., Melief, K., and Cantor, H. (1974). *Immunology* **27**, 989–1007.

van Elven, E., Agterberg, J., Sadal, S., and Gleichmann, E. (1981). *J. Immunol.* **126**, 1684–1691.

van Rappard-van der Veen, F., Rolink, A., and Gleichmann, E. (1982). *J. Exp. Med.* **155**, 1555–1560.

van Rappard-van der Veen, F., Radaszkiewicz, T., Terraneo, L., and Gleichmann, E. (1983). *J. Immunol.* **130**, 2693–2701.

Via, C., and Shearer, G. (1988). *Immunol. Today* **9**, 207–213.

Volk, H., Kopp, J., Korner, J., Jahn, S., Grunow, R., Barthelmes, H., and Fiebig, H. (1986). *Scand. J. Immunol.* **24**, 109–114.

Chapter 19

Assessment of Discomfort in Laboratory Animals

H. van Herck,[1] V. Baumans,[2] and S. F. de Boer[3]

[1]Central Laboratory Animal Institute (GDL) and [2]Department of Laboratory Animal Science, Veterinary Faculty, Utrecht University, 3508 TD Utrecht, The Netherlands and [3]Department of Animal Physiology, University of Groningen, 9750 AA Haren, The Netherlands

I. Introduction

Judgments of the ethical admissibility of animal experiments should be based on balancing the anticipated benefits for humans against the anticipated discomfort in the animals. To be able to judge the admissibility of experiments, investigators, animal caretakers, animal technicians, and animal welfare officers must be able to recognize signs of discomfort and situations which may cause discomfort in laboratory animals. In extreme cases of disturbed animal welfare, consensus as to the presence of discomfort and possibly also its degree will readily be reached. However, in less obvious cases, it can be very difficult to assess the degree of discomfort.

Before thinking about discomfort in animals, it is necessary to realize that discomfort is a human term, in which feelings play a role. We all know it is difficult to prove to someone else that we feel pain, for example. It is even impossible to give exact information about the amount of pain we feel. We

Autoimmune Disease Models:
A Guidebook

simply accept that someone can have pain because we know so from our own experience. In the same way, it is impossible to prove that animals have these states of mind. However, based on the principle of analogy between man and animal, we also have accepted the principle of analogy, which means that we assume that similar treatments cause similar pain in man and animals, unless the contrary has been proven.

II. Arguments for Assessing Discomfort

What are the reasons for assessing discomfort in laboratory animals? First, humane considerations demand that attempts be made to reduce discomfort in laboratory animals to an absolute minimum. Furthermore, one of the objectives of legislation concerning animal experimentation is to watch over animal welfare (Beynen et al., 1989). A survey of European and U.S. legislation and guidelines available on the protection of laboratory animals reveals that all texts include reference to at least one of the terms "pain," "distress," or "suffering" (Bennett et al., 1990; FELASA, 1994).

According to most of these regulations, precautions must be taken to avoid or minimize experiences like pain, distress, and suffering. This implies that if it is likely that animals will be in pain during an experiment, anesthetics must be used unless they jeopardize the objective of the experiment (Beynen et al., 1989). Furthermore, animals in pain must be euthanized as soon as the experiment allows it. Therefore, information about the degree of discomfort in laboratory animals in experiments is needed in order to judge the admissibility of experiments or the necessity for using anesthetics, but also for estimating the point at which animals should be euthanized. Such information could also be used to indicate priorities as to research on replacement, reduction, and refinement of animal experiments. For all these reasons, it is essential that objective information about discomfort be included when developing guidelines for the care and use of laboratory animals.

Also, from a scientific point of view, it is important to recognize discomfort in animals under study because discomfort can lead to physiological and behavioral changes which may render invalid experimental results (Fox, 1986). In the laboratory, situations may arise in which discomfort for the animal can be expected because of the husbandry or because of the experimental procedures to which the animal is subjected. As a consequence of this, discomfort frequently increases the variability of experimental results and may lead to biased results (Figure 1). This means that the greater the discomfort, the more animals are needed to get, at best, the same results. This involves costs to both the animals and the researcher: for the latter it means more work and higher financial requirements. In other words, an

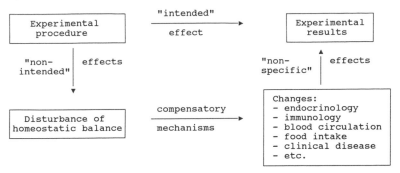

Figure 1. Intended and unintended effects of procedures on experimental results.

animal in pain or distress generally is a poor research object, unless pain itself is the subject of study. These practical features reinforce the ethical reasons for minimizing such responses in experimentation.

III. Stress and Discomfort

It is clear that the words "stress" and "discomfort" have several meanings, depending upon the context in which they are used. Because consensus upon the definitions does not exist, aspects of "stress" and "discomfort" need to be elucidated.

A. Stress

1. Definition

Despite a wide range of environmental conditions and metabolic needs, the *milieu interieur* of living individuals is adjusted to certain standards (homeostasis) (Dantzer and Mormède, 1985). In this context, stress can be considered to be the state resulting from stimuli (stressors) of external or internal origin that have the possibility for affecting homeostasis (Hadley, 1988) (Figure 2).

2. Behavioral Physiology

The organisms' response to stress is composed of a coordinated pattern of behavioral, endocrine, and autonomic responses (Table I). The behavioral responses to stressors include generally the facilitation of adaptive, and inhibition of nonadaptive neural pathways which enable the organism to cope more successfully with the stressful stimulus. These behavioral responses

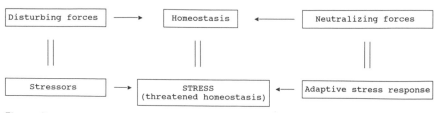

Figure 2. Concept of stress.

include suppression of feeding and reproductive behavior, and increased arousal, vigilance, and alertness. The hypothalamus–pituitary–adrenocortical (HPA) axis and the sympathetic–adrenomedullary (SA) system (Figure 3) are the main autonomic and neuroendocrine pathways that are activated in the response to environmental conditions which affect homeostasis (i.e., physical and psychological stressors).

Activation of these systems results in an increased release of the glucocorticoid corticosterone (from the adrenal cortex; HPA axis) and of the catecholamines noradrenaline (from sympathetic nerves) and adrenaline (from the adrenal medulla; SA system) into the bloodstream (Axelrod and Reisine, 1984; Bohus, 1984; Cannon, 1915; Selye, 1950). In addition to these classical stress hormones, several other hormones or neuropeptides (i.e., second-generation stress hormones) may be released from the pituitary, peripheral nerve endings, and the adrenal gland (Bohus, 1984a). Together, these agents appear to orchestrate the complex chain of biochemical processes underlying adequate physiological and behavioral adaptation to stressors by affecting cardiovascular, energy-producing, and immune systems (Bohus, 1984b; Moberg, 1985; Ursin, 1989).

3. Modes of Stress Response

In behavioral physiological stress research, two fundamental modes of stress response are suggested. The first is the fight-flight pattern, characterized by activation of mainly the SA system (Moberg, 1985; Stephens, 1980), and resulting in release of the catecholamines adrenaline and noradrenaline. Corresponding behavior is supposed to be characterized by enhanced activity (Dantzer and Mormède, 1985; Moberg, 1985). The second is the conservation withdrawal mode of stress response, associated with a pronounced increase in HPA activity. Immobility and suppression of environmentally directed activities are considered the primary behavioral characteristics. The relative expression of these generalized modes of stress response depends on a number of organismic and environmental factors.

Table I

Profile of Behavioral, Endocrine, and Autonomic Responses to Stress in Rats[a]

Behavioral responses		Endocrine responses		Autonomic responses	
Locomotor activity		Pituitary hormones		Sympathetic activity	↑
Novel environment	↓	β-endotrophin	↑	Blood-pressure	↑
Familiar environment	↑	Adrenocorticotropic hormone	↑	Temperature	↑
Withdrawal	↑	Prolactin	↑	Heart rate	↑
Immobility	↑	Vasopressin	↑	Plasma noradrenaline	↑
Grooming	↑	Growth hormone	↑	Plasma renin	↑
Burying	↑	Thyrotrophic hormone	↑	Plasma glucose	↑
Startle	↑	Follicle stimulating hormone	↑	Parasympathetic activity	↓
Ingestion	↓	Luteinizing hormone	↑	Gastric acid secretion	↓
Exploration	↓	Adrenal hormones		Gastric emptying	↓
Sexual activity	↓	Corticosteroids	↑	Gastric ulceration	↑
Social interaction	↓	Adrenaline	↑	Fecal excretion	↑
Operant responding	↓	Pancreatic hormones		Immune functions	↓
		Glucagon	↑		
		Insulin	↓/↑		

[a] ↑ = increase; ↓ = decrease.

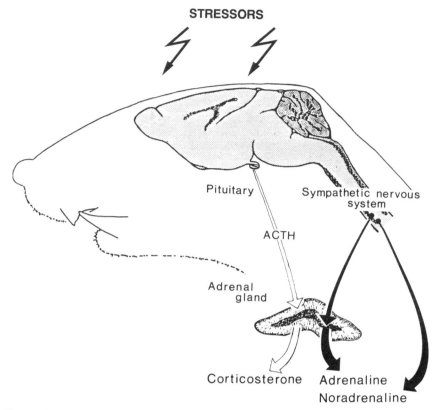

Figure 3. Stressors ranging from the mildly emotional to the intensely physical cause an increased activity of both the SA system and the HPA axis. This results in a discharge of the catecholamines noradrenaline and adrenaline, and of the glucocorticoid corticosterone into the bloodstream.

4. Factors Moderating the Stress Response in Rats

The qualitative and quantitative aspects of the behavioral and autonomic/neuroendocrine response to stressful stimuli are determined by a number of factors. Organismic characteristics such as sex, age, strain, and nutritional status (Bronson and Rissman, 1989; Levin *et al.*, 1984; Livezey *et al.*, 1985; McCarty *et al.*, 1984; McCarty and Stone, 1984; Sapolsky, 1986); and various physical stressor properties such as type, intensity, duration, and frequency of stimulation (Armario *et al.*, 1986; Bronson and Rissman, 1989; Cleroux *et al.*, 1985; Gärtner *et al.*, 1980; Kjaer *et al.*, 1987; Natelson *et al.*, 1987; Paris *et al.*, 1987) are of evident importance. However, the stress responses of brain and body seem to depend more strongly on prior experiences and on the type (active or passive) and degree of behavioral control or predictability over a stressful situation, whereas the noxious nature of the stressor seems to be of less importance. In general, it is assumed that an aversive or noxious situation becomes less stressful as it becomes more predictable and as the organism achieves control over it (Dantzer and Mormède, 1985; Levine, 1980; Steptoe, 1983; Weinberg and Levine, 1980).

Together, these factors are also termed coping factors. Coping can be defined as a psychological process or behavior (handling stressful information) that leads to a decreased physiological or hormonal activation (Dantzer and Mormède, 1985; Ursin, 1980). Repeated confrontation with the same stressor can both increase and decrease future responsiveness of the neuroendocrine systems.

In general, chronic intermittent or repeated exposure to a stressful event leads to adaptation in the form of a gradual attenuation of the neuroendocrine response to that stressor (Armario *et al.*, 1988; Cox *et al.*, 1985; Dobrakovova and Jurcovicova, 1984; Kant *et al.*, 1985; Konarska *et al.*, 1989; Muir and Pfister, 1986; Murison *et al.*, 1986; Ratner *et al.*, 1989; Thiagarajan *et al.*, 1989; Vogel and Jensh, 1988; Yelvington *et al.*, 1985). Although biochemical changes (i.e., adaptations) evidently do occur at various peripheral levels of the neuroendocrine response system involved (Kvetnansky *et al.*, 1984; McCarty and Stone, 1984), the decreased responsiveness appears to be mainly the result of a central nervous (psychological) process, that is, habituation (Armario *et al.*, 1988; Dobrakovova and Jurcovicova, 1984; Konarska *et al.*, 1989; McCarty and Stone, 1984).

5. (Pre)pathological State

External stressors may have such a severe impact that they bring an animal into a "prepathological state" (Moberg, 1985): the animal can only cope with the stressors (i.e., maintain homeostasis) at the risk of physical malfunctioning and/or abnormal behavior. Uncoordinated or unbalanced physiological reactions may eventually cause stress-related pathologies of the brain (i.e., affective disorders) and the body (i.e., cardiovascular, gastrointestinal, and immunological diseases) (Bohus, 1984; Moberg, 1985; Ursin, 1980).

The (risk of) physical and or mental disease is the real threat to the animal's well-being. However, the changes occurring much earlier during a stress response (behavior, biochemical processes, cardiovascular, gastrointestinal, and immune systems) may be a threat to the results of the researcher's work.

B. Discomfort

"Comfort is a state of physiologic, psychologic, and behavioral equilibrium in which an animal is accustomed to its environment and engages in normal activities" (National Research Council, 1992). Following this definition, discomfort can tentatively be described as any deviation from the state of comfort in the animal. Thus, discomfort covers a variety of unpleasant sensations. A selected number (pain, distress, and suffering) of the different aspects of discomfort are more concrete.

1. Pain

Pain may be defined as "an unpleasant sensory and emotional experience associated with actual or potential damage" (FELASA, 1994). A crucial aspect of this definition is that pain is an experience. This requires the animal to be conscious. It is also important to note that this definition of pain is mainly physical: it delimits pain to experiencing stimuli that (are capable of) injure or damage organs or tissues of the body. Thus, mental pain is excluded from this definition.

2. Distress

"Distress is a state where the animal has to put substantial efforts or resources into the adaptive response to challenges in the environmental situation" (FELASA, 1994). This means that distress may be considered as the emotional or mental equivalent of pain. Thus "distress" differs from "stress" by its chronicity or excessiveness of stress system activation. Examples of stimuli which may lead to distress are various environmental factors, such as housing and experimental conditions. The severity of the distress depends upon the extent to which the animal can cope with the situation. The better the animal is able to cope with the situation, the less severe the distress will be. If an animal can completely cope with it, there is no distress at all.

3. Suffering

"Suffering is a specific state of mind, which occurs when the amount of pain and/or distress has reached a level which is no longer tolerated by an individual animal" (FELASA, 1994). Distress and physical pain may result in suffering if their duration, intensity (Moberg, 1985), unpredictability and/or uncontrollability has reached or passed the level that the animal can cope with: the animal is in or passed the "prepathological state" (Moberg, 1985). Suffering may result in such clinical signs as abnormal behavior, retarded growth, impaired breeding, or inadequate care of the individual's own body (FELASA, 1994; Manser, 1992; Moberg, 1985).

IV. Assessment of Discomfort

A. Parameters for Assessing Discomfort

To be able to assess discomfort, it is important to know which signs may indicate discomfort in an animal. As stated before, by accepting the principle of analogy, conditions which cause discomfort in humans should be assumed to cause discomfort in animals as well, unless the contrary has been proven. Looking for parameters by which to assess discomfort, this statement can be modified as follows: signs as expressed by animals which are comparable to signs of discomfort in man are also indicative of discomfort in animals. This means that not only changes in behavior, but also results of clinical examinations and postmortem observations may provide clues concerning discomfort, especially when these variables have been shown to correlate with clinical signs of discomfort in man and/or in animals (Beynen *et al.*, 1989). In this way, generally accepted painful lesions and manifestations of disturbed homeostasis (e.g., of the anabolic/catabolic, neuroendocrine, immunological, and behavioral balance) are useful in assessing discomfort. Some of these can be assessed during life, others only after death (Table II) (FELASA, 1994; Farnell and Maronpot, 1987; LASA, 1990; Manser, 1992; Militzer, 1986; Walvoort, 1991). Needless to say, knowledge of the normal behavior and appearance of a given animal species and strain is a prerequisite without which assessment of discomfort is nearly impossible. Theoretically, all these parameters can be measured in an objective way. They can also be assessed just by looking at the animals during or after the performance of an experimental procedure.

Another source of information useful in estimating the amount of discomfort which animals might endure in an experimental procedure is to assess which organs and/or tissues might be affected by the procedure. Taking into account the sensitivity of these tissues, a rough estimation of the degree of discomfort can be made. A classification of tissues and organs in terms of a decreasing sensitivity can be generated: cornea, dental pulp, testis, nerves, spinal cord, skin, serous membranes, periosteum/blood vessels, viscera, joints, bones, encephalic tissue (FELASA, 1994).

B. Methods for Assessing Discomfort

Acknowledging that it is in the interest of both animal and man to inflict on animals as little discomfort as possible during experiments, the question arises: How can discomfort in experiments be assessed and prevented? As stated before, pain, distress, and suffering cannot be measured in an objective way. In general, discomfort can be assessed in a qualitative and a more-

Table II
Examples of *Intra Vitam* and Postmortem Parameters for Discomfort

	Intra Vitam	Postmortem
Painful lesions	Bone fracture	Pericarditis
	Arthritis	Intestinal obstruction
	Skin ulceration	Bone tissue metastasis of tumor
Clinical signs	Piloerection	
	Heart rate	
	Body temperature	
	Abnormal stances and posture	
	Gait (e.g., lameness)	
Disturbed homeostasis		
Behavioral	Activity	Abnormal length of toenails
	Crying	Chromorhino-dacryorroea
	Automutilation	Abortion
	Aggression	
	Decrease in body care/grooming	
Anabolic/catabolic	Reduced weight gain	Fatty depots
	Weight loss	Muscle volume
	Reduced food intake	Gastrointestinal contents
		Fluid balance
Neuroendocrine	Stress hormones	Gonad size
		Adrenal cortex size
		Gastric mucosal barrier
Immunological	Blood leukocytes	Lymphoid organ size
	Immunoglobulins	Opportunistic infections

or-less quantitative way. In both the qualitative and the quantitative way, assessment of discomfort contains two steps: collection of data, which can be regarded as an objective process, followed by "translation" into a degree of discomfort, which is a subjective process (Beynen *et al.*, 1989).

The main difference between the quantitative and the qualitative methods is that in the quantitative methods one tries to indicate the amount of discomfort with a numerical rating, whereas in qualitative methods only broad categories are used. Wright and Woodson (1990) use qualitative criteria from clinical examination and physiological signs. Buckwell (1992) listed physical signs for rodents that can be related to mild, moderate, and substantial severity, which are categories used in the legislation of several European countries.

In quantitative methods to assess discomfort as elaborated by Morton and Griffiths (1985), Beynen *et al.* (1987), Barclay *et al.* (1988), and LASA (1990), the approach is to assign numerical scores to signs of pain and discomfort.

An approach that assesses discomfort on the basis of the signs the animals show during and after experimental procedures implies that the estimated degree of discomfort depends on the experiences of the assessor and the experience of the person performing the technique. The main advantage is that one focuses on the animals. Morton and Griffiths (1985) were the first to assign a numerical rating to parameters scored during clinical investigation. Beynen *et al.* (1987) have modified this method. They assigned scores to selected *intravitam* as well as postmortem parameters for discomfort in an objective way by comparing nontreated control animals and test animals. Since several assessors examine the same animals, it is possible to average out variations in the scores assigned to a certain parameter.

A third method used to compare different experimental procedures or experiments is the "disturbance index," a behavioral method for assessing the severity of procedures on rodents. In this method, the degree of disturbance of a rodent's exploratory behavior caused by subjecting it to an experimental procedure is quantified. An animal is brought into a new environment, where—during a defined period of time—its movements are detected by an electronic monitor and converted to electrical pulses. The number of pulses of treated and control animals is used to calculate the disturbance index. Every deviation from normal animal activity, both an increase and a decrease, is interpreted as an indication of discomfort. The degree of the discomfort is thought to be related to the difference between test and control animals. Like the method developed by Beynen *et al.* (1987), this method is also time-consuming. Another drawback is that animal activity is the only parameter used to assess discomfort in the disturbance index.

For these reasons, it is not expected that all experimental procedures will be assessed in this way in the near future. For the time being, it will be more practical to assess discomfort by listing the experimental procedures to be used and estimating discomfort on the basis of the literature and personal experience with experimental procedures, for example, the method the "LASA working party on assessment and control of severity of pain and distress in laboratory animals" proposes with the severity index. They have proposed a system for developing an index of severity for scientific procedures. In this system, the components of severity common to many procedures are identified and given a numerical rating that reflects a potential range of severity (Table III). An experimental procedure is reviewed for the components of severity and each component is awarded a score that reflects the adverse effect upon the animal. Individual scores for each component are added to reach an index of severity for the experimental procedure. The higher the final score of the procedure (the severity index), the greater the potential severity of the procedure.

Table III
Parameters Used to Assess Discomfort Induced by an Experimental Procedure[a]

Parameter	Scale	Scores depend upon
Conscious	0–1	Possibility of animal experiencing discomfort: score 1
Anesthesia	0–4	Risk of mortality and unpleasant effects during induction and recovery
Preparation	0–2	Possible stressful preparatory manipulations (shaving, fasting, training)
Restraint	0–4	Method of restraint (if performed) varying from brief manual (score 1) to continuous, whole-body restraint (score 4)
Duration	0–2	Duration of application of physical, noxious, or aversive stimuli
Tissue sensitivity	0–2	The sensitivity of affected tissues to noxious stimuli applied
Organ risk	0–2	The risk of harm to specific tissues and organ systems
Mortality	0–4	Known or predictable risk to the survival of the animal
During procedure		
Pain	0–5	The nature, intensity, and duration of the pain caused
Distress	0–5	The risk of inducing conflict, frustration, fear, or anxiety
Deprivation	0–5	The risk and degree of depriving the animal of normal physiological function or activity, permanently or temporarily
After procedure		
Pain	0–5	See During procedure
Distress	0–5	See During procedure
Deprivation	0–5	See During procedure
Severity Index		(Sum of scores of parameters)

[a] From LASA (1990).

V. An Example of Assessing Discomfort in Practice

An assessment of discomfort has the risk of being mainly a theoretical issue. To illustrate the assessment (and possibility of diminishing) discomfort in practice, the adjuvant arthritis rat model is used as an example.

A. Step 1: Collection of Objective Information

The model of adjuvant arthritis is based upon the injection of complete Freund's adjuvant (CFA) in the base of the tail (or footpad) of a rat (see Chapter 13). During the experiment (especially during the phase of acute arthritis), generally a number of parameters are measured, among which are body weight and diameter of the (arthritic) joints. At the end of the experiment, the animals are euthanized and body organs and tissues collected for further research.

In this rat model, the animals develop arthritic changes which are already visible during superficial clinical inspection. The severity of the changes seen varies with the mycobacterial species, concentration and particle size of the mycobacteria in oil, the oily adjuvant, and the rat strain used. If the experiment includes testing possible therapeutics for the disease, these also may affect (increase or decrease) the severity of the changes. The lesions induced range from invisible (not present?) to fulminant arthritis with gross swelling, redness and deformity of the hind paws, front paws, and toes. When the arthritis becomes more chronic, ankylotic changes of the affected joints occur. Furthermore, an ulcerative dermatitis at the base of the tail (caused by the injection of CFA) is to be found during superficial clinical inspection of the animal. Closer examination may also reveal inflammation of the penis and conjunctiva (Butler, 1985). At necropsy, a poorly filled gastrointestinal tract and erosion and/or ulceration of the gastric wall may be observed during the acute phase of arthritis. Histology may, among other things, show nodular inflammatory reactions in the lungs and the spleen, and arthritic changes in the spinal column.

B. Step 2: Translation into Discomfort

Discomfort can be estimated by looking at the techniques used (before the experiment starts) or by evaluating the data collected from the animals during life and after death (during the experiment).

In this model, at a minimum the following techniques are applied to each animal during an experiment: (1) intracutaneous injection; (2) clinical investigations of each animal (body weight, diameter of joints); (3) euthanasia. With this information alone, it is not possible to make a realistic estimate of the degree of discomfort. Additional information is needed; this includes the number of animals that will be injected with CFA intracutaneously, the number of animals which are expected to develop arthritis and to what severity, the length of time the animals will live after the injection with CFA, the manipulations performed (or parameters measured) during clinical examination, and the method of euthanasia to be used.

During the experiment, the animals develop a number of lesions that are generally accepted to be painful: acute arthritis, ulcerative dermatitis, and conjunctivitis. Within the context of this experiment, the diminished food intake and growth, the diminished ambulation and very abnormal gait, the poorly filled gastrointestinal tract, and the erosion and/or ulceration of the gastric wall are to be interpreted, not as the cause, but as the consequence of the discomfort present. Both collection of the techniques to be applied and collection of the signs the animals show have disadvantages. Estimation of the discomfort caused by a technique is only possible if one knows the effects of the technique upon the animal. And even if they are known in general, the effects may be different during a given experiment, depending upon experiment-dependent variables (the antigen used, effectiveness of therapeutics to be tested) and experiment-independent variables (husbandry, animal technician, microbiological environment). Combining the results of the techniques (and their consequences) before and carefully looking for signs of discomfort (*intra vitam* and postmortem) during the experiment is the most reliable way to prevent unnecessary discomfort for the animals and to evaluate techniques and models both for their admissibility and for unexpected effects upon experimental results.

C. Step 3: "Quantifying" Discomfort

In the LASA system, the different procedures performed in an animal experiment are identified and reviewed for a total number of 14 parameters (Table III). For a given parameter, the range of the scores (scale) is limited and is related to the estimated impact of this parameter upon discomfort.

In the adjuvant arthritis rat model, a limited number of procedures may be performed: intracutaneous injection at the base of the tail, scoring of clinical parameters (e.g., body weight, diameter of joints), and finally euthanasia, followed by collection of tissues and/or organs (Table IV). The score assigned to a parameter depends upon the consequences of the procedure for the animal. For example, intracutaneous injection with CFA will cause pain (ulceration) afterward, in contrast to the intracutaneous injection of, for example, saline. If the injection induces arthritis (and other inflammatory reactions), there will be more pain. Furthermore, distress and deprivation (locomotion) are then to be expected and several organs and sensitive tissues may be affected. During clinical investigations, manipulation of the animal and especially of the joints (when arthritic) will be painful. Euthanasia by collecting organs while the animal is anesthetized will only cause minor effects on the animal's well-being, according to the LASA system.

The use of an "objective," quantitative system to assess discomfort in animal experiments encourages a structured approach at an operational level, leading to an increased awareness of the potential adverse effects of experimental procedures and the needs of animals.

VI. Possibilities for Diminishing Discomfort

Prior to considering the possibility of diminishing discomfort the benefits of the experiment should be balanced against the costs, both economical and ethical. If it is decided to perform the experiment, it is essential to use

Table IV

Tentative Interpretation of Discomfort Caused in the Adjuvant Arthritis Rat Model

Parameter	Scale	Intracutaneous injection, saline	Intracutaneous injection, CFA	Intracutaneous injection, CFA arthritis	Clinical Score	Ether anesthesia
Conscious	0–1	1	1	1	1	0
Anesthesia	0–4	0	0	0	0	1
Preparation	0–2	1	1	1	0	0
Restraint	0–4	2	2	2	2	0
Duration	0–2	0	0	0	1	0
Tissue sensitivity	0–2	0	1	1	0	0
Organ Risk	0–2	0	1	1	0	0
Mortality	0–4	0	0	0	0	0
During procedure						
Pain	0–5	1	1	1	2–3[a]	0
Distress	0–5	1	1	1	1–2[a]	0
Deprivation	0–5	0	0	0	0	0
After procedure						
Pain	0–5	1	4	5	0	0
Distress	0–5	0	0	3	0	0
Deprivation	0–5	0	0	3	0	0
Severity index		7	12	19	7–9	1

[a] Depending upon manipulations with and sensitivity of (arthritic) joints.

animals of "an appropriate species and quality and the minimum number required to obtain valid results. Methods such as mathematical models, computer simulation, and *in vitro* biological systems should be considered." (Mann *et al.*, 1991). Not only the use of too many, but also of too few animals in an experiment results in needless use of animals. In too many experiments, the results appear to be unreliable because of the use of an inadequate number of animals or an inappropriate statistical test (Festing, 1992). Thus, before an experiment is started, the number of animals required for the test should be estimated by performing a power analysis (Beynen *et al.*, 1993) and the statistical test to be used in analyzing the data should be decided upon (NIH, 1986). If the feasibility of an experiment(al procedure) or, for example, the effect of a therapy or drug is uncertain, a pilot test should precede the performance of the experiment (Toth and Olson, 1991).

During an adjuvant arthritis experiment, the use of analgesics is not common because the nonsteroid anti-inflammatory drugs (NSAIDs) which have an analgesic and presumably beneficial effect and lead to increased movement and mobility (Colpaert, 1987) may jeopardize the objectives of the experiment. The opioid drugs (such as buprenorphine) are not effective in reducing chronic pain caused by arthritis. Thus, discomfort can only be reduced by improving the physical environment of the animal. Housing two animals at a maximum in a macrolon type 3 cage (382×220 mm floor space) lowers the risk of their injuring each other. An ample amount of soft bedding material may diminish the discomfort of lying on the floor of the cage. The accessibility of food and drinking water can be improved by providing food not only in the food hopper but also on the cage floor, and by using long-spouted water bottles.

Staff members, animal technicians, and animal caretakers should be well informed about how the experiment will affect the animals to guarantee careful handling during clinical investigations and routine care. Last but not least, humane end points should be defined and clear agreements must be reached upon who is authorized to euthanize animals if calamities should occur.

References

Armario, A., Montero, J. L., and Balasch, J. (1986). *Physiol. Behav.* **37**, 559–561.

Armario, A., Hidalgo, G., and Giralt, M. (1988). *Neuroendocrinology* **47**, 263–267.

Axelrod, J., and Reisine, T. D. (1984). *Science* **224**, 452–459.

Barclay, R. J., Herbert, W. J., and Poole, T. B. (1988). "The Disturbance Index: A Behavioral Method of Assessing the Severity of Common Laboratory Procedures on Rodents." Universities Federation for Animal Welfare, Potters Bar, England.

Bennett, B. T., Brown, M. J., and Schofield, J. C. (1990). *In* "Essentials for Animal Research." pp. 3–12. National Agricultural Library, Beltsville, Maryland.

Beynen, A. C., Festing, M. F. W., and van Montfort, M. A. J. (1993). *In* "Laboratory Animal Science: A Contribution to the Humane Use and Care of Animals and the Quality of Experimental Results" (L. F. M. van Zutphen, V. Baumans, and A. C. Beynen, Eds.), pp. 209–239. Elsevier Science Publishers, Amsterdam.

Beynen, A. C., Stafleu, F. R., Baumans, V., and Herck, H. van (1989). *In* "Animal Experimentation: Legislation and Education" (L. F. M. van Zutphen, H. Rozemond, and A. C. Beynen, Eds.), pp. 139–149. Veterinary Public Health Inspectorate/Department of Laboratory Animal Science, Rijswijk/Utrecht.

Beynen, A. C., Baumans, V., Bertens, A. P. M. G., Havenaar, R., Hesp, A. P. M., and Zutphen, L. F. M. van (1987). *Lab. Anim.* **21**, 35–42.

Bohus, B. (1984a). *J. Psychosom. Res.* **28**, 429–438.

Bohus, B. (1984b). *In* "Breakdown in Human Adaptation to Stress: Towards a Multidisciplinary Approach" (R. E. Balliaux, J. F. Fielding, and A. L'Abbate, Eds.), pp. 638–652. M. Nijhoff, Gravenhage.

Bronson, F. H., and Rissman, E. F. (1989). *Physiol. Behav.* **45**, 185–189.

Buckwell, A. (1992). *LASA* (*Winter Newslett.*) 16–17.

Butler, S. H. (1985). *In* "Issues in Pain Measurement" (C. R. Chapman and J. D. Loeser, Eds.), pp. 473–479. Raven Press, New York.

Cannon, W. B. (1915). "Bodily Changes in Pain, Hunger, Fear and Anger." Appleton, New York.

Cleroux, J., Peronnet, F., and Champlain, J. de (1985). *Physiol. Behav.* **35**, 271–275.

Colpaert, F. C. (1987). *Pain* **28**, 201–222.

Cox, R. H., Hubbard, J. W., Lawler, J. E., Sanders, B. J., and Mitchell, V. P. (1985). *J. Appl. Physiol.* **58**, 1207–1214.

Dantzer, R., and Mormède, P. (1985). *In* "Animal Stress" (G. P. Moberg, Ed.), pp. 81–97. Waverly Press, Bethesda, Maryland.

Dobrakovova, M., and Jurcovicova, J. (1984). *Exp. Clin. Endocrinol.* **83**, 21–27.

Farnell, R., and Maronpot, R. R. (1987). *Proc. 6th Intern. Symp. on Gastrointestinal Tox. Path., Philadelphia.*

FELASA (Federation of European Laboratory Animal Science Associations) working group on pain and distress in laboratory animals (1994). *Lab. Anim.* **28**, 97–112.

Festing, M. F. W. (1992). *Lab. Anim.* **26**, 256–267.

Fox, M. W. (1986). *In* "Laboratory Animal Husbandry. Ethology, Welfare and Experimental Variables." (M. W. Fox, eds.), pp. 1–6, State University of New York Press, Albany.

Gärtner, K., Buttner, D., Dohler, K., Friedel, R., Lindena, J., and Trautschold, I. (1980). *Lab. Anim.* **14**, 267–274.

Hadley, M. E. (1988). "Endocrinology," 2nd ed. Prentice–Hall, Englewood Cliffs.

Kant, G. J., Nielsen, C. J., Olehansky, M. V., Mougey, E. H., Pennington, L. L., and Meyerhoff, J. L. (1985). *Life Sci.* **36**, 2421–2428.

Kjaer, M., Secher, N. H., and Galbo, H. (1987). *In* "Clinical Endocrinology and Metabolism: Neuroendocrinology of Stress" (A. Grossman, Ed.), pp. 279–329. Balliere Tindall, London.

Konarska, M., Stewart, R. E., and McCarty, R. (1989). *Physiol. Behav.* **45**, 255–261.

Kvetnansky, R., Nemeth, S., Vigas, M., Oprsalova, Z., Jurcovicova, J. (1984). *In* "Stress: Role of Catecholamines and Other Neurotransmitters" (E. Usdin, R. Kvetnansky, and J. Axelrod, Eds.), pp. 537–562. Gordon Breach, New York.

LASA (Laboratory Animals Science Association) working group on the assessment and control of the severity of scientific procedures on laboratory animals. (1990). *Lab. Anim.* **24**, 97–130.

Levin, B. E., Stoddard-Apter, S., and Sullivan, A. C. (1984). *Physiol. Behav.* **32**, 295–299.

Levine, S. (1980). *In* "Animal Stress" (G. P. Moberg, Ed.), pp. 51–69. Waverly Press, Baltimore.

Livezey, G. T., Miller, J. M., and Vogel, W. H. (1985). *Neurosci. Lett.* **62**, 51–56.

Mann, M. D., Crouse, D. A., and Prentice, E. D. (1991). *Lab. Anim. Sci.* **41**, 6–14.

Manser, C. E. (1992). "The Assessment of Stress in Laboratory Animals" (C. E. Manser, Ed.), pp. 1–207. Royal Society for the Prevention of Cruelty to Animals. Horsham, West Sussex.

McCarty, R., and Stone, E. (1984). *In* "Stress: Role of Catecholamines and Other Neurotransmitters" (E. Usdin, R. Kvetnansky, and J. Axelrod, Eds.), pp. 563–576. Gordon Breach, New York.

McCarty, R., Kirby, R. F., and Garn, P. G. (1984). *Behav. Neural Biol.* **40**, 98–113.

Militzer, K. (1986). "Wege zur Beurteilung tiergerechter Haltung bei Labor-, Zoo-, und Haustieren" (M. Merkenschlager, and K. Gärtner, Eds.), pp. 33–77. Verlag Paul Parey. Berlin and Hamburg.

Moberg, G. P. (1985). *In* "Animal Stress" (G. P. Moberg, Ed.), pp. 27–49. Waverly Press, Baltimore.

Morton, D. B., and Griffiths, P. H. M. (1985). *Vet. Rec.* **116**, 431–436.

Muir, J. L., and Pfister, H. P. (1986). *Physiol. Behav.* **37**, 285–288.

Murison, R., Overmier, J. B., and Skoglund, E. J. (1986). *Behav. Neural Biol.* **45**, 185–195.

Natelson, B. H., Creighton, D., McCarty, R., Tapp, W. N., Pitman, D., and Ottenweller, J. E. (1987). *Physiol. Behav.* **39**, 117–125.

National Research Council, Commission on Life Sciences, Institute of Laboratory Animal Resources, Committee on Pain and Distress in Laboratory Animals (1992). "Recognition and Alleviation of Pain and Distress in Laboratory Animals." National Academy Press, Washington, D.C.

NIH (National Institutes of Health) Office for Protection from Research Risks. (1986). "Public Health Service Policy on Humane Use of Laboratory Animals." NIH, Bethesda, Maryland.

Paris, J. M., Lorens, S. A., vander Kar, L. D., Urban, J. H., Richardson-Morton, K. D., and Bethea, C. L. (1987). *Physiol. Behav.* **39**, 33–43.

Ratner, A., Yelvington, D. B., and Rosenthal, M. (1989). *Psychoneuroendocrinology* **14**, 393–396.

Sapolsky, R. M., Krey, L. C., and McEwen, B. S. (1986). *Endocrine Rev.* **7**, 284–301.

Selye, H. (1950). "Stress: The Physiology and Pathology of Exposure to Stress." Acta Medica Publ., Montreal.

Stephens, D. B. (1980). *Adv. Vet. Sci. Comp. Med.* **24**, 179–210.

Steptoe, A. (1983). *In* "The Scientific Basis of Psychiatry" (M. Weller, Ed.), pp. 378–388. Balliere Tindall, London.

Thiagarajan, A. B., Mefford, I. N., and Eskay, R. L. (1989). *Neuroendocrinology* **50**, 427–432.

Toth, L. A., and Olson, G. A. (1991). *Lab. Anim.* **20**, 33–39.

Ursin, H. (1980). *In* "Coping and Health" (S. Levine and H. Ursin, Eds.), pp. 259–279. Plenum Press, New York.

Vogel, W. H., and Jensh, R. (1988). *Neurosci. Lett.* **87**, 183–188.

Walvoort, H. C. (1991). *In* "Animals in Biomedical Research. Replacement, Reduction and Refinement: Present Possibilities and Future Prospects" (C. F. M. Hendriksen and H. B. W. M. Koëter, Eds.), pp. 265–271. Elsevier Science Publishers, Amsterdam.

Weinberg, J., and Levine, S. (1980). *In* "Coping and Health" (S. Levine and H. Ursin, Eds.), pp. 39–61. Plenum Press, New York.

Wright, E. M. J., and Woodson, J. F. (1990). *In* "The Experimental Animal in Biomedical Research" (B. E. Rollin and M. L. Kesel, Eds.), pp. 205–215. CRC Press, Boca Raton.

Yelvington, D. B., Weiss, G. K., and Ratner, A. (1985). *Psychoneuroendocrinology* **10**, 95–102.

Index